Renal Involvement in Rheumatic Diseases

Editors

ANDREW S. BOMBACK
MEGHAN E. SISE

RHEUMATIC DISEASE CLINICS OF NORTH AMERICA

www.rheumatic.theclinics.com

Consulting Editor
MICHAEL H. WEISMAN

November 2018 • Volume 44 • Number 4

ELSEVIER

1600 John F. Kennedy Boulevard • Suite 1800 • Philadelphia, Pennsylvania, 19103-2899
http://www.theclinics.com

RHEUMATIC DISEASE CLINICS OF NORTH AMERICA Volume 44, Number 4
November 2018 ISSN 0889-857X, ISBN 13: 978-0-323-64173-9

Editor: Lauren Boyle
Developmental Editor: Casey Potter

Rheumatic Disease Clinics of North America (ISSN 0889-857X) is published quarterly by Elsevier Inc., 360 Park Avenue South, New York, NY 10010-1710. Months of issue are February, May, August, and November. Business and editorial offices: 1600 John F. Kennedy Boulevard, Suite 1800, Philadelphia, PA 19103-2899. Periodicals postage paid at New York, NY and additional mailing offices. Subscription prices are USD 355.00 per year for US individuals, USD 706.00 per year for US institutions, USD 100.00 per year for US students and residents, USD 419.00 per year for Canadian individuals, USD 880.00 per year for Canadian institutions, USD 465.00 per year for international individuals, USD 880.00 per year for international institutions, and USD 230.00 per year for Canadian and foreign students/residents. To receive student/resident rate, orders must be accompanied by name of affiliated institution, date of term, and the *signature* of program/residency coordinator on institution letterhead. Orders will be billed at individual rate until proof of status received. Foreign air speed delivery is included in all *Clinics* subscription prices. All prices are subject to change without notice. **POSTMASTER:** Send address changes to *Rheumatic Disease Clinics of North America,* Elsevier Health Sciences Division, Subscription Customer Service, 3251 Riverport Lane, Maryland Heights, MO 63043. **Customer Service: 1-800-654-2452 (US and Canada). From outside of the US and Canada: 314-447-8871. Fax: 314-447-8029. For print support, e-mail: JournalsCustomerService-usa@elsevier.com. For online support, e-mail: JournalsOnline Support-usa@elsevier.com.**

Reprints. For copies of 100 or more of articles in this publication, please contact the Commercial Reprints Department, Elsevier Inc., 360 Park Avenue South, New York, New York, 10010-1710; Tel.: +1-212-633-3874, Fax: +1-212-633-3820, and E-mail: reprints@elsevier.com.

Rheumatic Disease Clinics of North America is covered in *MEDLINE/PubMed (Index Medicus), Current Contents/Clinical Medicine, Science Citation Index, ISI/BIOMED,* and *EMBASE/Excerpta Medica.*

Contributors

CONSULTING EDITOR

MICHAEL H. WEISMAN, MD
Cedars-Sinai Chair in Rheumatology, Director, Division of Rheumatology, Professor of Medicine, Cedars-Sinai Medical Center, Distinguished Professor, David Geffen School of Medicine at UCLA, Los Angeles, California, USA

EDITORS

ANDREW S. BOMBACK, MD, MPH
Assistant Professor, Department of Medicine, Division of Nephrology, Columbia University Vagelos College of Physicians & Surgeons, New York, New York, USA

MEGHAN E. SISE, MD, MS
Instructor, Department of Medicine, Division of Nephrology, Massachusetts General Hospital, Boston, Massachusetts, USA

AUTHORS

JOSEPHINE M. AMBRUZS, MD, MPH
Nephropathology, Arkana Laboratories, Little Rock, Arkansas, USA

RUPALI S. AVASARE, MD
Oregon Health & Science University, Portland, Oregon, USA

FAIZAN BABAR, MD
Division of Renal Diseases and Hypertension, Department of Medicine, The George Washington University, Washington, DC, USA

JOAN BATHON, MD
Professor, Department of Medicine, Division of Rheumatology, Columbia University Vagelos College of Physicians & Surgeons, New York, New York, USA

ANDREW S. BOMBACK, MD, MPH
Assistant Professor, Department of Medicine, Division of Nephrology, Columbia University Vagelos College of Physicians & Surgeons, New York, New York, USA

KIRK N. CAMPBELL, MD
Division of Nephrology, Icahn School of Medicine at Mount Sinai, New York, New York, USA

MIRIAM CHUNG, MD
Division of Nephrology, Icahn School of Medicine at Mount Sinai, New York, New York, USA

SCOTT D. COHEN, MD, MPH, FASN
Division of Renal Diseases and Hypertension, Department of Medicine, The George Washington University, Washington, DC, USA

FRANK B. CORTAZAR, MD
Instructor in Medicine, Harvard Medical School, Division of Nephrology, Vasculitis and Glomerulonephritis Center, Massachusetts General Hospital, Boston, Massachusetts, USA

KAVITA GULATI, MB BCh, BAO, BSc
Doctor, NIHR Academic Clinical Fellow, Renal and Vascular Inflammation Section, Department of Medicine, Imperial College London, Vasculitis Clinic, Imperial College Healthcare NHS Trust, London, United Kingdom

TEJA KAPOOR, MD
Assistant Professor, Department of Medicine, Division of Rheumatology, Columbia University Vagelos College of Physicians & Surgeons, New York, New York, USA

HELEN J. LACHMANN, MD, FRCP, FRCPath
National Amyloidosis Centre, Royal Free Campus, University College Medical School, London, United Kingdom

CHRISTOPHER P. LARSEN, MD
Nephropathology, Arkana Laboratories, Little Rock, Arkansas, USA

JOSHUA D. LONG, BA
Department of Medicine, Division of Nephrology, Massachusetts General Hospital, Boston, Massachusetts, USA

STEPHEN P. MCADOO, MBBS, PhD
Doctor, Clinician Researcher and Consultant Nephrologist, Renal and Vascular Inflammation Section, Department of Medicine, Imperial College London, Vasculitis Clinic, Imperial College Healthcare NHS Trust, London, United Kingdom

KRISTIN MELIAMBRO, MD
Division of Nephrology, Icahn School of Medicine at Mount Sinai, New York, New York, USA

JOHN L. NILES, MD
Assistant Professor of Medicine, Harvard Medical School, Division of Nephrology, Vasculitis and Glomerulonephritis Center, Massachusetts General Hospital, Boston, Massachusetts, USA

ELENA OLIVA-DAMASO, MD, PhD
Department of Medicine, Division of Nephrology, Hospital Doctor Negrin, Las Palmas de Gran Canaria, Spain

NESTOR OLIVA-DAMASO, MD
Department of Medicine, Division of Nephrology, Hospital Costa del Sol, Marbella, Malaga, Spain

RICCARDO PAPA, MD
Autoinflammatory Diseases and Immunodeficiencies Centre, Pediatric and Rheumatology Clinic, Giannina Gaslini Institute, University of Genoa, Genova, Italy

JUAN PAYAN, MD
Department of Medicine, Division of Nephrology, Hospital Costa del Sol, Marbella, Malaga, Spain

STEPHANIE M. RUTLEDGE, MBBS
Department of Medicine, Massachusetts General Hospital, Boston, Massachusetts, USA

MEGHAN E. SISE, MD, MS
Instructor, Department of Medicine, Division of Nephrology, Massachusetts General Hospital, Boston, Massachusetts, USA

TYLER WOODELL, MD
Oregon Health & Science University, Portland, Oregon, USA

REZA ZONOZI, MD
Clinical and Research Fellow, Harvard Medical School, Division of Nephrology, Vasculitis and Glomerulonephritis Center, Massachusetts General Hospital, Boston, Massachusetts, USA

Contents

Antineutrophil cytoplasmic antibody (ANCA)–associated vasculitis (AAV) is the most common cause of rapidly progressive glomerulonephritis. ANCAs play an important role in the pathogenesis and diagnosis of AAV. The classic renal lesion in AAV is a pauci-immune necrotizing and crescentic glomerulonephritis. Treatment is divided into 2 phases: (1) induction of remission to eliminate disease activity and (2) maintenance of remission to prevent disease relapse. Patients with AAV with end-stage renal disease require modification of immunosuppressive strategies and consideration for kidney transplant. An improved understanding of disease pathogenesis has led to new treatment strategies being tested in clinical trials.

Proliferative lupus nephritis requires prompt diagnosis and treatment with immunosuppressive therapy. Cyclophosphamide is the longest studied agent, but mycophenolate mofetil has recently emerged as an efficacious induction and maintenance treatment that does not impart the risk of infertility. However, overall remission rates remain suboptimal and there is a need for improved therapeutic options. To this end, ongoing clinical studies are focusing on agents that target key molecules and pathways implicated in the pathogenesis of lupus nephritis based on previous animal and human studies. This article reviews key findings of trials supporting established induction and maintenance treatment regimens along with novel therapeutic investigations.

Most of the attention paid to lupus nephritis, in the medical literature and in clinical trials, has primarily focused on proliferative forms of lupus nephritis (class III and IV lesions), but with lower thresholds to biopsy and rebiopsy patients with lupus, clinicians are encountering more cases with purely mesangial disease (classes I and II) or membranous nephropathy patterns (class V). These lesions often are associated with milder disease courses but still require dedicated follow-up by a nephrologist and focused therapeutic strategies that, at times, include immunosuppression.

Renal manifestations in rheumatoid arthritis (RA) have evolved as RA management has improved. In the past, older disease-modifying antirheumatic drugs, uncontrolled systemic inflammation, and chronic nonsteroidal anti-inflammatory drug (NSAID) use contributed to kidney disease. Over time, the use of methotrexate and biologic medications, decrease in NSAID use, and a treat-to-target strategy have contributed to a decrease in renal manifestations. Chronic kidney disease in RA now is more likely to be caused by cardiovascular risk factors than uncontrolled RA disease severity. In patients with renal dysfunction, NSAIDs, methotrexate, and tofacitinib may need to be adjusted or avoided to prevent adverse events.

Secondary, AA, amyloidosis is a rare systemic complication that can develop in any long-term inflammatory disorder and is characterized by the extracellular deposition of fibrils derived from serum amyloid A (SAA) protein. SAA is an acute-phase reactant synthetized largely by hepatocytes under the transcriptional regulation of proinflammatory cytokines. The kidney is the major involved organ, with proteinuria as the first clinical manifestation; renal biopsy is the most common diagnostic investigation. Targeted anti-inflammatory treatment promotes normalization of circulating SAA levels preventing amyloid deposition and renal damage. Novel therapies aimed at promoting clearance of existing amyloid deposits soon may be an effective treatment approach.

Several drugs commonly used in the management of rheumatic diseases may lead to nephrotoxicity, electrolyte disturbances, and hypertension. Here the authors focus on nonsteroidal anti-inflammatory drugs, uric acid–lowering therapy, and commonly used immunosuppressant therapies. The authors include a drug dosing table for patients with kidney disease.

Tubulointerstitial nephritis (TIN) is the second most common cause of acute intrinsic kidney injury after acute tubular necrosis. Although drug-induced forms of TIN represent the vast majority, rheumatic disease is another common cause and often underdiagnosed. Early diagnosis of acute interstitial nephritis and prompt withdrawal of the culprit medication or a correct treatment can avoid chronic damage and progressive chronic kidney disease. This article highlights the recent updates, clinical features, and treatment in TIN in autoimmune rheumatic disease.

Thrombotic microangiopathies are heterogeneous disorders characterized by microangiopathic hemolytic anemia with thrombocytopenia and renal injury. There are a variety of causes, including metabolic disorders, infections, medications, complement disorders, pregnancy, malignancy, and autoimmune disorders. This article focuses on renal thrombotic microangiopathy in the setting of rheumatologic diseases. Systemic lupus erythematosus is the most common autoimmune disease associated with thrombotic microangiopathy. Other causes include scleroderma renal crisis and antiphospholipid antibody syndrome, which can be primary or secondary to autoimmune diseases, including systemic lupus erythematosus. There have also been case reports of thrombotic microangiopathy in the setting of rheumatoid arthritis and dermatomyositis.

Kavita Gulati and Stephen P. McAdoo

Anti–glomerular basement membrane (anti-GBM) disease is a rare autoimmune small vessel vasculitis characterized by autoreactivity to antigens in type IV collagen chains expressed in glomerular and alveolar basement membrane. The detection of circulating anti-GBM antibodies, which are shown to be directly pathogenic, is central to disease diagnosis. Clinically, anti-GBM disease usually presents with rapidly progressive glomerulonephritis with or without alveolar hemorrhage. Rapid diagnosis and early treatment are required to prevent mortality and to preserve renal function. Relapse in anti-GBM disease is uncommon. Variant and atypical forms of anti-GBM disease are increasingly recognized.

Joshua D. Long, Stephanie M. Rutledge, and Meghan E. Sise

Autoimmune kidney diseases triggered by viruses are an important cause of kidney disease in patients affected by chronic viral infection. Hepatitis B virus (HBV) infection is associated with membranous nephropathy and polyarteritis nodosa. Hepatitis C virus (HCV) infection is a major cause of cryoglobulinemic glomerulonephritis. Patients with human immunodeficiency virus (HIV) may develop HIV-associated nephropathy, a form of collapsing focal segmental glomerulosclerosis, or various forms of immune-complex–mediated kidney diseases. This article summarizes what is known about the pathogenesis, diagnosis, and management of immune-mediated kidney diseases in adults with chronic HBV, HCV, and HIV infections.

Josephine M. Ambruzs and Christopher P. Larsen

Renal and urinary involvement has been reported to occur in 4% to 23% of patients with inflammatory bowel disease (IBD). Parenchymal renal disease is rare and most commonly affects glomerular and tubulointerstitial compartments. The most common findings on renal biopsy of patients with IBD are IgA nephropathy and tubulointerstitial nephritis. Overall morbidity of IBD-related renal manifestations is significant, and there is often only a short window of injury reversibility. This, along with subtle clinical presentation, requires a high index of suspicion and routine monitoring of renal function. There are no established guidelines for the optimal screening and monitoring of renal function in patients with IBD.

RHEUMATIC DISEASE CLINICS OF NORTH AMERICA

SERIES OF RELATED INTEREST

Physical Medicine and Rehabilitation Clinics
Medical Clinics
Primary Care Clinics
Dermatologic Clinics
Neurologic Clinics

THE CLINICS ARE AVAILABLE ONLINE!
Access your subscription at:
www.theclinics.com

Foreword

Renal Involvement in Rheumatic Diseases

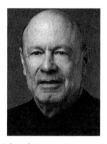

Michael H. Weisman, MD
Consulting Editor

For the strictly basic science-based or for the practicing rheumatologist, this issue is unique. It represents the coming together of two specialties (Rheumatology, Nephrology) that generally only meet when there is a diagnostic crisis with a patient or when there is a controversial issue to address in patient management. However, here is a different approach for the *Rheumatic Disease Clinics of North America*. We are trying to understand what one or the other specialty is thinking about these conditions from a mechanistic standpoint. We can see, in one issue, the various molecular mechanisms, immune and thrombotic dysregulated pathways, and the adaptive and immune responses as they affect the kidney. This issue is especially well referenced and highly current. Three conditions: lupus, rheumatoid arthritis, and inflammatory bowel disease, are an integral part of our rheumatologic patient care targets today, and these reviews give us chapter and verse of the most current thinking about diagnosis, pathogenesis, and management. Furthermore, the issue addresses antineutrophil cytoplasmic antibody–associated vasculitis, secondary amyloidosis, kidney toxicity of rheumatic disease medications, antiglomerular basement membrane disease, and viral diseases with renal manifestations. We are especially proud of the efforts of our editors in putting this highly topical and comprehensive issue together.

Michael H. Weisman, MD
Director, Division of Rheumatology
Professor of Medicine, Cedars-Sinai Medical Center
8700 Beverly Boulevard
Los Angeles, CA 90048, USA

E-mail address:
Michael.Weisman@cshs.org

Rheum Dis Clin N Am 44 (2018) xi
https://doi.org/10.1016/j.rdc.2018.08.002
0889-857X/18/© 2018 Published by Elsevier Inc.

rheumatic.theclinics.com

Preface

A Three-Headed Approach to Kidney Involvement in Rheumatic Diseases

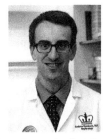
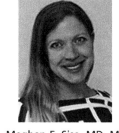

Andrew S. Bomback, MD, MPH   Meghan E. Sise, MD, MS
Editors

This issue of *Rheumatic Disease Clinics of North America* is devoted to renal involvement in rheumatic diseases. Not surprisingly, the authors of the included reviews are all nephrologists and rheumatologists, as these clinicians usually comanage cases of the diagnoses discussed herein. However, a third group of physicians, while not represented in the author list, clearly contributes to virtually every topic covered in this issue. Renal pathologists represent the third head in approaching most of the rheumatologic diseases that have kidney involvement, as biopsies have become a mainstay not only for diagnosing such conditions but also for providing the most reliable data for prognosis.

A question that often arises is whether a renal biopsy is "needed" in cases of kidney disease with positive serologic testing, which extends to many of the diseases discussed in this issue, including antiglomerular basement membrane disease, antineutrophil cytoplasmic antibody (ANCA)-associated glomerulonephritis, and lupus nephritis. As nephrologists, we almost always answer with a resounding "yes." A thorough kidney biopsy report not only suggests or confirms a pathologic diagnosis but can also provide information on the severity of the injury, activity versus chronicity of the lesion, and the presence of other, significant renal or vascular abnormalities. In other words, a well-read kidney biopsy can tell the nephrologist and rheumatologist what the patient has and whether there is a reasonable chance of recovery with successful therapy. There is no serologic test that can impart that degree of information.

Renal pathologists will admit that a biopsy never truly "makes" the diagnosis. The histopathology, rather, presents a pattern of injury that in turn allows the treating physicians to seek out a cause behind that pattern. Using ANCA-associated glomerulonephritis as an example, the kidney biopsy may show a necrotizing and crescentic

Rheum Dis Clin N Am 44 (2018) xiii–xiv
https://doi.org/10.1016/j.rdc.2018.08.001
0889-857X/18/© 2018 Published by Elsevier Inc.

glomerulonephritis with pauci-immune staining on immunofluorescence and no electron dense deposits on electron microscopy. This information is then combined with the clinical history and physical findings elicited by the nephrologist and rheumatologist, alongside the results of serologic testing for anti-myeloperoxidase and anti-proteinase 3 antibodies, to give the patient a diagnosis of ANCA-associated disease. And the nephrologist and rheumatologist will then rely heavily on what the biopsy shows to decide on a treatment plan. In many kidney diseases with rheumatologic components, a second or even third kidney biopsy can improve long-term management decisions.

As our understanding of the pathophysiology behind kidney and rheumatologic diseases has grown, the armamentarium of serologic tests at our disposal has expanded. However, we should not expect biopsies to fall out of favor or decline in importance just because a new test is available. The information gleaned from a biopsy will continue to complement the clinical and serologic data, guiding diagnostic and treatment decisions. In other words, the optimal approach to renal involvement in rheumatic diseases will remain a 3-headed one that includes a nephrologist, a rheumatologist, and a renal pathologist.

Andrew S. Bomback, MD, MPH
Department of Medicine
Division of Nephrology
Columbia University College of Physicians and Surgeons
622 West 168th Street, PH 4-124
New York, NY 10032, USA

Meghan E. Sise, MD, MS
Department of Medicine
Division of Nephrology
Massachusetts General Hospital
55 Fruit Street
Boston, MA 02114, USA

E-mail addresses:
asb68@cumc.columbia.edu (A.S. Bomback)
msise@partners.org (M.E. Sise)

Renal Involvement in Antineutrophil Cytoplasmic Antibody–Associated Vasculitis

Reza Zonozi, MD, John L. Niles, MD, Frank B. Cortazar, MD*

KEYWORDS

- ANCA-associated vasculitis • Granulomatosis with polyangiitis
- Microscopic polyangiitis • Rapidly progressive glomerulonephritis

KEY POINTS

- Antineutrophil cytoplasmic antibody (ANCA)-associated vasculitis (AAV) is the most common cause of rapidly progressive glomerulonephritis (RPGN).
- ANCAs play an important pathogenic role in the development of AAV via the activation of neutrophils.
- The hallmark pathologic renal lesion in AAV is pauci-immune necrotizing and crescentic glomerulonephritis presenting as RPGN. In many cases, however, the disease course can be indolent with a slow deterioration of renal function.
- Early initiation of treatment is paramount to prevent irreversible organ damage.
- Enhanced understating of the pathogenesis of AAV has provided the rationale for novel targeted therapies.

INTRODUCTION

Antineutrophil cytoplasmic antibody (ANCA)-associated vasculitis (AAV) is a small-vessel vasculitis, which is the most common cause of rapidly progressive glomerulonephritis (RPGN).[1] If diagnosis or therapy is delayed, there are organ-threatening and life-threatening implications. Thus, the practicing clinician should pay special heed to this entity. This article reviews the renal involvement of AAV.

DEFINITIONS, NOMENCLATURE, AND CLASSIFICATION

AAV has traditionally been classified based on clinical and pathologic features into 4 entities: granulomatosis with polyangiitis (GPA), microscopic polyangiitis (MPA),

Disclosure Statement: F.B. Cortazar and J.L. Niles have served as consultants for ChemoCentryx. R. Zonozi has no disclosures.
Division of Nephrology, Vasculitis and Glomerulonephritis Center, Massachusetts General Hospital, 101 Merrimac Street, Boston, MA 02114, USA
* Corresponding author.
E-mail address: FCORTAZAR@PARTNERS.ORG

Rheum Dis Clin N Am 44 (2018) 525–543
https://doi.org/10.1016/j.rdc.2018.06.001
0889-857X/18/© 2018 Elsevier Inc. All rights reserved.

rheumatic.theclinics.com

renal limited vasculitis, and eosinophilic GPA (EGPA).[2] During the active phase of disease, greater than 90% of AAV patients with glomerulonephritis are ANCA positive.[3,4]

GPA is characterized by extravascular necrotizing granulomatous inflammation and necrotizing vasculitis with a proclivity for the upper and lower respiratory tract in addition to the kidney. GPA is more commonly associated with proteinase 3 (PR3)-ANCA than myeloperoxidase (MPO)-ANCA. MPA is distinguished from GPA by the lack of extravascular granulomatous inflammation and is more frequently associated with MPO-ANCA. Likewise, renal limited vasculitis is predominantly an MPO-ANCA disease (>75% of cases) and is defined by the lack of extrarenal manifestations of vasculitis.[5]

EGPA, like GPA, leads to necrotizing granulomatous inflammation of the respiratory tract and is distinguished from other causes of AAV by the presence of eosinophilia and asthma. Unlike the other AAV syndromes, only approximately 50% of patients with EGPA have a positive ANCA, typically MPO-ANCA.[6] ANCA-positive and ANCA-negative cases, however, have different clinical phenotypes. ANCA-positive EGPA more commonly causes glomerulonephritis and mononeuritis multiplex, whereas ANCA-negative EGPA is more commonly associated with cardiac involvement.[7]

In clinical practice, the distinction between GPA and MPA is rarely definitive, because granulomatous inflammation is apt to be missed by sampling error and biopsy is often foregone in the setting of a positive ANCA and a characteristic presentation. Rather, a presumptive diagnosis is made based on apparent clinical features. For example, patients with destructive upper airway disease or cavitary pulmonary nodules are given a diagnosis of GPA, whereas those presenting with pulmonary hemorrhage and RPGN are generally labeled as MPA. From a practical standpoint, classifying a patient as GPA versus MPA is somewhat subjective and may not add significant value to disease management.

Another way to classify AAV patients is by ANCA serotype. There is a geographic variation of the frequency of ANCA specificity, with PR3-ANCA more common in northern Europe and MPO-ANCA more common in southern Europe and Asia.[8] Genome-wide studies have demonstrated that key predisposing genetic variants correlate with ANCA serotype more strongly than clinical diagnosis (eg, GPA).[9]

In the clinical setting, ANCA serotype better predicts disease prognosis and the propensity for relapse than clinical syndrome, with PR3-ANCA patients more likely to have refractory disease and a relapsing course.[10] Finally, ANCA specificity can be associated with certain disease manifestations and clinical scenarios. For example, ANCA with interstitial lung disease, which can occur in isolation of other clinical features and masquerade as idiopathic interstitial lung disease, is essentially always an MPO-ANCA disease.[11] Similarly, drug-associated AAV occurs with MPO-ANCA with or without PR3-ANCA but virtually never with PR3-ANCA alone.[12] Due to genetic and pathophysiologic underpinnings and the superior clinical utility, many experts now propose classifying AAV patients as having simply PR3-ANCA or MPO-ANCA rather than having GPA or MPA.

PATHOGENESIS
Risk Factors for Antineutrophil Cytoplasmic Antibody Production

Although the exact mechanisms leading to the genesis of ANCA autoantibodies remain unclear, several risk factors have been implicated, including genetic predispositions, infectious insults, and medication exposures.

Given the central role of antigen presentation in the initiation of an adaptive immune response that ultimately leads to antibody production, it is conceivable that different

HLA molecules may predispose an individual to develop autoantibodies to MPO or PR3. Genome-wide association studies have demonstrated an association between ANCA serotype and HLA status.[9,13] PR3-ANCA seropositivity associates with HLA-DP, whereas MPO-ANCA seropositivity associates with HLA-DQ.[9] In addition to HLA molecules, PR3-ANCA is associated with the genes encoding PR3 itself and α_1-antitrypsin, a serine protease inhibitor whose target includes PR3.

The development of ANCA, specifically MPO-ANCA, can be linked to the prolonged exposure of certain medications.[14] The implicated medications in clinical use include hydralazine, minocycline, propylthiouracil, allopurinol, and sulfasalazine.[12,14–16] Hydralazine-associated disease is particularly aggressive, often manifesting as RPGN and pulmonary hemorrhage. MPO titters in hydralazine-associated cases are characteristically markedly elevated compared with patients who have idiopathic MPO-ANCA vasculitis.[14] More recently, cocaine adulterated with levamisole has been found to cause a unique form of ANCA vasculitis among chronic cocaine users.[17] Characteristically, patients present with arthralgias, necrotic skin lesions, and often double positivity for MPO-ANCA and PR3-ANCA. The mechanism by which medications induce ANCA vasculitis is unclear, although certain hypotheses have been proposed. For example, hydralazine acts as a methylation inhibitor in addition to a vasodilator, and may prevent epigenetic silencing of the gene encoding MPO.[14]

Role of Antineutrophil Cytoplasmic Antibody

There is a preponderance of evidence that ANCA play a key pathogenic role in the development of pauci-immune necrotizing vasculitis. In a classic animal model, passive transfer of MPO-ANCA into a RAG-2–deficient mouse (which lacks B cells and T cells) is sufficient to recapitulate the hallmark necrotizing and crescentic glomerulonephritis characteristic of AAV.[18] In a natural human model, a newborn developed pulmonary hemorrhage and RPGN after placental transfer of MPO-ANCA from the mother.[19]

In in vitro studies, ANCA has been demonstrated to activate neutrophils that have been primed with inflammatory mediators, such as tumor necrosis factor and C5a.[20,21] Neutrophil priming allows MPO and PR3, which are typically sequestered in the cytosol, to migrate to or near the cell surface, where they can bind ANCA. Activation via engagement of the Fc receptor or cross-linking of antigen at the cell surface leads to a respiratory burst and the degranulation of cytotoxic enzymes that cause tissue injury.[22–24]

The importance of ANCA in the pathogenesis of AAV can also be inferred from the success of current therapeutic strategies. As discussed later, removal of ANCA via plasma exchange (PLEX) and inhibition of ANCA production via B-cell depletion are important components of therapy in AAV.

Role of Complement

Historically, complement was not believed to play an important pathophysiologic role in AAV due to the normal serum complement levels during active disease and the paucity of deposited complement in cases of necrotizing crescentic glomerulonephritis. More recently, it has been appreciated that neutrophil stimulation with ANCA leads to activation of the alternative complement pathway.[25] Observational data in humans have shown that AAV patients with lower C3 levels have worse patient and renal survival.[26] The anaphylatoxin C5a, which serves to recruit and prime neutrophils, has been identified as a key pathogenic mediator. In animal models, mice lacking the C5a receptor are protected from developing vasculitis, as are mice treated with a drug that inhibits the C5a receptor.[21,27] A drug targeting the C5a receptor is currently being tested in clinical trial for AAV (**Table 1**).

CLINICOPATHOLOGIC SPECTRUM OF RENAL INVOLVEMENT IN ANTINEUTROPHIL CYTOPLASMIC ANTIBODY–ASSOCIATED VASCULITIS
Rapidly Progressive Glomerulonephritis

The classic renal presentation of AAV is RPGN, which is characterized by a progressive and rapid decline in kidney function over days to a few months. AAV is the most common cause of RPGN worldwide.[28] Patients typically present with subnephrotic proteinuria, microscopic hematuria, hypertension, and edema. In rare cases, the patient reports a history of gross hematuria. Examination of the urinary sediment typically reveals dysmorphic red blood cells and occasionally red blood cell casts (**Fig. 1**).

The pathologic correlate of RPGN in AAV is pauci-immune necrotizing and crescentic glomerulonephritis. Light microscopy reveals areas of segmental fibrinoid necrosis and cellular crescents (**Fig. 2**A, B). The hallmark immunofluorescence shows little or no glomerular staining for immunoglobulins or complement, the so-called pauci-immune staining pattern (**Fig. 2**C).[29] Likewise, electron microscopy typically reveals few or no deposits within the glomerular basement membrane (GBM) (**Fig. 2**D).[28]

Although AAV is classically known for being pauci-immune, on occasion more prominent immune complex deposition may be observed. It is possible that this is

Table 1		
Ongoing clinical trials in antineutrophil cytoplasmic antibody–associated vasculitis		
Trial	**CTI**	**Treatment Tested**
ADVOCATE	NCT02994927	AVACOPAN (C5aR antagonist) vs prednisone in patients receiving cyclophosphamide or RTX for remission induction
ABROGATE	NCT02108860	Abatacept vs placebo in patients with GPA receiving remission maintenance with azathioprine, methotrexate, or MMF
PEXIVAS	NCT00987389	PLEX vs no PLEX AND low-dose glucocorticoids vs standard glucocorticoids in patients with severe renal involvement or pulmonary hemorrhage
LoVAS	NCT02198248	Low-dose glucocorticoids vs standard glucocorticoids in patients receiving remission induction with RTX
RITAZAREM	NCT01697267	Rituximab vs azathioprine for maintenance of remission
MAINRITSAN 2	NCT01731561	Maintenance RTX dosing based on B cells or ANCA vs conventional RTX dosing (every 6 mo)
MAINRITSAN 3	NCT02433522	Long-term RTX maintenance treatment (46 mo) vs conventional RTX maintenance treatment (18 mo)
MAINTANCAVAS	NCT02749292	Dosing RTX based on B cells vs serologic ANCA flare for long-term maintenance of remission
TAPIR	NCT01940094	Extended low-dose glucocorticoids vs glucocorticoid cessation for maintenance of remission
MAINEPSAN	NCT03290456	Extended low-dose glucocorticoids vs glucocorticoid cessation for maintenance of remission
MASTER-ANCA	NCT03323476	Maintenance immunosuppression vs no maintenance immunosuppression for AAV patients with ESRD

Abbreviations: C5aR, complement component 5a receptor; CTI, Clinicaltrials.gov identifier; RTX, rituximab.
From www.clinicaltrials.gov. Accessed April 1, 2018.

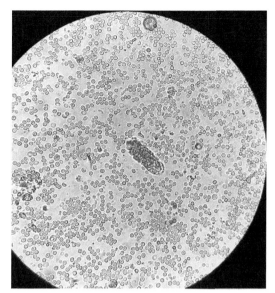

Fig. 1. Urine sediment in AAV. High-powered (×40) light microscopic view of urinary sediment of a 34-year-old man presenting to the Massachusetts General Hospital with RPGN and pulmonary hemorrhage. Demonstration of a red blood cell cast surrounded by dysmorphic and nondysmorphic red blood cells. (*Courtesy of* Reza Zonozi, MD, Boston, MA.)

particularly true in drug-induced cases, which are often associated with other autoantibodies (**Fig. 3**A, B). Two reports determined that the presence of immune deposits in AAV are associated with greater proteinuria.[30,31]

Indolent Glomerulonephritis

Although conventionally associated with RPGN, in a subset of patients AAV leads to an indolent and protracted deterioration of renal function more akin to IgA nephropathy.[32,33] In retrospect, these patients are often noted to have a long history of microscopic hematuria and a slow decline in glomerular filtration rate (GFR) over months to years. This phenotype is almost exclusively observed in patients with MPO-ANCA, many of whom have renal-limited disease. Pathologically, patients with MPO-ANCA have more chronic damage as manifested by greater interstitial fibrosis, tubular atrophy, glomerulosclerosis, and fibrous or fibrocellular rather than cellular crescents.[5,33] Consequently, the magnitude of GFR improvement with treatment is less in patients with MPO-ANCA.[34]

Concomitant Glomerular Lesions

Five percent of patients with a positive ANCA have concurrent anti-GBM disease, whereas approximately one-third of patients with anti-GBM disease have concurrent ANCA positivity, more commonly MPO-ANCA.[35] These cases of double-positive disease can have varying degrees of clinical presentation consistent with anti-GBM disease and AAV. ANCA may appear in sera prior to anti-GBM, which suggests that the damage from ANCA may lead to the exposure of GBM antigens with subsequent anti-GBM autoantibody formation.[36] Patients with isolated anti-GBM disease essentially never relapse. Among patients with double-positive disease, the potential for relapse of AAV seems similar to patients with AAV alone.[37]

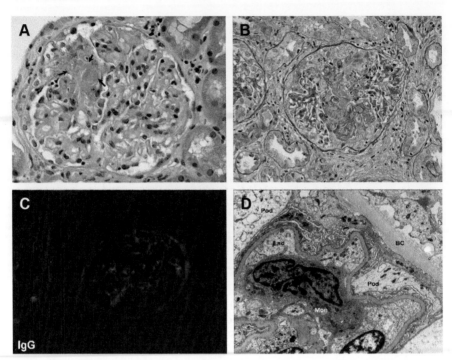

Fig. 2. Pauci-immune crescentic glomerulonephritis. Demonstration of classic histology with light microscopy, immunofluorescence, and electron microscopy from a kidney biopsy in a patient presenting with RPGN from AAV. (*A*) Focal necrotizing glomerulitis with early cellular crescent (hematoxylin-eosin, original magnification x 160). The glomerulus revels segmental fibrinoid necrosis of the tuft (*arrows*) and limited karyorrhexis (nuclear fragmentation), with formation of an early cellular crescent (*white asterisk*). (*B*) Focal necrotizing glomerulitis with early crescent formation (periodic acid-Schiff, original magnification x 135). There is also mild periglomerular interstitial inflammation. (*C*) ANCA-associated diseases are usually pauci-immune, and significant immunoglobulin or complement deposits are not seen in the glomeruli. The glomerulus depicted here shows background staining for IgG, similar in intensity to the staining with antialbumin reagents (not shown) (FITC-labeled human IgG antibodies, original magnification x 120). (*D*) ANCA-associated glomerular lesions are usually pauci-immune, showing few or no deposits on electron microscopy (hematoxylin-eosin, original magnification X 3500). BC, Bowman capsule; End, endothelial cell; Mon, monocyte occupying the capillary lumen; Pod, podocyte. (*Courtesy of* Helmut Rennke, MD, Boston, MA.)

AAV has been described occurring simultaneously with other glomerular diseases, notably membranous nephropathy and lupus nephritis.[38–40]

Nonglomerular Lesions

Interstitial nephritis caused by AAV is often found in association with glomerular lesions, but can also occur without glomerular involvement. Rare patients with AAV have a prominent tubulointerstitial nephritis, which can be associated with vasculitis of the vasa recta (**Fig. 3**C).[41] Alternatively, a patient with necrotizing glomerulonephritis from AAV may develop a superimposed interstitial nephritis related to a drug (eg, azathioprine).[42]

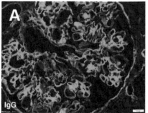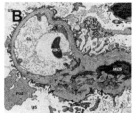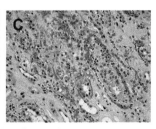

Fig. 3. Variable spectrum of renal pathology in AAV. (*A*) This glomerulus reveals scattered and predominantly mesangial deposits of IgG in a patient with hydralazine-induced AAV with focal necrotizing and crescentic glomerulonephritis (immunofluorescence, original magnification X 180). (*B*) Electron microscopy in the same patient shows prominent electron dense deposits in a predominantly mesangial distribution (*arrows*, original magnification x 2000). (*C*) ANCA-associated interstitial nephritis with medullary angiitis (capillaritis) (hematoxylin-eosin, magnification 90x). The outer medulla shows a hemorrhagic interstitial nephritis with prominent neutrophilic capillaritis. CL, capillary lumen; MES, mesangial cell; Pod, podocyte; RBC, red blood cell; US, urinary space. (*Courtesy of* Helmut Rennke, MD, Boston, MA.)

DIAGNOSIS

A diagnosis of AAV incorporates the integration of clinical features, ANCA serology, and tissue pathology as needed. Patients with a clinical syndrome compatible with AAV should have peripheral blood sent for ANCA testing. Testing for ANCA involves 2 distinct assays: an indirect immunofluorescence assay and an enzyme-linked immunosorbent assay (ELISA).

Indirect immunofluorescence generally reveals a perinuclear staining pattern (p-ANCA) in patients with MPO-ANCA and a cytoplasmic staining pattern (c-ANCA) in patients with PR3-ANCA (**Fig. 4**). Indirect immunofluorescence alone, however, is not sufficiently specific for diagnosis because autoantibodies to other antigens not associated with vasculitis (eg, lactoferrin and human leukocyte elastase) can result in a positive staining pattern.[43] Importantly, only ANCAs specific for MPO or PR3 are associated with vasculitis.[44–46] Thus, in many laboratories indirect immunofluorescence is used as a screening test. If a p-ANCA or c-ANCA pattern is detected, antigen-specific testing with ELISA must be performed to confirm the presence of autoantibodies against MPO or PR3.

The need for a confirmatory tissue diagnosis in patients with clinical features of vasculitis and autoantibodies to MPO or PR3 depends on the clinical scenario. As with any diagnostic test, the positive predictive value of a positive ANCA is dependent on the sensitivity and specificity of the test and the prevalence of the disease in the population tested. In a patient with a clinical syndrome of RPGN, a positive ANCA is virtually diagnostic of AAV, with a positive predictive value of approximately 99%.[47,48] In such patients, the authors generally forgo biopsy. Many other centers, however, routinely biopsy all patients, particularly in settings where results of ANCA testing are not rapidly available. In patients who have less characteristic or atypical presentations, the diagnosis should be confirmed with biopsy of an affected organ, when possible. Importantly, in patients with acute organ-threatening or life-threatening disease (eg, RPGN or pulmonary hemorrhage), treatment should not be delayed while a diagnosis is confirmed with ANCA testing or biopsy.

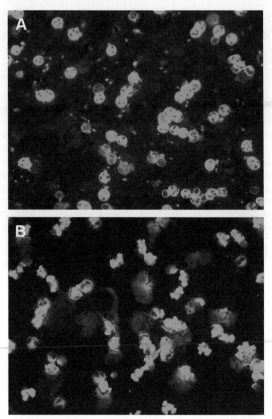

Fig. 4. Indirect immunofluorescence. Indirect immunofluorescence is performed after incubation of serum with ethanol-fixed human neutrophils to assess for the presence of ANCAs. (*A*) A cytoplasmic staining pattern (c-ANCA) usually corresponds to antibodies directed against proteinase 3. (*B*) A perinuclear staining pattern usually corresponds to the presence of autoantibodies to myeloperoxidase. (*Courtesy of* ANCA Laboratory of the Massachusetts General Hospital, Boston, MA; with permission.)

TREATMENT

Treatment of AAV consists of 2 phases: (1) induction of remission and (2) maintenance of remission. The goal of induction therapy is to rapidly quell disease activity with the intention of preventing irreversible organ damage. Maintenance therapy is used to prevent disease relapse after a remission has been achieved. The following sections review standard treatment regimens for AAV and highlight new potential therapies currently being evaluated in clinical trials.

Induction of Remission

Standard therapy for life-threatening or organ-threatening AAV, which includes cases with renal involvement, is glucocorticoids in combination with either cyclophosphamide or rituximab.[49,50] The Rituximab for the Treatment of Wegener's Granulomatosis and Microscopic Polyangiitis (RAVE) trial compared a cyclophosphamide-based regimen to a rituximab-based regimen and found no difference in efficacy.[50] In addition, the rate of adverse events, including serious infections, was similar across the 2 groups.

Cyclophosphamide

If cyclophosphamide is used, it can be administered orally or intravenously (IV). The Randomized Trial of Daily Oral Versus Pulse Cyclophosphamide as Therapy for ANCA-associated Systemic Vasculitis (CYCLOPS) found no difference in remission rate between oral and IV therapy.[51] IV therapy had the advantage of reduced cumulative dose and fewer episodes of leukopenia. Conversely, oral therapy affords greater titratability and was associated with a lower risk of relapse than IV therapy.[52] Regardless of the administration route, cyclophosphamide is generally continued for 3 months to 6 months.

Oral cyclophosphamide is administered at 1.5 mg/kg to 2 mg/kg daily. During treatment with oral cyclophosphamide, a complete blood cell count should be checked approximately every 2 weeks and the daily dose adjusted to maintain the leukocyte count greater than 3.5 cells/L $\times 10^9$ cells/L. Many different dosing strategies for IV cyclophosphamide exist. Some experts use the regimen used in the CYCLOPS trial: 15 mg/kg every 2 weeks for 3 doses, then 15 mg/kg every 3 weeks to complete a 3-month to 6-month course.[51] Another commonly used regimen is to administer 0.5 mg/m^2 to 0.75 mg/m^2 of body surface area (BSA) every 2 weeks to 3 weeks. In either case, the cyclophosphamide dose should be modified as needed to maintain a nadir leukocyte count (checked approximately 10–14 days after each IV dose) above 3.5 cells/L $\times 10^9$ cells/L. Patients receiving IV cyclophosphamide are pretreated with IV saline and instructed to drink liberally after the infusion. Although convincing data are lacking, 2-mercaptoethane sodium sulfonate (mesna) is routinely used with IV dosing to protect the bladder from acrolein, a toxic metabolite of cyclophosphamide.[53]

Regardless of route of administration, it is paramount to adjust the cyclophosphamide dose for renal impairment because renal clearance is a primary route of elimination for both active metabolites and the parent compound.[54] Failure to do so leads to a high rate of leukopenia and increases the risk of serious infections. Currently, there are no established guidelines for cyclophosphamide dosing in the setting of renal impairment. The authors' practice is to reduce both the daily oral and IV cyclophosphamide dose as follows: 10% if the estimated GFR (eGFR) is 60 mL/min to 89 mL/min per 1.73 m^2; 25% if the eGFR is 45 mL/min to 59 mL/min per 1.73 m^2, 33% if the eGFR is 30 mL/min to 44 mL/min per 1.73 m^2, 40% if the eGFR is 15 mL/min to 29 mL/min per 1.73 m^2, and 50% if the eGFR is less than or equal to15 mL/min per 1.73 m^2 or the patient is on dialysis.[34]

Cyclophosphamide is associated with a dose-dependent risk of infertility and secondary malignancies, in particular bladder cancer.[55,56] Therefore, care should be taken to limit the cumulative cyclophosphamide exposure to the greatest extent possible. In general, the duration of cyclophosphamide exposure should be limited to 3 months in most patients and should not exceed 6 months.

Rituximab

If rituximab is used for remission induction, the standard dosing protocol is that used in the RAVE trial: 375 mg/m^2 BSA IV weekly for 4 weeks. Another option is to administer two 1000-mg IV doses separated by approximately 2 weeks as is traditionally done for rheumatoid arthritis.[57] When used in AAV, this dosing protocol produces similar outcomes to the standard dosing regimen, reliably induces complete B-cell depletion, affords greater convenience to patients, and is more cost effective.[34,58]

The dosing of rituximab must be modified in patients receiving PLEX because the procedure removes the drug from circulation. One approach is to administer 1 g early in the PLEX course immediately after a treatment session and delay the next PLEX for 48 hours. The second 1-g rituximab dose is then administered on completion of the final PLEX.[34] A detailed discussion on unique complications of rituximab is provided in the section on maintenance therapy.

Glucocorticoids

The optimal glucocorticoid regimen for remission induction in AAV remains unknown. In patients with RPGN, therapy is typically commenced with high dose IV methylprednisolone (500–1000 mg daily) for 3 days. Thereafter, prednisone is commenced at 1 mg/kg daily (maximum dose 60–80 mg), which is continued for approximately 2 weeks to 4 weeks based on disease response. The prednisone dose is then tapered with the goal of reaching 20 mg daily by 2 months and low dose ($\leq$7.5 mg daily) or complete discontinuation by 6 months.[49,50] As discussed later, the choice of maintenance therapy often dictates whether prednisone can be weaned to discontinuation.[59]

Glucocorticoids can lead to a significant array of adverse events, including infection, weight gain, diabetes mellitus, cataracts, and osteoporosis.[60,61] As discussed later, novel strategies are being used to attenuate glucocorticoid exposure.

Plasma exchange

PLEX is added to remission induction immunosuppression to facilitate rapid removal of ANCA in the setting of severe RPGN and/or pulmonary hemorrhage.[62,63] The Methylprednisolone versus Plasma Exchange (MEPEX) trial examined the role of PLEX in patients with RPGN and a serum creatinine greater than 5.7 mg/dL. All patients received a standard remission induction regimen with cyclophosphamide and prednisone and were randomized to PLEX or pulse IV methylprednisolone (1000 mg daily for 3 days).[63] Patients randomized to PLEX had a lower rate of dialysis dependence at 1 year.

The results of the MEPEX trial are difficult to apply in clinical practice given that pulse steroids and PLEX are often given simultaneously. Moreover, no data are provided on patients with a serum creatinine less than 5.7 mg/dL. The ongoing Plasma Exchange and Glucocorticoids for Treatment of Anti-Neutrophil Cytoplasm Antibody (ANCA) - Associated Vasculitis (PEXIVAS) trial is evaluating the role of PLEX in patients with RPGN and an eGFR less than 50 mL/min/1.73 m^2 in the context of a glucocorticoid regimen than commences with pulse methylprednisolone.[64] Until the results of this trial are available, the authors' practice is to use PLEX in patients with rapidly deteriorating renal function, even if the serum creatinine has not reached 5.7 mg/dL.

The authors typically administer 7 sessions of a 1 to 1.2 plasma volume exchange with 5% albumin over 2 weeks. In cases where bleeding is a concern, such as in patients with pulmonary hemorrhage or a recent kidney biopsy, fresh frozen plasma can be substituted as a portion of the exchange volume to prevent coagulopathy. PLEX is also indicated in all cases of AAV with concomitant anti-GBM membrane autoantibodies. In these cases, a more aggressive PLEX regimen is typically used as for anti-GBM disease (see article in this issue).

Maintenance of Remission

After remission has been achieved, maintenance therapy is initiated to prevent disease relapse. Maintenance therapy is commenced immediately after completion of oral cyclophosphamide or 2 weeks to 4 weeks after the last dose of IV cyclophosphamide, provided the total leukocyte count and absolute neutrophil count are near normal in both scenarios. If rituximab was used for remission induction, maintenance therapy is initiated 4 months to 6 months after the final rituximab dose. Some practitioners forgo maintenance therapy in patients who received rituximab for remission induction and await relapse prior to additional treatment. This strategy is associated with a high relapse rate, with approximately one-third of patients sustaining a disease flare by 18 months.[65]

Until recently, azathioprine and methotrexate were the maintenance agents of choice for AAV.[66–68] Methotrexate is associated with an increased rate of adverse events in the setting of renal insufficiency, and azathioprine has thus been used preferentially in patients with renal involvement. Rituximab has emerged, however, as an extremely effective maintenance agent with a favorable side-effect profile and low risk of disease relapse.[69,70] The Maintenance of Remission using Riuximab in Systemic ANCA-associated Vasculitis (MAINRITSAN) trial directly compared azathioprine with rituximab for maintenance of remission. At 28 months, the relapse rate was significantly lower in patients treated with rituximab (5%) than with azathioprine (29%), with a similar rate of adverse events across the 2 groups. A majority of patients in the MAINRITSAN trial had PR3-ANCA, raising questions about the generalizability of the results to patients with MPO-ANCA. Due to the higher costs, rituximab is restricted to patients with a history of relapsing disease in some practice settings. In addition, azathioprine is the treatment of choice for pregnant women given the extensive experience and low rate of fetal complications with the medication.[71]

Azathioprine

Azathioprine is typically administered as 2 mg/kg initially.[49,66] The relapse rate in patients treated with azathioprine is significantly lower when low-dose glucocorticoids are continued as part of the maintenance regimen.[59,66] Thus, when using azathioprine, the authors' practice is to continue low-dose glucocorticoids (eg, prednisone, 7.5 mg daily) in most patients. In select patients, a higher dose of prednisone may be needed to maintain remission.

The major side effects of azathioprine are gastrointestinal complaints and bone marrow suppression.[72] A complete blood cell count should be checked 2 weeks after initiating azathioprine and after any dose escalation to ensure significant leukopenia has not developed. Thereafter, periodic monitoring is needed to document stability of leukocyte count with the azathioprine dose titrated to maintain a white blood cell count above the lower limit of normal. Patients on long-term azathioprine maintenance should be referred to dermatology for routine skin checks given the high rate of squamous cell carcinoma in this population.[73]

Rituximab

When used as maintenance therapy, rituximab is generally dosed as 500 mg to 1000 mg IV every 4 months to 6 months.[69,70] In contrast to maintenance with azathioprine, glucocorticoids can be tapered to discontinuation in a vast majority of patients treated with rituximab maintenance.[34,69,74] During the initial stages of maintenance therapy, the authors administer 1000 mg IV every 4 months with the aim of achieving continuous B-cell depletion.[69,74] B-cell depletion is confirmed at a given dosing interval with flow cytometry as an undetectable population of $CD19^+CD20^+$ lymphocytes. If remission is maintained, the dosing interval can subsequently be extended to 6 months or longer. One strategy is to extend the interval to the point where B cell reconstitution occurs. Trials evaluating the optimal rituximab dosing strategy for maintenance of remission are ongoing (see **Table 1**).

Unique side effects of rituximab need to be considered, particularly when used for long-term maintenance therapy. Not surprisingly, B-cell depletion can lead to varying degrees of hypogammaglobulinemia.[74,75] This effect is partially mitigated, however, by established populations of long-lived plasma cells that are resistant to rituximab and serve to maintain the IgG pool. The largest decline in IgG levels occurs after the induction doses of rituximab. Thereafter, IgG levels remain relatively constant despite prolonged B-cell depletion, declining at a rate of approximately 0.6% annually.[74] Serious infections are associated with significant hypogammaglobulinemia (IgG level <400 mg/dL).[74,76] Thus, IgG levels should be monitored in patients whose IgG level falls close to 400 mg/dL after the first round of rituximab therapy. IV immunoglobulin supplementation can be administered to patients with significant hypogammaglobulinemia who develop infectious complications.

Late-onset neutropenia is a rare but important side effect of rituximab that manifests as abrupt and often severe neutropenia.[77,78] This phenomenon can occur anytime after rituximab administration until B-cell reconstitution occurs. In many cases, patients come to clinical attention because of fever.[34,78] A complete blood cell count should be checked promptly in any febrile patient on rituximab. Patients with confirmed neutropenic fever should be referred to the hospital for an infectious work-up and empiric antibiotics. The neutropenia itself is readily reversible with filgrastim in most cases. The authors' practice is to administer filgrastim to asymptomatic patients with an absolute neutrophil count less than 750 and febrile patients with an absolute neutrophil count less than 1000. Patients who require ongoing maintenance therapy and have sustained an episode of late-onset neutropenia can be cautiously rechallenged with rituximab.

Duration of maintenance therapy

The optimal duration of maintenance therapy is unknown and must be individualized after integrating several patient-specific factors: (1) risk of relapse, (2) existing disease damage and risk of end-stage renal disease (ESRD) or other irreversible organ damage if a recurrent flare occurred, (3) ability to tolerate reinduction therapy, and (4) risk of complications from continued maintenance therapy. Important risk factors for disease relapse include a history of prior relapse, PR3 seropositivity, and upper airway disease.[10,79] In patients presenting with de novo disease, maintenance therapy is often continued for at least 2 years.[49,80] Longer courses of maintenance therapy are used in patients at high risk for relapse and in those who have accrued significant disease damage (eg, advanced chronic kidney disease). In patients with a history of multiple relapses, maintenance therapy is often continued indefinitely.

Special Scenarios in Patients with Renal Disease

Treatment of patients with end-stage renal disease

There is a paucity of data regarding the optimal management of patients who become dialysis dependent despite remission induction therapy. The rate of relapse is lower and the rate of infectious complications is greater in patients with AAV on dialysis compared with AAV patients not on dialysis.[81] Therefore, in patients on dialysis without evidence of active extrarenal disease, the duration of maintenance therapy is often abridged to approximately 6 months. Renal recovery after this duration of treatment is unlikely.[82] Patients who relapse while on dialysis are treated similar to other relapsing AAV patients. The ongoing Maintaining or Stopping Immunosuppressive Therapy in Patients with ANCA Vasculitis and End-stage Renal Disease (MASTER-ANCA) trial is assessing the utility of maintenance treatment for patients with AAV and ESRD (see **Table 1**).

Kidney transplantation in antineutrophil cytoplasmic antibody–associated vasculitis
In patients with ESRD from AAV, kidney transplantation results in patient and graft survival rates comparable with those in other kidney transplant recipients.[83] As such, kidney transplantation is the treatment of choice for all eligible AAV patients with ESRD. Importantly, clinically active disease is a contraindication to kidney transplantation. Patients should generally be in clinical remission for 1 year (minimum 6 months) prior to preceding with transplantation.[84,85] A stable positive ANCA titer in the setting of sustained clinical remission is not a contraindication to transplant.[86] Relapse rates of AAV are lower in patients who have undergone transplantation compared with those on dialysis, probably due to the immunosuppressive regimen of the transplant recipient.[87–89]

Novel Treatment Strategies

Combination rituximab and cyclophosphamide
Some centers routinely combine cyclophosphamide with rituximab in an attempt to more rapidly induce remission and reduce exposure to glucocorticoids.[34,90,91] In the largest series, 129 patients were treated with rituximab, 8 weeks of low-dose oral cyclophosphamide, and an accelerated steroid taper. By 6 months, 91% of patients were in complete remission on less than 10 mg of prednisone with a low rate of serious adverse events. Combination therapy is particularly appealing in patients at high risk for glucocorticoid intolerance and in patients with aggressive renal or pulmonary disease. Importantly, the RAVE trial excluded patients with a serum creatinine greater than 4 mg/dL, and there remains concern about the slow onset of action of rituximab in this subset of patients. More data, in particular randomized controlled trials comparing combination therapy to standard regimens, are needed before combination therapy can be broadly recommended.

Complement inhibition
The alternative complement pathway, in particular C5a, is an important mediator of disease activity in AAV (discussed previously). In a phase II clinical trial, treatment with an oral C5a receptor antagonist seemed capable of effectively replacing glucocorticoids in patients receiving remission induction with either cyclophosphamide or rituximab.[92] Moreover, treatment with the C5a antagonist was associated with more rapid resolution of proteinuria and greater improvement in health-related quality-of-life outcomes. The A Phase 3 Clinical Trial of CCX168 (Avacopan) in Patients with ANCA-Associated Vasculitis (ADVOCATE) trial is currently being conducted to confirm these findings in a large multinational population. If successful, the ability to reliably induce remission without the use of glucocorticoids will be a landmark advancement in the treatment of AAV.

Rituximab dosing strategies
Rituximab has proved an extremely effective remission maintenance agent for AAV. Many important questions remain, however, about the optimal rituximab dosing interval and the overall duration of rituximab therapy. Fortunately, multiple randomized clinical trials are currently under way to address some of these questions. The MAINRITSAN 2 trial is evaluating whether dosing rituximab based on an ANCA titer rise and/or B-cell reconstitution is superior to dosing rituximab at a fixed interval (ie, every 6 months). The MAINRITSAN 3 trial is testing whether extending the duration of fixed-interval maintenance rituximab (ie, every 6 months) beyond 18 months results in a lower relapse rate without significantly increasing the rate of adverse events. Finally, the Maintenance of ANCA Vasculitis Remission by Intermittent Rituximab Dosing Based on B-cell Reconstitution vs a Serologic ANCA

Flare (MAINTANCAVAS) trial is comparing 2 strategies for long-term maintenance of remission: (1) dosing rituximab based on B-cell reconstitution and (2) dosing rituximab based on a significant rise in ANCA titer. In aggregate, the results of these trials should assist in refining the use rituximab for maintenance therapy in AAV.

SUMMARY

The morbidity and mortality from AAV primarily relate to damage that occurs before or at the beginning of induction therapy. Early suspicion of disease with rapid diagnosis and initiation of treatment remains the most essential steps to minimize damage. Refinements of treatment regimens are leading to improved remission rates and a reduction of adverse events. Long-term follow-up and balanced use of maintenance treatments are essential to prevent recurrences and minimize toxicity. New therapies and strategies are emerging that may further expand and consolidate the gains.

ACKNOWLEDGMENTS

The authors thank Helmut Rennke, MD, for providing the renal pathology images.

REFERENCES

1. Rutgers A, Sanders JS, Stegeman CA, et al. Pauci-immune necrotizing glomerulonephritis. Rheum Dis Clin North Am 2010;36(3):559–72.
2. Niles M, John L. Antineutrophil cytoplasmic antibodies in the classification of vasculitis. Annu Rev Med 1996;47(1):303–13.
3. Guillevin L, Durand-Gasselin B, Cevallos R, et al. Microscopic polyangiitis: clinical and laboratory findings in eighty-five patients. Arthritis Rheum 1999;42(3):421–30.
4. Finkielman JD, Lee AS, Hummel AM, et al. ANCA are detectable in nearly all patients with active severe Wegener's granulomatosis. Am J Med 2007;120(7):643.e9-14.
5. Hauer HA, Bajema IM, Van Houwelingen HC, et al. Renal histology in ANCA-associated vasculitis: differences between diagnostic and serologic subgroups. Kidney Int 2002;61(1):80–9.
6. Sinico RA, Di Toma L, Maggiore U, et al. Prevalence and clinical significance of antineutrophil cytoplasmic antibodies in Churg-Strauss syndrome. Arthritis Rheumatol 2005;52(9):2926–35.
7. Guillevin L, Cohen P, Gayraud M, et al. Churg-Strauss syndrome. Clinical study and long-term follow-up of 96 patients. Medicine 1999;78(1):26–37.
8. Ntatsaki E, Watts RA, Scott DG. Epidemiology of ANCA-associated vasculitis. Rheum Dis Clin North Am 2010;36(3):447–61.
9. Lyons PA, Rayner TF, Trivedi S, et al. Genetically distinct subsets within ANCA-associated vasculitis. N Engl J Med 2012;367(3):214–23.
10. Hogan SL, Falk RJ, Chin H, et al. Predictors of relapse and treatment resistance in antineutrophil cytoplasmic antibody–associated small-vessel vasculitis. Ann Intern Med 2005;143(9):621–31.
11. Ando M, Miyazaki E, Ishii T, et al. Incidence of myeloperoxidase anti-neutrophil cytoplasmic antibody positivity and microscopic polyangitis in the course of idiopathic pulmonary fibrosis. Respir Med 2013;107(4):608–15.
12. Choi HK, Merkel PA, Walker AM, et al. Drug-associated antineutrophil cytoplasmic antibody–positive vasculitis: Prevalence among patients with high titers of antimyeloperoxidase antibodies. Arthritis Rheumatol 2000;43(2):405–13.

13. Merkel PA, Xie G, Monach PA, et al. Identification of functional and expression polymorphisms associated with risk for antineutrophil cytoplasmic autoantibody–associated vasculitis. Arthritis Rheumatol 2017;69(5):1054–66.

14. Pendergraft WF III, Niles JL. Trojan horses: drug culprits associated with antineutrophil cytoplasmic autoantibody (ANCA) vasculitis. Curr Opin Rheumatol 2014; 26(1):42–9.

15. Chen M, Gao Y, Guo X-H, et al. Propylthiouracil-induced antineutrophil cytoplasmic antibody-associated vasculitis. Nat Rev Nephrol 2012;8(8):476–83.

16. Dobre M, Wish J, Negrea L. Hydralazine-induced ANCA-positive pauci-immune glomerulonephritis: a case report and literature review. Ren Fail 2009;31(8): 745–8.

17. McGrath MM, Isakova T, Rennke HG, et al. Contaminated cocaine and antineutrophil cytoplasmic antibody-associated disease. Clin J Am Soc Nephrol 2011; 6(12):2799–805.

18. Xiao H, Heeringa P, Hu P, et al. Antineutrophil cytoplasmic autoantibodies specific for myeloperoxidase cause glomerulonephritis and vasculitis in mice. J Clin Invest 2002;110(7):955–63.

19. Schlieben DJ, Korbet SM, Kimura RE, et al. Pulmonary-renal syndrome in a newborn with placental transmission of ANCAs. Am J Kidney Dis 2005;45(4): 758–61.

20. Van Rossum AP, Limburg PC, Kallenberg CG. Human anti-neutrophil cytoplasm autoantibodies to proteinase 3 (PR3-ANCA) bind to neutrophils. Kidney Int 2005;68(2):537–41.

21. Schreiber A, Xiao H, Jennette JC, et al. C5a receptor mediates neutrophil activation and ANCA-induced glomerulonephritis. J Am Soc Nephrol 2009;20(2): 289–98.

22. Falk RJ, Terrell RS, Charles LA, et al. Anti-neutrophil cytoplasmic autoantibodies induce neutrophils to degranulate and produce oxygen radicals in vitro. Proc Natl Acad Sci U S A 1990;87(11):4115–9.

23. Porges AJ, Redecha PB, Kimberly WT, et al. Anti-neutrophil cytoplasmic antibodies engage and activate human neutrophils via Fc gamma RIIa. J Immunol 1994;153(3):1271–80.

24. Kettritz R, Jennette JC, Falk RJ. Crosslinking of ANCA-antigens stimulates superoxide release by human neutrophils. J Am Soc Nephrol 1997;8(3):386–94.

25. Xiao H, Schreiber A, Heeringa P, et al. Alternative complement pathway in the pathogenesis of disease mediated by anti-neutrophil cytoplasmic autoantibodies. Am J Pathol 2007;170(1):52–64.

26. Augusto J-F, Langs V, Demiselle J, et al. Low serum complement C3 levels at diagnosis of renal ANCA-associated vasculitis is associated with poor prognosis. PLoS One 2016;11(7):e0158871.

27. Xiao H, Dairaghi DJ, Powers JP, et al. C5a receptor (CD88) blockade protects against MPO-ANCA GN. J Am Soc Nephrol 2014;25(2):225–31.

28. Berden AE, Ferrario F, Hagen EC, et al. Histopathologic classification of ANCA-associated glomerulonephritis. J Am Soc Nephrol 2010;21(10):1628–36.

29. Jennette JC, Wilkman AS, Falk R. Anti-neutrophil cytoplasmic autoantibody-associated glomerulonephritis and vasculitis. Am J Pathol 1989;135(5):921–30.

30. Haas M, Eustace JA. Immune complex deposits in ANCA-associated crescentic glomerulonephritis: a study of 126 cases. Kidney Int 2004;65(6):2145–52.

31. Neumann I, Regele H, Kain R, et al. Glomerular immune deposits are associated with increased proteinuria in patients with ANCA-associated crescentic nephritis. Nephrol Dial Transplant 2003;18(3):524–31.

32. Baldwin DS, Neugarten J, Feiner HD, et al. The existence of a protracted course in crescentic glomerulonephritis. Kidney Int 1987;31(3):790–4.

33. Franssen CF, Gans RO, Arends B, et al. Differences between anti-myeloperoxidase-and anti-proteinase 3-associated renal disease. Kidney Int 1995;47(1):193–9.

34. Cortazar FB, Muhsin SA, Pendergraft WF III, et al. Combination therapy with rituximab and cyclophosphamide for remission induction in ANCA vasculitis. Kidney Int Rep 2017;3(2):394–402.

35. Levy JB, Hammad T, Coulthart A, et al. Clinical features and outcome of patients with both ANCA and anti-GBM antibodies. Kidney Int 2004;66(4):1535–40.

36. Olson SW, Arbogast CB, Baker TP, et al. Asymptomatic autoantibodies associate with future anti-glomerular basement membrane disease. J Am Soc Nephrol 2011;22(10):1946–52.

37. McAdoo SP, Tanna A, Hrušková Z, et al. Patients double-seropositive for ANCA and anti-GBM antibodies have varied renal survival, frequency of relapse, and outcomes compared to single-seropositive patients. Kidney Int 2017;92(3): 693–702.

38. Nasr SH, Said SM, Valeri AM, et al. Membranous glomerulonephritis with ANCA-associated necrotizing and crescentic glomerulonephritis. Clin J Am Soc Nephrol 2009;4(2):299–308.

39. Tse W, Howie A, Adu D, et al. Association of vasculitic glomerulonephritis with membranous nephropathy: a report of 10 cases. Nephrol Dial Transplant 1997; 12(5):1017–27.

40. Sen D, Isenberg DA. Antineutrophil cytoplasmic autoantibodies in systemic lupus erythematosus. Lupus 2003;12(9):651–8.

41. Jennette JC, Falk RJ. The pathology of vasculitis involving the kidney. Am J kidney Dis 1994;24(1):130–41.

42. Bir K, Herzenberg AM, Carette S. Azathioprine induced acute interstitial nephritis as the cause of rapidly progressive renal failure in a patient with Wegener's granulomatosis. J Rheumatol 2006;33(1):185–7.

43. Locht H, Skogh T, Wiik A. Characterisation of autoantibodies to neutrophil granule constituents among patients with reactive arthritis, rheumatoid arthritis, and ulcerative colitis. Ann Rheum Dis 2000;59(11):898–903.

44. Niles JL, Pan G, Collins AB, et al. Antigen-specific radioimmunoassays for anti-neutrophil cytoplasmic antibodies in the diagnosis of rapidly progressive glomerulonephritis. J Am Soc Nephrol 1991;2(1):27–36.

45. Fienberg R, Mark EJ, Goodman M, et al. Correlation of antineutrophil cytoplasmic antibodies with the extrarenal histopathology of Wegener's (pathergic) granulomatosis and related forms of vasculitis. Hum Pathol 1993;24(2):160–8.

46. Merkel PA, Polisson RP, Chang Y, et al. Prevalence of antineutrophil cytoplasmic antibodies in a large inception cohort of patients with connective tissue disease. Ann Intern Med 1997;126(11):866–73.

47. Jennette JC, Wilkman AS, Falk RJ. Diagnostic predictive value of ANCA serology. Kidney Int 1998;53(3):796–8.

48. Choi HK, Liu S, Merkel PA, et al. Diagnostic performance of antineutrophil cytoplasmic antibody tests for idiopathic vasculitides: metaanalysis with a focus on antimyeloperoxidase antibodies. J Rheumatol 2001;28(7):1584–90.

49. Yates M, Watts R, Bajema I, et al. EULAR/ERA-EDTA recommendations for the management of ANCA-associated vasculitis. Ann Rheum Dis 2016;75(9): 1583–94.

50. Stone JH, Merkel PA, Spiera R, et al. Rituximab versus cyclophosphamide for ANCA-associated vasculitis. N Engl J Med 2010;363(3):221–32.

51. de Groot K, Harper L, Jayne DR, et al. Pulse versus daily oral cyclophosphamide for induction of remission in antineutrophil cytoplasmic antibody—associated vasculitis: a randomized trial. Ann Intern Med 2009;150(10):670–80.

52. Harper L, Morgan MD, Walsh M, et al. Pulse versus daily oral cyclophosphamide for induction of remission in ANCA-associated vasculitis: long-term follow-up. Ann Rheum Dis 2012;71(6):955–60.

53. Yilmaz N, Emmungil H, Gucenmez S, et al. Incidence of cyclophosphamide-induced urotoxicity and protective effect of mesna in rheumatic diseases. J Rheumatol 2015;42(9):1661–6.

54. Haubitz M, Bohnenstengel F, Brunkhorst R, et al. Cyclophosphamide pharmaco-kinetics and dose requirements in patients with renal insufficiency. Kidney Int 2002;61(4):1495–501.

55. van den Brand JA, van Dijk PR, Hofstra JM, et al. Cancer risk after cyclophospha-mide treatment in idiopathic membranous nephropathy. Clin J Am Soc Nephrol 2014;9(6):1066–73.

56. Talar-Williams C, Hijazi YM, Walther MM, et al. Cyclophosphamide-induced cystitis and bladder cancer in patients with Wegener granulomatosis. Ann Intern Med 1996;124(5):477–84.

57. Edwards JC, Szczepański L, Szechiński J, et al. Efficacy of B-cell–targeted ther-apy with rituximab in patients with rheumatoid arthritis. N Engl J Med 2004; 350(25):2572–81.

58. Jones RB, Ferraro AJ, Chaudhry AN, et al. A multicenter survey of rituximab ther-apy for refractory antineutrophil cytoplasmic antibody–associated vasculitis. Arthritis Rheumatol 2009;60(7):2156–68.

59. Walsh M, Merkel PA, Mahr A, et al. Effects of duration of glucocorticoid therapy on relapse rate in antineutrophil cytoplasmic antibody–associated vasculitis: a meta-analysis. Arthritis Care Res 2010;62(8):1166–73.

60. Saag KG, Koehnke R, Caldwell JR, et al. Low dose long-term corticosteroid ther-apy in rheumatoid arthritis: an analysis of serious adverse events. Am J Med 1994;96(2):115–23.

61. Tesar V, Hruskova Z. Limitations of standard immunosuppressive treatment in ANCA-associated vasculitis and lupus nephritis. Nephron Clin Pract 2014; 128(3–4):205–15.

62. Klemmer PJ, Chalermskulrat W, Reif MS, et al. Plasmapheresis therapy for diffuse alveolar hemorrhage in patients with small-vessel vasculitis. Am J kidney Dis 2003;42(6):1149–53.

63. Jayne DR, Gaskin G, Rasmussen N, et al. Randomized trial of plasma exchange or high-dosage methylprednisolone as adjunctive therapy for severe renal vascu-litis. J Am Soc Nephrol 2007;18(7):2180–8.

64. Walsh M, Merkel PA, Peh CA, et al. Plasma exchange and glucocorticoid dosing in the treatment of anti-neutrophil cytoplasm antibody associated vasculitis (PEX-IVAS): protocol for a randomized controlled trial. Trials 2013;14(1):73.

65. Specks U, Merkel PA, Seo P, et al. Efficacy of remission-induction regimens for ANCA-associated vasculitis. N Engl J Med 2013;369(5):417–27.

66. Jayne D, Rasmussen N, Andrassy K, et al. A randomized trial of maintenance therapy for vasculitis associated with antineutrophil cytoplasmic autoantibodies. N Engl J Med 2003;349(1):36–44.

67. Hiemstra TF, Walsh M, Mahr A, et al. Mycophenolate mofetil vs azathioprine for remission maintenance in antineutrophil cytoplasmic antibody–associated vasculitis: A randomized controlled trial. JAMA 2010;304(21):2381–8.
68. Pagnoux C, Mahr A, Hamidou MA, et al. Azathioprine or methotrexate maintenance for ANCA-associated vasculitis. N Engl J Med 2008;359(26):2790–803.
69. Pendergraft WF, Cortazar FB, Wenger J, et al. Long-term maintenance therapy using rituximab-induced continuous B-cell depletion in patients with ANCA vasculitis. Clin J Am Soc Nephrol 2014;9(4):736–44.
70. Guillevin L, Pagnoux C, Karras A, et al. Rituximab versus azathioprine for maintenance in ANCA-associated vasculitis. N Engl J Med 2014;371(19):1771–80.
71. Østensen M, Khamashta M, Lockshin M, et al. Anti-inflammatory and immunosuppressive drugs and reproduction. Arthritis Res Ther 2006;8(3):209.
72. Whisnant J, Pelkey J. Rheumatoid arthritis: treatment with azathioprine (IMURAN (R)). Clinical side-effects and laboratory abnormalities. Ann Rheum Dis 1982; 41(Suppl 1):44–7.
73. Van den Reek J, van Lümig P, Janssen M, et al. Increased incidence of squamous cell carcinoma of the skin after long-term treatment with azathioprine in patients with auto-immune inflammatory rheumatic diseases. J Eur Acad Dermatol Venereol 2014;28(1):27–33.
74. Cortazar FB, Pendergraft WF, Wenger J, et al. Effect of continuous B cell depletion with rituximab on pathogenic autoantibodies and total IgG levels in antineutrophil cytoplasmic antibody–associated vasculitis. Arthritis Rheumatol 2017; 69(5):1045–53.
75. Roberts DM, Jones RB, Smith RM, et al. Rituximab-associated hypogammaglobulinemia: incidence, predictors and outcomes in patients with multi-system autoimmune disease. J Autoimmun 2015;57:60–5.
76. Florescu D, Kalil A, Qiu F, et al. What is the impact of hypogammaglobulinemia on the rate of infections and survival in solid organ transplantation? A meta-analysis. Am J Transplant 2013;13(10):2601–10.
77. Wolach O, Bairey O, Lahav M. Late-onset neutropenia after rituximab treatment: case series and comprehensive review of the literature. Medicine 2010;89(5): 308–18.
78. Tesfa D, Ajeganova S, Hägglund H, et al. Late-onset neutropenia following rituximab therapy in rheumatic diseases: association with B lymphocyte depletion and infections. Arthritis Rheumatol 2011;63(8):2209–14.
79. Pagnoux C, Hogan SL, Chin H, et al. Predictors of treatment resistance and relapse in antineutrophil cytoplasmic antibody–associated small-vessel vasculitis: comparison of two independent cohorts. Arthritis Rheumatol 2008;58(9): 2908–18.
80. Springer J, Nutter B, Langford CA, et al. Granulomatosis with polyangiitis (Wegener's): impact of maintenance therapy duration. Medicine 2014;93(2):82–90.
81. Lionaki S, Hogan SL, Jennette CE, et al. The clinical course of ANCA small-vessel vasculitis on chronic dialysis. Kidney Int 2009;76(6):644–51.
82. Lee T, Gasim A, Derebail VK, et al. Predictors of treatment outcomes in ANCA-associated vasculitis with severe kidney failure. Clin J Am Soc Nephrol 2014; 9(5):905–13.
83. Moran S, Little MA. Renal transplantation in antineutrophil cytoplasmic antibody-associated vasculitis. Curr Opin Rheumatol 2014;26(1):37–41.
84. Beck L, Bomback AS, Choi MJ, et al. KDOQI US commentary on the 2012 KDIGO clinical practice guideline for glomerulonephritis. Am J Kidney Dis 2013;62(3): 403–41.

85. Knoll G, Cockfield S, Blydt-Hansen T, et al. Canadian Society of Transplantation: consensus guidelines on eligibility for kidney transplantation. Can Med Assoc J 2005;173(10):S1–25.
86. Nachman PH, Segelmark M, Westman K, et al. Recurrent ANCA-associated small vessel vasculitis after transplantation: a pooled analysis. Kidney Int 1999;56(4): 1544–50.
87. Hruskova Z, Geetha D, Tesar V. Renal transplantation in anti-neutrophil cytoplasmic antibody-associated vasculitis. Nephrol Dial Transplant 2014; 30(suppl_1):i159–63.
88. Geetha D, Eirin A, True K, et al. Renal transplantation in antineutrophil cytoplasmic antibody-associated vasculitis: a multicenter experience. Transplantation 2011;91(12):1370–5.
89. Cattran DC, Feehally J, Cook HT, et al. Kidney disease: improving global outcomes (KDIGO) glomerulonephritis work group. KDIGO clinical practice guideline for glomerulonephritis. Kidney Int Suppl 2012;2(2):139–274.
90. Mansfield N, Hamour S, Habib A-M, et al. Prolonged disease-free remission following rituximab and low-dose cyclophosphamide therapy for renal ANCA-associated vasculitis. Nephrol Dial Transplant 2011;26(10):3280–6.
91. McAdoo SP, Medjeral-Thomas N, Gopaluni S, et al. Long-term follow-up of a combined rituximab and cyclophosphamide regimen in renal anti-neutrophil cytoplasm antibody-associated vasculitis. Nephrol Dial Transplant 2018;33(5):899.
92. Jayne D, Bruchfeld AN, Harper L, et al. Randomized trial of C5a receptor inhibitor avacopan in ANCA-associated vasculitis. J Am Soc Nephrol 2017;28(9): 2756–67.

Therapy for Proliferative Lupus Nephritis

Kristin Meliambro, MD, Kirk N. Campbell, MD, Miriam Chung, MD*

KEYWORDS

- Lupus nephritis • Proliferative • Treatment • SLE • Immunosuppressive

KEY POINTS

- Overall remission rates for proliferative LN remain suboptimal, with up to 30% of LN patients progressing to ESRD. Proliferative LN requires prompt treatment with immunosuppressive agents.
- Recent studies have shown that mycophenolate mofetil (MMF) is as effective as cyclophosphamide (CYC) as an induction agent.
- There are fewer studies evaluating maintenance therapies, but existing literature favors the use of MMF with azathioprine as an acceptable alternative.
- Newly developed drugs target key molecules/pathways implicated in the pathogenesis of LN, including B-cell/T-cell costimulation, INF-α, the immunoproteasome, TWEAK, and IL-6.
- Ongoing clinical trials will further evaluate the efficacy of established and novel anti-B-cell and anti-T-cell therapies when added to standard of care induction and maintenance treatment regimens.

INTRODUCTION

Lupus nephritis (LN) is an immune complex–mediated glomerulonephritis that affects nearly 50% of patients with systemic lupus erythematosus (SLE).[1,2] Prompt diagnosis and treatment initiation are essential because renal involvement in lupus imparts high morbidity and mortality.[3–5] Recent literature has shed light on racial and ethnic differences in the incidence of LN, with people of African, Asian, and Hispanic descent having a significantly higher risk of LN compared with white persons.[1,6] Along these same lines, African-American and Hispanic patients with LN had a significantly higher rate of progression to end-stage renal disease (ESRD) compared with their white counterparts according to US Renal Data System data recorded between 1996 and 2004.[7]

The immune-complex LN classification system using the 2003 International Society of Nephrology/Renal Pathology Society nomenclature divides lupus-associated

Division of Nephrology, Icahn School of Medicine at Mount Sinai, Box 1243, One Gustave L. Levy Place, New York, NY 10029, USA
* Corresponding author.
E-mail address: miriam.chung@mountsinai.org

Rheum Dis Clin N Am 44 (2018) 545–560
https://doi.org/10.1016/j.rdc.2018.06.002
0889-857X/18/© 2018 Elsevier Inc. All rights reserved.

rheumatic.theclinics.com

glomerulonephritis into six different classes based on kidney pathology. Proliferative LN, characterized by endocapillary and/or extracapillary glomerulonephritis, encompasses classes III and IV of the International Society of Nephrology/Renal Pathology Society LN classification scheme.[8] Class III refers to focal disease, affecting less than 50% of the glomeruli, and Class IV is defined by diffuse glomerular involvement affecting greater than 50% of the glomeruli. Both class III and IV are further characterized by the presence of active lesions (A), chronic lesions (C), or both active and chronic lesions simultaneously in the same biopsy sample (A/C). Class IV is further divided in to segmental (S) or global (G) glomerular involvement.

Because proliferative LN is an aggressive disease that may lead to ESRD, treatment relies on the use of intensive immunosuppressive medications. Before 1970, the 5-year survival rate was reported to be a dismal 20% for patients with diffuse LN.[9,10] Although current treatment regimens have improved renal outcomes and survival rates beyond those reported historically, recent studies of either intravenous (IV) cyclophosphamide (CYC) or mycophenolate mofetil (MMF) for LN induction therapy still demonstrate overall remission rates of 50% to 55%.[11–13] This highlights a pressing need for development of targeted therapies with greater efficacy than those currently in use while maintaining acceptable safety profiles.

In this review, we explore the key findings of clinical studies centered on induction and maintenance treatment regimens for proliferative LN, and review novel therapeutic agents and regimens that are currently under investigation.

EVIDENCE BEHIND INDUCTION THERAPIES

Induction therapy refers to the use of immunosuppressive agents to treat the renal-immune-complex-mediated injury responsible for producing the primary manifestations of LN flares (reduced renal function, hematuria, and proteinuria). Induction treatment is standard of care in active proliferative LN (class III and IV LN) and also in membranous LN (class V LN) with persistent nephrotic range proteinuria. The first major study to demonstrate the superiority of cytotoxic therapy compared with corticosteroids alone involved 111 patients, mainly with class IV or membranoproliferative LN, who were randomized to one of five groups: (1) high-dose prednisone only; (2) oral CYC; (3) oral azathioprine (AZA); (4) oral CYC and AZA; and (5) IV CYC, dosed 0.5 to 1 g/m^2 every 3 months.[14] The CYC and AZA groups all additionally received low-dose prednisone. Therapy was continued for a minimum of 18 months after achievement of complete remission or until completion of 4 years of protocol therapy. After a 5-year period of observation, patients who received high-dose oral prednisone were less likely than the other groups to have preserved renal function. After a median 7-year follow-up period, IV CYC therapy achieved significantly better renal outcomes compared with oral prednisone overall, especially among a subgroup of high-risk patients characterized by either fibrosis or glomerulosclerosis on renal biopsy. There were notable differences in rates of adverse events: all CYC-containing regimens were associated with increased rates of herpes zoster infection and premature ovarian failure, whereas the risk of hemorrhagic cystitis was increased only in those patients receiving oral CYC.

The superiority of CYC to glucocorticoids as induction therapy for proliferative LN was later solidified by another National Institutes of Health (NIH)-sponsored trial that evaluated renal outcomes in patients receiving extended courses of IV methylprednisolone and IV CYC.[15] This study randomized 82 participants, most of whom were white persons, with hematuria, at least 1 g of proteinuria, and an average serum creatinine of 1.6 to 2 mg/dL, to one of three treatment groups (all given in conjunction with oral prednisone): (1) 12 monthly infusions of IV methylprednisolone, (2) 6 monthly infusions of IV CYC followed by quarterly infusions for a total of 2 years, or (3) combination therapy. After a minimum follow-up period of 5 years, renal remission rates were significantly higher in the IV CYC (62%) and combination therapy (85%) groups than in the IV methylprednisolone group (29%), although differences between the groups did not become apparent until 2 to 3 years after treatment initiation. Common adverse events across all groups included avascular necrosis, herpes zoster, and other infections, but only amenorrhea was found to occur at significantly higher rate in the IV CYC and combination therapy arms. An extended 11-year follow-up of this trial revealed that both CYC-containing groups were significantly less likely to reach a composite study end point that included need for additional treatment, doubling of serum creatinine concentration, or death.[16] Similar to the delay in observed differences in remission rates, differences in the risk of reaching ESRD were not seen until after a treatment period of 5 years, at which point the risk was found to be significantly higher for the methylprednisolone group.

The results of a 2004 Cochrane Database meta-analysis that included 25 trials (randomized controlled and quasi randomized controlled) and a total of 915 patients with active proliferative LN further supported the greater efficacy of CYC in preserving renal function as compared with steroids alone.[17] CYC therapy was found again to impart a greater risk of infertility, yet the risks of infections and malignancies did not differ between CYC and steroid-only groups. Adjunctive agents, such as AZA and plasma exchange, did not provide improve the therapeutic efficacy of CYC. Interestingly, this meta-analysis found no differences in either efficacy or adverse events with different formulations of CYC, specifically IV versus oral administration, high versus low dose, or long versus short duration.

Dosing and duration of CYC were directly addressed in the Euro-Lupus Nephritis Trial,[11] which included 90 patients with proliferative LN, most of whom were white persons with normal baseline serum creatinine levels. Participants were either administered IV CYC high dose (0.5 mg/m^2 monthly for 6 months then two additional doses quarterly) or low dose (500 mg every 2 weeks for six total doses), in addition to steroid pulse followed by prednisone taper. Once renal remission was achieved, both groups transitioned to AZA as maintenance therapy until 30 months post-treatment initiation. At a median follow-up of about 41 months, low-dose IV CYC was found to be equally efficacious in inducing renal remission as was high-dose IV CYC (71% renal remission for low-dose group vs 54% renal remission for high-dose group), with a trend toward lower rate of severe infection in the low-dose group, although this difference was not statistically significant. Although a reduced-dose CYC regimen was well-received by nephrologists and patients alike at the time, the generalizability of this regimen to a diverse patient population or those with impaired renal function remained in question.

Despite the beneficial renal outcomes afforded by IV CYC therapy, the toxicities, especially infection and infertility, remained a concern particularly for this disease with highest prevalence among young women. This led investigators in Hong Kong to conduct a randomized, prospective trial comparing efficacy and side effects of oral CYC and prednisolone and MMF and prednisolone.[18] The study included 42 patients with diffuse proliferative LN, randomized to either prednisolone and MMF for 12 months (2 g/d × 6 months, then 1 g/d × 6 months), or prednisolone and oral CYC for 6 months followed by prednisolone and AZA for 6 months (CYC 2.5 mg/kg/d, then AZA 1.5 mg/kg/d). At 12 months, MMF therapy had similar efficacy as the CYC-AZA regimen (MMF with 81% complete remission vs CYC-AZA with 76% complete remission). Infections were seen in 19% of the MMF group and 33% in the CYC-AZA group ($P = .29$), whereas only the CYC-AZA group had other adverse outcomes including amenorrhea (23%), hair loss (19%), and death (10%).

MMF was also compared with CYC for induction treatment of proliferative LN in a multicenter trial in the United States, which was designed as open label noninferiority trial of oral MMF (initial dose 1 g/d, increased to 3 g/d) versus monthly IV CYC (initial dose 0.5 g/m^2, increased to 1 g/m^2).[13] Similar to the Euro-Lupus Nephritis Trial, the 140 enrolled patients were predominantly females with preserved renal function; however, more than half the patients in both treatment arms were African-American. After 24 weeks of induction therapy, significantly more patients in the MMF group achieved a complete renal remission than did the CYC group (22.5% for MMF and 6% for CYC), which drove a significantly higher overall remission rate (complete + partial remission) for MMF (51%) in contrast to CYC therapy (30%). There were no significant differences, however, in the rates of renal or overall survival between the groups after a follow-up period of about 3 years. The risk of pyogenic infections was higher in the CYC group, and two patients receiving CYC experienced amenorrhea, whereas none of the MMF patients did.

Given that the aforementioned MMF trial was only powered to demonstrate noninferiority, the Aspreva Lupus Management (ALMS) trial followed shortly thereafter to answer the question of whether MMF was a superior induction agent to CYC.[12] ALMS was a multinational trial that randomized 370 patients with class III or class IV ± class V LN to receive either MMF (up to 3 g/d) or monthly IV CYC (up to 1 g/m^2). Enrolled patients were more racially and ethnically diverse compared with the older NIH and Euro-Lupus trials, with approximately one-third of the study population classified as Asian, one-third as Hispanic, and 40% as white. Additionally, about 18% of study subjects had an estimated glomerular filtration rate (GFR) less than 60 mL/min, with approximately 9% having an estimated GFR less than 30 mL/min. After 24 weeks of induction therapy, the MMF and CYC groups demonstrated similar rates of renal response, which was specified by degree of reduction in proteinuria and stabilization/improvement in serum creatinine (response rate 56% for MMF vs 53% for CYC). Rates of total and serious adverse events also did not differ significantly between the two groups. Although this first phase of the ALMS trial did not meet its primary goal of demonstrating superiority of MMF over IV CYC, there were key secondary findings. First, although primary response rates did not differ between treatment arms overall, there were significantly higher renal response rates for nonwhite patients/non-Asian patients who received MMF (60.4%) as opposed to CYC (38.5%). This is important to note in light of the previously described higher incidence of LN and decreased renal survival reported for African-American and Hispanic patients. Another interesting finding highlighted in a post hoc analysis of ALMS was that response rates were similarly low in patients with estimated GFR less than 30 mL/min (20% for MMF group and 17% for IV CYC group), whereas serious adverse events rates were significantly higher (52%) compared with the overall study population (25%).[19] This finding emphasizes the need to strongly consider the treatment risk-to-benefit ratio in LN patients presenting with severe renal insufficiency.

In summary, although response rates to induction therapy remain suboptimal, the landmark studies described here and shown in **Table 1** established a lower-toxicity regimen for CYC and supported MMF as an equally efficacious alternative to CYC, with potential added benefit for African-American and Hispanic patients who are at the highest risk for complications of LN. Of note, more data are needed for treatment of severe LN with low estimated GFR.

The goal of induction therapy with immunosuppressive agents is to achieve renal remission. The aforementioned trials used different criteria for renal remission. In general, remission is defined as improvement in proteinuria (ie, <3 g/d with baseline nephrotic range, or by >50% with subnephrotic baseline), improvement or stabilization

Table 1 Induction therapy		
Current Standard of Care Treatment	**CYC**	**MMF**
Dose/duration	*NIH trial*: IV 0.5–1 g/m^2 q mo × 6 mo *Euro LN trial*: (low dose) IV 500 mg q 2 wk × 6 doses	*NEJM (Ginzler et al) trial*: initial 1 g/d, increased to 3 g/d × 6 mo *ALMS trial*: initial 1 g/d, increased to 3 g/d × 6 mo
Response rate	*NIH trial*: renal remission = 62% CYC vs 29% methylprednisolone (CYC significantly better) *Euro LN trial*: renal remission = 71% low-dose CYC vs 54% high-dose CYC (no significant difference)	*NEJM trial*: overall renal remission = 51% MMF vs 30% CYC (MMF significantly better, although noninferiority trial) *ALMS trial*: response rate = 56.2% MMF vs 53% CYC (no significant difference)

All trial regimens also included glucocorticoids: NIH trial: PO prednisone 0.5 mg/kg/d × 4 wk, then tapered. Euro LN trial: IV 750 mg methylprednisolone × 3 d + PO prednisone 0.5 mg/kg/d × 4 wk, then tapered. NEJM (Ginzler et al.) trial: PO prednisone 1 mg/kg/d, then tapered. ALMS trial: PO prednisone max starting dose 60 mg/d, then tapered.

of creatinine or estimated GFR, and improvement of urine sediment. If a patient is resistant to initial therapy (ie, fails to achieve remission after 6 months), then one can switch to the alternative standard of care induction agent. For example, MMF-resistant patients can be treated with CYC, and CYC-resistant patients can be treated with MMF.

EVIDENCE BEHIND MAINTENANCE THERAPIES

The theory behind a maintenance treatment phase for LN is to foster achievement of complete remission in patients who had only partial remission with induction therapy and to prevent disease relapses and flares. Earlier studies highlighted the need for a maintenance regimen following induction therapy for proliferative LN, because shorter courses of IV CYC were associated with higher risk of renal relapse than were prolonged courses.[20] Although the optimal induction regimen was still being evaluated in the early 2000s, investigators at the University of Miami turned their attention to maintenance therapy options.[21] Fifty-nine patients with proliferative LN received induction therapy with IV CYC (0.5–1 g/m^2) for 4 to 7 months and then were randomized to either receive quarterly infusions of IV CYC, oral MMF (500 mg–3 g/d), or oral AZA (1–3 mg/kg/d) plus low-dose steroids for a maintenance period of 1 to 3 years. Similar to the ALMS trial, the patient population was racially diverse, and there was also baseline renal impairment among study subjects, with a mean creatinine value of 1.6 mg/dL. At conclusion of the study follow-up period, MMF and AZA were found to be superior maintenance agents to CYC with significantly higher event-free survival rates for the composite end point of death or chronic renal failure. Although renal survival rates were found to be similar among all three agents (74% for CYC, 80% for AZA, 95% for MMF), the relapse-free survival rate was significantly greater for MMF, whereas patient survival rate was higher for AZA as compared with IV CYC. Importantly, the rates of infections and amenorrhea were significantly lower for the MMF and AZA groups compared with the IV CYC group.

Because the University of Miami trial demonstrated that IV CYC was inferior as a maintenance therapy, European investigators sought to establish whether MMF or

AZA was more efficacious. The MAINTAIN trial enrolled 105 patients with proliferative LN, all of whom were treated with IV CYC and steroids according to the Euro-Lupus trial protocol and then randomized to either receive MMF (total 2 g/d) or AZA (2 mg/kg/d).[22] After 5 years, there was no significant difference in the incidence of the primary end point, which was time to renal flare (renal flare rate 19% for MMF vs 25% for AZA; $P = .48$). The rates of adverse events were similar for both agents during the study period, with the exception of hematologic cytopenias occurring more frequently in the AZA group. The MAINTAIN trial possessed similar drawbacks to the Euro-Lupus Trial in that the patient population was small in size and included mostly white patients with baseline preserved renal function, limiting the widespread application of study results to the broader international population of LN patients. Some of these remaining issues were addressed with the publication of the maintenance phase of the ALMS trial in 2011, which randomized 227 patients who completed the ALMS induction phase to receive either MMF (2 g/d) or AZA (2 mg/kg/d) with low-dose steroids in a double-blind, double-dummy fashion.[23] After 36 months of maintenance therapy, MMF was found to be superior to AZA with respect to the primary end point of time to treatment failure, defined as death, ESRD, doubling of the serum creatinine level, renal flare, or rescue therapy for LN (hazard ratio, 0.44; 95% confidence interval, 0.25–0.77; $P = .003$). Individually, the times to renal flare and rescue therapy were significantly longer for MMF as compared with AZA (hazard ratio, <1.00; $P<.05$). The benefits of MMF were seen regardless of patient characteristics, including the type of induction therapy received, geographic region, or race. The incidence of adverse events was similar between the treatment arms, including infections, although a greater proportion of patients in the AZA group withdrew from the study because of adverse events (39.6%) than for the MMF group (25.2%; $P = .02$) (**Table 2**).

The University of Miami and ALMS trials favor MMF as the agent of choice for the maintenance phase of treatment of LN. However, when these trials were subsequently analyzed in conjunction with earlier studies in meta-analyses and systematic reviews, the clear benefit of MMF over AZA was diminished.[24,25] This highlights a need still for extended study follow-up periods to determine the optimal long-term management for patients with proliferative LN.

NOVEL THERAPIES CURRENTLY IN TRIALS OR UNDER DEVELOPMENT

Complete and overall remission rates for LN have remained suboptimal over the 30 years since publication of the initial NIH Lupus trials. Furthermore, up to 30% of patients with LN still progress to ESRD.[7,26] Research into the pathogenesis of LN over the past few decades has resulted in investigative studies of novel therapies, including

Table 2 Maintenance therapy		
Current Standard of Care Treatment	**MMF**	**AZA**
Dose/duration	*MAINTAIN*: 0.5–2 g/d × 1–3 y *ALMS*: 2 g/d × ≥3 y	*MAINTAIN*: 1–2 mg/kg/d × 1–3 y *ALMS*: 2 mg/kg/d × ≥3 y
Response rate	*MAINTAIN*: renal flare rate = 19% AZA vs 25% MMF (no significant difference) *ALMS*: time to composite primary end point (MMF vs AZA) = hazard ratio, 0.44 (MMF significantly better)	

repurposed immunosuppressive and biologic agents from other disease entities, and new targeted antilupus treatments (**Table 3**).

Anti-B-Cell Therapy

Because B cells have been implicated in the inflammatory injury that characterizes LN, the efficacy of anti-B-cell therapy is being investigated.[27] The LUNAR trial randomized 140 patients with either class III or class IV ($\pm$ class V) LN to receive MMF and corticosteroids either with or without rituximab, an anti-CD20 monoclonal antibody.[28] After 52 weeks of therapy, there was no significant difference in the rates of renal response (complete and partial remissions) between the two groups, though the rituximab group did show greater improvement in serologic disease markers, including serum complement C3, C4, and anti-double-stranded DNA levels. Although superior results were not achieved with rituximab, several issues have been raised with LUNAR, including perhaps a limited follow-up period for the effects of rituximab to be seen and failure of rituximab to actually achieve adequate B-cell depletion. Some answers may be provided by an ongoing trial of obinutuzumab, a chimeric, anti-CD20 monoclonal antibody that may cause more efficient B-cell depletion than rituximab, in patients with LN.[29] Similar to LUNAR, experimental groups will receive MMF and corticosteroids with or without obinutuzumab and complete renal response will be measured at 52 weeks (identifier: NCT02550652). Furthermore, the ongoing RING (Rituximab for Lupus Nephritis with Remission as a Goal) trial will evaluate rituximab as a rescue agent in patients who failed to achieve complete remission after 6 months of standard of care induction therapy (either IV CYC or MMF and corticosteroids) (identifier: NCT01673295).

Rituximab is also being investigated as part of a maintenance corticosteroid-sparing regimen. A small study from the United Kingdom used rituximab with two doses of IV methylprednisolone as induction therapy and then MMF sans corticosteroids as maintenance therapy in 20 patients with proliferative LN. The total remission rate was 78%, with 67% of patients in sustained remission at 1 year.[30] A multicenter phase III trial, RITUXILUP, sought to compare this steroid-sparing approach with a standard of care regimen of MMF, methylprednisolone, and prednisone, but this study was recently terminated early (identifier: NCT01773616). Although the question of rituximab's ability to supplant long-term steroid use remains open, the prospect of eliminating steroids and their numerous associated side effects remains an exciting one.

In addition to CD20 receptor blockade, another therapeutic target is B-cell activating factor (BAFF) or B-lymphocyte stimulator (BLyS), which is a soluble ligand of the tumor necrosis factor (TNF) cytokine family that promotes B-cell differentiation, homeostasis, and selection. Increased levels of BLyS have been implicated in the autoantibody production that spurs lupus exacerbations.[31] To this effect, a humanized monoclonal anti-BLyS antibody, belimumab, was demonstrated to reduce SLE exacerbations and flares when added to standard therapy in a phase 3 randomized clinical trial of 819 patients with SLE.[32] Post hoc analysis of patients with renal involvement in belimumab trials (which excluded severe LN) showed trends toward reduced renal flares and higher renal remission rates at 52 weeks of therapy, particularly in patients on MMF, although these did not reach statistical significance.[33] However, another anti-BAFF/BLyS antibody, tabalumab, did not improve renal outcomes when added to standard therapy for 52 weeks in two recent phase 3 randomized clinical trials.[34] Additionally, blisibmod, a BAFF inhibitor, did not reach its primary efficacy/safety end points in a phase 3 trial of patients with SLE, although the drug was associated with improved proteinuria and successful reduction in steroids.[35] Importantly, there is an ongoing trial (BLISS-LN) to directly examine renal outcomes in patients with

Table 3
Investigational therapies

Class or Category	Target	Drug	Trial in LN	Outcome
Anti-B-cell therapy	Anti-CD20	Rituximab Obinutuzumab	*Rituximab*: LUNAR, RITUXILUP (completed); RING (ongoing phase III) *Obinutuzumab*: ongoing phase II	LUNAR: no benefit to MMF induction therapy RITUXILUP: terminated
	Anti-BLyS/BAFF	Belimumab Tabalumab Blisbimod	*Belimumab*: Bliss-LN (ongoing phase III); CALIBRATE (ongoing phase II, + rituximab)	No published trial in severe active LN *Belimumab*: trend toward higher renal remission *Tabalumab*: no renal benefit *Blisbimod*: improved proteinuria and successful steroid reduction
Proteasome/immunoproteasome inhibitors	Proteasome inhibition Immunoproteasome inhibition	Bortezomib KZR-616	No Ongoing phase I	No published trial in LN
Anti-T-cell therapy	Calcineurin inhibitor	Cyclosporine Tacrolimus (FK) Voclosporin	*Cyclosporine*: Cyclofa-Lune FK: FK vs MMF induction; multitarget trial (FK + MMF vs IV CYC) *Voclosporin*: AURA-LV (ongoing phase II)	*Cyclosporine*: similar response rates vs IV CYC FK: similar CR rate but higher relapse rate vs MMF FK + MMF (multitarget): higher renal remission rate and similar relapse rates vs IV CYC
Costimulatory blockade	CD28/CD80 inhibition CD40L antagonist	Abatacept BI 655064	Adjunct to MMF and IV CYC Ongoing phase II	No renal benefit when added to MMF or CYC
INF-α inhibitors	Anti-INF-α Anti-INF-α receptor	Rontalizumab Sifalimumab Anifrolumab	No Tulip-LN1 (ongoing phase II)	No published trial in LN *Sifalimumab* and *anifrolumab* reduced SLE activity; *rontalizumab* did not
Nonsteroidal anti-inflammatory agents	Anti-TWEAK Anti-IL-6	BIIB023 Sirukumab	Phase II, terminated Phase II	Terminated; did not show efficacy vs MMF induction No benefit when added to MMF or AZA, higher adverse event
	NF-κB inhibitor Synthetic corticotropin	Laquinimod Acthar	Ongoing phase II Ongoing phase IV	

Abbreviations: BAFF, B-cell activating factor; BLyS, B-lymphocyte stimulator; IFN, interferon; IL, interleukin; NF, nuclear factor; TWEAK, tumor necrosis factor–like weak inducer of apoptosis.

LN receiving belimumab or placebo with standard of care induction and maintenance therapies over at least a 2-year period (identifier: NCT01639339). It is hoped that this dedicated trial in LN with an extended follow-up period will shed light on the future efficacy of anti-BAFF/BLyS therapy. Furthermore, a dual-targeted anti-B-cell approach will be undertaken by the CALIBRATE study, which will primarily evaluate safety end points after sequential administration of IV CYC plus rituximab followed by belimumab in patients with LN (identifier: NCT02260934). The rationale for this study is to prevent the increase in BAFF levels that is seen after B-cell depletion, which is suspected to subsequently promote the production of autoreactive B cells.[36,37]

Proteasome and Immunoproteasome Inhibition

Anti-B-cell therapies do not destroy the long-lived plasma cells that are responsible for producing pathogenic autoantibodies in LN.[38,39] Therefore, plasma cells, although derived from B cells, are separate potential targets of therapy. Proteasome inhibitors, the mainstay of treatment of multiple myeloma, can interfere with plasma cell stimulation via inflammatory cytokines and also increase T-regulatory cells in experimental LN.[40] Indeed proteasome inhibitors were demonstrated to attenuate LN in murine models, but they have not yet been well studied in clinical disease. In a small trial of 12 patients with active, refractory SLE, proteasome inhibitor bortezomib reduced disease activity; yet treatment was discontinued in seven patients because of suspected adverse events.[41] A potentially rectifying treatment strategy has focused on selective inhibition of the immunoproteasome, a proteasome variant that yields degraded peptides with MHC1 binding affinity and plays a role in T-cell survival, differentiation, and proliferation.[42] A phase I trial of a selective immunoproteasome inhibitor KZR-616 recently demonstrated an acceptable safety profile in healthy volunteers without the traditional hematologic and neurologic toxicities ascribed to bortezomib use.[43] An ongoing phase 1b/2 trial will examine the safety, tolerability, and efficacy of KZR-616 when added to an induction regimen with MMF/corticosteroids in proliferative LN (identifier: NCT03393013).

Anti-T-Cell Therapy

Given that calcineurin inhibitors (CNIs) inhibit T-cell activation and have been successfully used to treat several glomerulopathies, they are reasonable candidates for LN therapy.[44] A direct comparison of cyclosporine with IV CYC in 40 patients from the Czech Republic with proliferative LN showed similar remission and renal response rates at 18 months and similar relapse rates at 40 months.[45] A larger recent trial from China comparing a 6-month induction course of tacrolimus to MMF found similar complete remission rates among the two study groups, but there was a nonsignificant trend toward higher rates of renal relapse in the tacrolimus group during the maintenance phase, during which all patients had been switched to AZA.[46] Although it remains to be seen whether CNIs can serve as an equivalent induction monotherapy to MMF or CYC, another experimental strategy has been to simultaneously target different arms of the immune response via CNI adjunctive therapy. The effects of tacrolimus (4 mg/d) added to MMF (1 g/d) and corticosteroids were compared with induction with IV CYC ($0.5-1$ g/m^2 monthly $\times$ 6) and corticosteroids in a large population of Chinese patients (n = 368) with proliferative LN.[47] After 24 weeks of follow-up, significantly more patients in the tacrolimus + MMF group achieved complete remission compared with the CYC group. An 18-month follow-up study in which continuation of multitarget therapy (tacrolimus + MMF) as maintenance therapy was compared with AZA maintenance therapy (for those who had received CYC induction) demonstrated similar renal relapse rates but more adverse effects in the AZA maintenance group.[48] However, the lack of identical comparison groups (ie, tacrolimus added to only the MMF induction group), homogeneous study population, and the fact that CNIs can also reduce proteinuria via nonimmune effects (ie, stabilization of the podocyte actin cytoskeleton and vasoconstriction of the renal afferent arteriole)[49] represent some important limitations to this study. A recently completed multinational trial of a new-generation CNI, voclosporin, for induction therapy will address some of these issues, in that MMF will be used as the induction agent in both study groups, and remission rates at 48 weeks will be a secondary end point, although remission rates at 24 weeks remains the primary end point (identifier: NCT02141672).

Costimulatory Blockade

A combined anti-immune approach involves blockade of the costimulatory pathways that lead to B- and T-cell activation. CD40 ligand (CD40L) is a costimulatory molecule on T cells that binds the CD40 receptor on B cells, resulting in B-cell activation.[50] Direct blockade of CD40L by the humanized monoclonal antibody BG9588 was found to decrease hematuria and double-stranded DNA antibody levels and normalize serum C3 levels in an older clinical trial; however, the study was terminated early because of the occurrence of thromboembolic events in patients receiving BG9588.[51] Recruitment is currently ongoing, however, for two trials that will evaluate the efficacy of another CD40L antagonist, BI 655064, as added to standard of care induction and maintenance therapies for LN (identifiers: NCT02770170 and NCT03385564). CD40L also upregulates CD80 on B cells, resulting in the interaction of CD80 with CD28 on T cells.[50] The CD28/CD80 signaling pathway has been targeted by abatacept, a fusion protein composed of the Fc portion of the immunoglobulin IgG1 linked to cytotoxic T-lymphocyte-associated antigen 4. Abatacept is approved for use in rheumatoid arthritis and juvenile inflammatory arthritis. Two trials using abatacept as an induction agent for LN failed to show any significant renal benefit of adding abatacept to standard therapy with either CYC or MMF and corticosteroids; however, abatacept may still have efficacy as a maintenance therapy.[52,53]

Interferon-α Inhibition

Interferon-α (IFN-α) also may play a central role in the pathogenesis of LN. High IFN-α activity has been associated with increased Ro and double stranded-DNA antibodies in patients with SLE across different racial and ethnic backgrounds.[54] Additionally, SLE-associated IgG antibodies can induce release of IFN-α by plasmacytoid dendritic cells.[55] Furthermore, adenovector-mediated-IFN-α expression was shown to induce glomerulonephritis in certain mouse strains[56] and accelerate the development of LN in murine models of SLE.[57] IFN-α and other type I IFNs bind to the IFN-α receptor, leading to transcription of IFN-stimulated genes, which is known as the "IFN gene signature."[58,59] IFN-α-inducible genes have been shown to be upregulated in the peripheral blood cells of patients with SLE and in the kidneys of patients with LN.[60,61] In light of these data, monoclonal antibodies targeting IFN-α and the IFN-α receptor are currently under clinical investigation. Rontalizumab, a human anti-IFN-α monoclonal antibody, failed to meet the primary end point of reduced SLE disease activity in a recent phase 2 clinical trial,[59] whereas sifalimumab, another human anti-IFN-α monoclonal antibody, did improve response rates in moderate to severe SLE when added to standard of care treatment.[62] Anifrolumab, a human monoclonal antibody targeting IFN-α receptor, was similarly shown to reduce SLE disease activity[63] and provided the added benefit of a greater and more sustained suppression of the IFN gene signature in a population of Japanese SLE patients compared with sifalimumab.[64] There is currently an ongoing phase 2 trial (Tulip-LN1; identifier: NCT02547922) to evaluate the efficacy of anifrolumab as an adjunct to current standard of care therapy with MMF/corticosteroids in class III or IV (± class V) LN. A sophisticated feature of this trial is that patients will be stratified based on their IFN gene signature levels thus allowing for evaluation of a targeted therapeutic response.

Anti-inflammatory Agents

Other inflammatory signaling pathways implicated in the pathogenesis of LN have been the targets of newly developed therapeutic molecules that are currently being explored in phase 1 and 2 trials. Driving these studies of novel anti-inflammatory molecules is an overall desire to minimize or eliminate the use of high-dose corticosteroids that are the mainstay of LN induction therapy and are unfortunately fraught with significant side effects. The cytokine TNF-like weak inducer of apoptosis (TWEAK) is a member of the TNF superfamily that has been demonstrated in murine lupus models to promote inflammation, renal cell proliferation and apoptosis, vascular activation, and fibrosis.[65] Additionally, TWEAK is being studied as a candidate urinary biomarker for LN.[66] A recent phase 2 trial of an anti-TWEAK monoclonal antibody, however, failed to show efficacy as an adjunct to MMF/corticosteroid therapy (identifier: NCT01499355). There is also evidence that interleukin (IL)-6 plays a pathogenic role in LN. Elevated urine IL-6 levels were found in patients with class IV LN as compared with those with nonproliferative LN subtypes and healthy control subjects, and urine IL-6 levels were also shown to correlate with SLE disease activity.[67,68] Additionally, inhibition of IL-6 prevented development of murine models of LN.[69,70] A phase 2 trial using monoclonal IL-6 antibody sirukumab in patients who had persistently active LN despite induction and maintenance therapy with standard of care immunosuppressive regimens failed to demonstrate overall improvement in proteinuria and also had a significantly higher rate of infections compared with placebo.[71] Another agent being investigated is the immunomodulatory drug laquinimod, an inhibitor of nuclear factor-κB, which was demonstrated to reduce renal macrophage/monocyte and lymphocyte infiltration and proinflammatory cytokine levels in murine LN models.[72] A phase 2 trial to explore the safety and efficacy of laquinimod when added to MMF/corticosteroid induction therapy in active LN is underway (identifier: NCT01085097). Finally, following the reported successes of Acthar gel (synthetic corticotropin) in treating a variety of glomerulopathies in case series or small prospective studies,[73–76] Acthar is currently being evaluated in a phase 4 trial as an additive to MMF induction therapy alone, without corticosteroids. Although Acthar can have a similar side effect profile to corticosteroids, its utility in steroid-resistant nephrosis[74] suggests that Acthar mediates some antiproteinuric effects by an independent mechanism from its steroidogenic actions, perhaps by direct activation of the melanocortin-1 receptor recently identified on podocytes.[77]

SUMMARY

In patients with proliferative LN, the preferred immunosuppressive therapy for induction of renal remission consist of either MMF with glucocorticoid or CYC with glucocorticoid. The preferred regimen for maintenance therapy is either MMF or AZA at lower dose. Data for LN therapy trials are limited by suboptimal complete response rates. The investigational studies described here are the result of a targeted approach to treatment based on the key molecular pathways that potentially drive the initial inflammation and sequelae of LN. Although some agents have failed to demonstrate efficacy, these methods provide the best opportunity for discovery of a drug or regimen that will improve remission rates and patient and renal survival. Furthermore, an individualized focus, such as with recognition of varying IFN gene signature patterns in the investigation of anifrolumab, represents an advanced and specific therapeutic program.

REFERENCES

1. Seligman VA, Lum RF, Olson JL, et al. Demographic differences in the development of lupus nephritis: a retrospective analysis. Am J Med 2002;112(9):726–9.
2. Al Arfaj AS, Khalil N, Al Saleh S. Lupus nephritis among 624 cases of systemic lupus erythematosus in Riyadh, Saudi Arabia. Rheumatol Int 2009;29(9):1057–67.
3. Campbell R Jr, Cooper GS, Gilkeson GS. Two aspects of the clinical and humanistic burden of systemic lupus erythematosus: mortality risk and quality of life early in the course of disease. Arthritis Rheum 2008;59(4):458–64.
4. Danila MI, Pons-Estel GJ, Zhang J, et al. Renal damage is the most important predictor of mortality within the damage index: data from LUMINA LXIV, a multiethnic US cohort. Rheumatology (Oxford) 2009;48(5):542–5.
5. Font J, Ramos-Casals M, Cervera R, et al. Cardiovascular risk factors and the long-term outcome of lupus nephritis. QJM 2001;94(1):19–26.
6. Bastian HM, Roseman JM, McGwin G Jr, et al. Systemic lupus erythematosus in three ethnic groups. XII. Risk factors for lupus nephritis after diagnosis. Lupus 2002;11(3):152–60.
7. Ward MM. Changes in the incidence of endstage renal disease due to lupus nephritis in the United States, 1996-2004. J Rheumatol 2009;36(1):63–7.
8. Weening JJ, D'Agati VD, Schwartz MM, et al. The classification of glomerulonephritis in systemic lupus erythematosus revisited. J Am Soc Nephrol 2004; 15(2):241–50.
9. Cameron JS. Lupus nephritis. J Am Soc Nephrol 1999;10(2):413–24.
10. Cameron JS. Lupus nephritis: an historical perspective 1968-1998. J Nephrol 1999;12(Suppl 2):S29–41.
11. Houssiau FA, Vasconcelos C, D'Cruz D, et al. Immunosuppressive therapy in lupus nephritis: the Euro-Lupus Nephritis Trial, a randomized trial of low-dose versus high-dose intravenous cyclophosphamide. Arthritis Rheum 2002;46(8): 2121–31.
12. Appel GB, Contreras G, Dooley MA, et al. Mycophenolate mofetil versus cyclophosphamide for induction treatment of lupus nephritis. J Am Soc Nephrol 2009;20(5):1103–12.
13. Ginzler EM, Dooley MA, Aranow C, et al. Mycophenolate mofetil or intravenous cyclophosphamide for lupus nephritis. N Engl J Med 2005;353(21):2219–28.
14. Austin HA 3rd, Klippel JH, Balow JE, et al. Therapy of lupus nephritis. Controlled trial of prednisone and cytotoxic drugs. N Engl J Med 1986;314(10):614–9.
15. Gourley MF, Austin HA 3rd, Scott D, et al. Methylprednisolone and cyclophosphamide, alone or in combination, in patients with lupus nephritis. A randomized, controlled trial. Ann Intern Med 1996;125(7):549–57.
16. Illei GG, Austin HA, Crane M, et al. Combination therapy with pulse cyclophosphamide plus pulse methylprednisolone improves long-term renal outcome without adding toxicity in patients with lupus nephritis. Ann Intern Med 2001; 135(4):248–57.
17. Flanc RS, Roberts MA, Strippoli GF, et al. Treatment for lupus nephritis. Cochrane Database Syst Rev 2004;(1):CD002922.

18. Chan TM, Li FK, Tang CS, et al. Efficacy of mycophenolate mofetil in patients with diffuse proliferative lupus nephritis. Hong Kong-Guangzhou Nephrology Study Group. N Engl J Med 2000;343(16):1156–62.

19. Walsh M, Solomons N, Lisk L, et al. Mycophenolate mofetil or intravenous cyclophosphamide for lupus nephritis with poor kidney function: a subgroup analysis of the Aspreva Lupus Management Study. Am J Kidney Dis 2013;61(5):710–5.

20. Boumpas DT, Austin HA 3rd, Vaughn EM, et al. Controlled trial of pulse methylprednisolone versus two regimens of pulse cyclophosphamide in severe lupus nephritis. Lancet 1992;340(8822):741–5.

21. Contreras G, Pardo V, Leclercq B, et al. Sequential therapies for proliferative lupus nephritis. N Engl J Med 2004;350(10):971–80.

22. Houssiau FA, D'Cruz D, Sangle S, et al. Azathioprine versus mycophenolate mofetil for long-term immunosuppression in lupus nephritis: results from the MAINTAIN nephritis trial. Ann Rheum Dis 2010;69(12):2083–9.

23. Dooley MA, Jayne D, Ginzler EM, et al. Mycophenolate versus azathioprine as maintenance therapy for lupus nephritis. N Engl J Med 2011;365(20):1886–95.

24. Feng L, Deng J, Huo DM, et al. Mycophenolate mofetil versus azathioprine as maintenance therapy for lupus nephritis: a meta-analysis. Nephrology (Carlton) 2013;18(2):104–10.

25. Tian SY, Feldman BM, Beyene J, et al. Immunosuppressive therapies for the maintenance treatment of proliferative lupus nephritis: a systematic review and network metaanalysis. J Rheumatol 2015;42(8):1392–400.

26. Ortega LM, Schultz DR, Lenz O, et al. Review: lupus nephritis: pathologic features, epidemiology and a guide to therapeutic decisions. Lupus 2010;19(5): 557–74.

27. Chang A, Henderson SG, Brandt D, et al. In situ B cell-mediated immune responses and tubulointerstitial inflammation in human lupus nephritis. J Immunol 2011;186(3):1849–60.

28. Rovin BH, Furie R, Latinis K, et al. Efficacy and safety of rituximab in patients with active proliferative lupus nephritis: the Lupus Nephritis Assessment with Rituximab study. Arthritis Rheum 2012;64(4):1215–26.

29. Reddy V, Klein C, Isenberg DA, et al. Obinutuzumab induces superior B-cell cytotoxicity to rituximab in rheumatoid arthritis and systemic lupus erythematosus patient samples. Rheumatology (Oxford) 2017;56(7):1227–37.

30. Pepper R, Griffith M, Kirwan C, et al. Rituximab is an effective treatment for lupus nephritis and allows a reduction in maintenance steroids. Nephrol Dial Transplant 2009;24(12):3717–23.

31. Cancro MP, D'Cruz DP, Khamashta MA. The role of B lymphocyte stimulator (BLyS) in systemic lupus erythematosus. J Clin Invest 2009;119(5):1066–73.

32. Furie R, Petri M, Zamani O, et al. A phase III, randomized, placebo-controlled study of belimumab, a monoclonal antibody that inhibits B lymphocyte stimulator, in patients with systemic lupus erythematosus. Arthritis Rheum 2011;63(12): 3918–30.

33. Dooley MA, Houssiau F, Aranow C, et al. Effect of belimumab treatment on renal outcomes: results from the phase 3 belimumab clinical trials in patients with SLE. Lupus 2013;22(1):63–72.

34. Rovin BH, Dooley MA, Radhakrishnan J, et al. The impact of tabalumab on the kidney in systemic lupus erythematosus: results from two phase 3 randomized, clinical trials. Lupus 2016;25(14):1597–601.

35. Merrill JT, Shanahan WR, Scheinberg M, et al. Phase III trial results with blisibimod, a selective inhibitor of B-cell activating factor, in subjects with systemic

lupus erythematosus (SLE): results from a randomised, double-blind, placebo-controlled trial. Ann Rheum Dis 2018;77(6):883–9.

36. Pollard RP, Abdulahad WH, Vissink A, et al. Serum levels of BAFF, but not APRIL, are increased after rituximab treatment in patients with primary Sjogren's syndrome: data from a placebo-controlled clinical trial. Ann Rheum Dis 2013;72(1): 146–8.

37. Tsuiji M, Yurasov S, Velinzon K, et al. A checkpoint for autoreactivity in human IgM+ memory B cell development. J Exp Med 2006;203(2):393–400.

38. Espeli M, Bokers S, Giannico G, et al. Local renal autoantibody production in lupus nephritis. J Am Soc Nephrol 2011;22(2):296–305.

39. Hiepe F, Dorner T, Hauser AE, et al. Long-lived autoreactive plasma cells drive persistent autoimmune inflammation. Nat Rev Rheumatol 2011;7(3):170–8.

40. Seavey MM, Lu LD, Stump KL, et al. Novel, orally active, proteasome inhibitor, delanzomib (CEP-18770), ameliorates disease symptoms and glomerulonephritis in two preclinical mouse models of SLE. Int Immunopharmacol 2012;12(1):257–70.

41. Alexander T, Sarfert R, Klotsche J, et al. The proteasome inhibitor bortezomib depletes plasma cells and ameliorates clinical manifestations of refractory systemic lupus erythematosus. Ann Rheum Dis 2015;74(7):1474–8.

42. Kaur G, Batra S. Emerging role of immunoproteasomes in pathophysiology. Immunol Cell Biol 2016;94(9):812–20.

43. Lickliter J, Anderl J, Kirk CJ. KZR-616, a selective inhibitor of the immunoproteasome, shows a promising safety and target inhibition profile in a phase I, double-blind, single (SAD) and multiple ascending dose (MAD) study in healthy volunteers [abstract]. Arthritis Rheumatol 2017;69(suppl 10).

44. Crabtree GR, Olson EN. NFAT signaling: choreographing the social lives of cells. Cell 2002;109(Suppl):S67–79.

45. Zavada J, Pesickova S, Rysava R, et al. Cyclosporine A or intravenous cyclophosphamide for lupus nephritis: the Cyclofa-Lune study. Lupus 2010;19(11): 1281–9.

46. Mok CC, Ying KY, Yim CW, et al. Tacrolimus versus mycophenolate mofetil for induction therapy of lupus nephritis: a randomised controlled trial and long-term follow-up. Ann Rheum Dis 2016;75(1):30–6.

47. Liu Z, Zhang H, Liu Z, et al. Multitarget therapy for induction treatment of lupus nephritis: a randomized trial. Ann Intern Med 2015;162(1):18–26.

48. Zhang H, Liu Z, Zhou M, et al. Multitarget therapy for maintenance treatment of lupus nephritis. J Am Soc Nephrol 2017;28(12):3671–8.

49. Faul C, Donnelly M, Merscher-Gomez S, et al. The actin cytoskeleton of kidney podocytes is a direct target of the antiproteinuric effect of cyclosporine A. Nat Med 2008;14(9):931–8.

50. Elgueta R, Benson MJ, de Vries VC, et al. Molecular mechanism and function of CD40/CD40L engagement in the immune system. Immunol Rev 2009;229(1): 152–72.

51. Boumpas DT, Furie R, Manzi S, et al. A short course of BG9588 (anti-CD40 ligand antibody) improves serologic activity and decreases hematuria in patients with proliferative lupus glomerulonephritis. Arthritis Rheum 2003;48(3):719–27.

52. Furie R, Nicholls K, Cheng TT, et al. Efficacy and safety of abatacept in lupus nephritis: a twelve-month, randomized, double-blind study. Arthritis Rheumatol 2014;66(2):379–89.

53. ACCESS Trial Group. Treatment of lupus nephritis with abatacept: the Abatacept and Cyclophosphamide Combination Efficacy and Safety Study. Arthritis Rheumatol 2014;66(11):3096–104.

54. Weckerle CE, Franek BS, Kelly JA, et al. Network analysis of associations between serum interferon-alpha activity, autoantibodies, and clinical features in systemic lupus erythematosus. Arthritis Rheum 2011;63(4):1044–53.
55. Lovgren T, Eloranta ML, Bave U, et al. Induction of interferon-alpha production in plasmacytoid dendritic cells by immune complexes containing nucleic acid released by necrotic or late apoptotic cells and lupus IgG. Arthritis Rheum 2004;50(6):1861–72.
56. Mathian A, Weinberg A, Gallegos M, et al. IFN-alpha induces early lethal lupus in preautoimmune (New Zealand Black x New Zealand White) F1 but not in BALB/c mice. J Immunol 2005;174(5):2499–506.
57. Fairhurst AM, Mathian A, Connolly JE, et al. Systemic IFN-alpha drives kidney nephritis in B6.Sle123 mice. Eur J Immunol 2008;38(7):1948–60.
58. Ivashkiv LB, Donlin LT. Regulation of type I interferon responses. Nat Rev Immunol 2014;14(1):36–49.
59. Kalunian KC, Merrill JT, Maciuca R, et al. A phase II study of the efficacy and safety of rontalizumab (rhuMAb interferon-alpha) in patients with systemic lupus erythematosus (ROSE). Ann Rheum Dis 2016;75(1):196–202.
60. Baechler EC, Batliwalla FM, Karypis G, et al. Interferon-inducible gene expression signature in peripheral blood cells of patients with severe lupus. Proc Natl Acad Sci U S A 2003;100(5):2610–5.
61. Feng X, Wu H, Grossman JM, et al. Association of increased interferon-inducible gene expression with disease activity and lupus nephritis in patients with systemic lupus erythematosus. Arthritis Rheum 2006;54(9):2951–62.
62. Khamashta M, Merrill JT, Werth VP, et al. Sifalimumab, an anti-interferon-alpha monoclonal antibody, in moderate to severe systemic lupus erythematosus: a randomised, double-blind, placebo-controlled study. Ann Rheum Dis 2016; 75(11):1909–16.
63. Furie R, Khamashta M, Merrill JT, et al. Anifrolumab, an anti-interferon-alpha receptor monoclonal antibody, in moderate-to-severe systemic lupus erythematosus. Arthritis Rheumatol 2017;69(2):376–86.
64. Morehouse C, Chang L, Wang L, et al. Target modulation of a type I interferon (IFN) gene signature with sifalimumab or anifrolumab in systemic lupus erythematosus (SLE) patients in two open label phase 2 Japanese Trials. Boston (MA): 2014 ACR/ARHP Annual Meeting; 2014.
65. Michaelson JS, Wisniacki N, Burkly LC, et al. Role of TWEAK in lupus nephritis: a bench-to-bedside review. J Autoimmun 2012;39(3):130–42.
66. Schwartz N, Rubinstein T, Burkly LC, et al. Urinary TWEAK as a biomarker of lupus nephritis: a multicenter cohort study. Arthritis Res Ther 2009;11(5):R143.
67. Iwano M, Dohi K, Hirata E, et al. Urinary levels of IL-6 in patients with active lupus nephritis. Clin Nephrol 1993;40(1):16–21.
68. Peterson E, Robertson AD, Emlen W. Serum and urinary interleukin-6 in systemic lupus erythematosus. Lupus 1996;5(6):571–5.
69. Kiberd BA. Interleukin-6 receptor blockage ameliorates murine lupus nephritis. J Am Soc Nephrol 1993;4(1):58–61.
70. Cash H, Relle M, Menke J, et al. Interleukin 6 (IL-6) deficiency delays lupus nephritis in MRL-Faslpr mice: the IL-6 pathway as a new therapeutic target in treatment of autoimmune kidney disease in systemic lupus erythematosus. J Rheumatol 2010;37(1):60–70.
71. Rovin BH, van Vollenhoven RF, Aranow C, et al. A multicenter, randomized, double-blind, placebo-controlled study to evaluate the efficacy and safety of

treatment with sirukumab (CNTO 136) in patients with active lupus nephritis. Arthritis Rheumatol 2016;68(9):2174–83.

72. Lourenco EV, Wong M, Hahn BH, et al. Laquinimod delays and suppresses nephritis in lupus-prone mice and affects both myeloid and lymphoid immune cells. Arthritis Rheumatol 2014;66(3):674–85.

73. Ponticelli C, Passerini P, Salvadori M, et al. A randomized pilot trial comparing methylprednisolone plus a cytotoxic agent versus synthetic adrenocorticotropic hormone in idiopathic membranous nephropathy. Am J Kidney Dis 2006;47(2): 233–40.

74. Berg AL, Arnadottir M. ACTH-induced improvement in the nephrotic syndrome in patients with a variety of diagnoses. Nephrol Dial Transplant 2004;19(5):1305–7.

75. Hogan J, Bomback AS, Mehta K, et al. Treatment of idiopathic FSGS with adrenocorticotropic hormone gel. Clin J Am Soc Nephrol 2013;8(12):2072–81.

76. Bomback AS, Canetta PA, Beck LH Jr, et al. Treatment of resistant glomerular diseases with adrenocorticotropic hormone gel: a prospective trial. Am J Nephrol 2012;36(1):58–67.

77. Lindskog A, Ebefors K, Johansson ME, et al. Melanocortin 1 receptor agonists reduce proteinuria. J Am Soc Nephrol 2010;21(8):1290–8.

Nonproliferative Forms of Lupus Nephritis: An Overview

Andrew S. Bomback, MD, MPH

KEYWORDS

• Lupus • Lupus nephritis • Nephrotic syndrome • Podoctyopathy

KEY POINTS

- Class I and class II lupus nephritis do not require immunosuppressive therapy but are prone to class switching to more aggressive lesions. A low threshold for repeat biopsy should be used in these patients.
- Class V lupus nephritis with preserved renal function and subnephrotic proteinuria usually has a good prognosis and can be treated conservatively with blockade of the renin angio-tensin aldosterone system.
- If immunosuppressive therapy is warranted for class V lupus nephritis, as with proliferative lupus nephritis, mycophenolate mofetil has emerged as the most commonly used first-line therapy.

INTRODUCTION

Kidney involvement in systemic lupus erythematosus (SLE), generally termed lupus nephritis, is a major contributor to SLE-associated morbidity and mortality. Up to 50% of SLE patients will have clinically evident kidney disease at presentation, and, during follow-up, kidney involvement occurs in up to 75% of patients, with an even greater representation among children and young adults.[1] Lupus nephritis has been shown to impact clinical outcomes in SLE both directly via target organ damage and indirectly through complications of therapy. Most of the attention paid to lupus nephritis, in the medical literature as well as in past and ongoing clinical trials, has primarily focused on proliferative forms of lupus nephritis. This review highlights the importance of recognizing and treating nonproliferative forms of lupus nephritis.

DISEASE PRESENTATION

Most patients with SLE will have laboratory evidence of kidney involvement at some point in their disease. In about one-third of SLE patients, kidney involvement first

Disclosure Statement: Nothing to disclose.
A.S. Bomback was supported by National Institutes of Health/National Institute on Minority Health and Health Disparities grant R01MD009223.
Department of Medicine, Division of Nephrology, Columbia University College of Physicians and Surgeons, 622 West 168th Street, PH 4-124, New York, NY 10032, USA
E-mail address: asb68@columbia.edu

Rheum Dis Clin N Am 44 (2018) 561–569
https://doi.org/10.1016/j.rdc.2018.06.003
0889-857X/18/© 2018 Elsevier Inc. All rights reserved.

rheumatic.theclinics.com

manifests with proteinuria and/or microhematuria on urinalysis; this eventually progresses to reduction in kidney function. Whereas the proliferative forms of lupus nephritis can sometimes present with renal dysfunction at the time of diagnosis, the nonproliferative forms of disease will most commonly manifest in low-level hematuria and varying degrees of proteinuria with preserved kidney function. Indeed, if a patient with a nonproliferative form of lupus nephritis presents with significantly reduced glomerular filtration rate, the clinician should suspect either long-standing undiagnosed disease or a second form of renal injury (eg, diabetic kidney disease, focal segmental glomerulosclerosis [FSGS]) alongside the lupus lesion.

Many urine and serologic tests have been studied as biomarkers for SLE and, specifically, lupus nephritis disease activity. These tests include standard laboratory values used to assess patients with lupus nephritis, such as measurement of kidney function (creatinine and/or cystatin C), urinary abnormalities (proteinuria and urinalysis with microscopic sediment), and immunologic markers of disease activity, including antinuclear antibodies, anti-double-stranded DNA antibody, antiphospholipid antibody, anti-Smith antibody, and serum complement levels (C3, C4, CH50). In addition, ongoing research has aimed to identify novel biomarkers of lupus nephritis using molecules specific to lupus (eg, anti-C1q antibodies), mediators of chronic inflammation (eg, tumor necrosis factor-like weak inducer of apoptosis), and generalized markers of kidney injury (urinary neutrophil gelatinase–associated lipocalin).[2,3] However, no serum or urine disease markers are able to provide as much information as a kidney biopsy. Hence, virtually all patients with SLE with suspected kidney involvement undergo one or more kidney biopsies at some point during their care.

KIDNEY BIOPSY FINDINGS: DISTINGUISHING PROLIFERATIVE FROM NONPROLIFERATIVE LUPUS NEPHRITIS

The 2012 American College of Rheumatology (ACR) Guidelines for Screening, Treatment, and Management of Lupus Nephritis recommended that all patients with clinical evidence of active lupus nephritis, previously untreated, undergo renal biopsy so that glomerular disease can be accurately classified according to the International Society of Nephrology and the Renal Pathology Society (ISN/RPS) classification.[4] Neither the ACR guidelines nor the guidelines put out 1 year earlier by the ISN provided specific parameters for what constitutes "clinical evidence" of active lupus nephritis.[5] Most centers, however, will recommend kidney biopsy for patients with SLE who have microscopic hematuria and proteinuria greater than 500 mg/d if renal function is preserved. The threshold to biopsy will often be lowered (eg, at any degree of proteinuria) if serum complement levels (C3 and/or C4) are depressed or if there is any evidence of renal dysfunction.

The classic pattern of lupus nephritis is an immune complex–mediated glomerulonephritis that usually demonstrates the following features: (1) glomerular deposits that stain dominantly for immunoglobulin G (IgG) with codeposits of IgA, IgM, C3, and C1q, the so-called full-house immunofluorescence pattern; (2) extraglomerular immune–type deposits within tubular basement membranes, the interstitium, and blood vessels; (3) the ultrastructural finding of coexistent mesangial, subendothelial, and subepithelial electron-dense deposits; and (4) the ultrastructural finding of tubuloreticular inclusions, which represent "interferon footprints" in the glomerular endothelial cell cytoplasm.

The ISN/RPS classification recognizes 6 different classes of immune complex–mediated lupus glomerulonephritis based on biopsy findings.[6] Class I represents the mildest possible glomerular lesion of immune deposits limited to the mesangium, without associated mesangial hypercellularity. In class II, the mesangial deposits detected by immunofluorescence and/or electron microscopy are accompanied by mesangial hypercellularity of any degree. In class III, there is focal and predominantly segmental endocapillary proliferation and/or sclerosis affecting less than 50% of glomeruli sampled. The active endocapillary lesions typically include infiltrating monocytes and neutrophils and may exhibit necrotizing features, including fibrinoid necrosis, rupture of glomerular basement membrane, and nuclear apoptosis. In class IV, the endocapillary lesions involve ≥50% of glomeruli sampled, typically in a diffuse and global distribution. Class V denotes membranous lupus nephritis. Subepithelial deposits are the defining feature, usually superimposed on a base of mesangial hypercellularity and/or mesangial immune deposits. In those patients with combined membranous and endocapillary lesions, a diagnosis of both class V and class III or IV is made. These mixed classes carry a worse prognosis than pure class V lupus nephritis. Class VI identifies advanced chronic disease exhibiting greater than 90% sclerotic glomeruli, without residual activity. Although there can be some degree of mesangial proliferation in class II cases, this review discusses the class I, II, and V lesions as examples of nonproliferative lupus nephritis.

CLASS I AND CLASS II LUPUS NEPHRITIS

Class I and class II lupus nephritis, which represent purely mesangial disease, carry a better prognosis than proliferative forms of lupus nephritis (ie, class III or IV) or the membranous form of lupus nephritis (ie, class V). In general, patients with class I and II lesions require no therapy directed at the kidney. Most patients will have good long-term renal outcomes, and the potential toxicity of any immunosuppressive regimen will negatively alter the risk-benefit ratio of treatment. An exception is the group of lupus patients with lupus podocytopathy (discussed later), who respond to a short course of high-dose corticosteroids in a fashion similar to patients with minimal change disease (MCD).

Optimal control of blood pressure through the renin angiotensin aldosterone system (RAAS) blockade is a cornerstone of conservative therapy in all forms of lupus nephritis and is the only required therapy for class I and class II lesions. The National Kidney Foundation's Kidney Disease Outcomes Quality Initiative guidelines recommend interruption of the RAAS with angiotensin-converting enzyme (ACE) inhibitors or angiotensin receptor blockers as first-line antihypertensive therapy in the management of proteinuric kidney diseases such as lupus nephritis.[7] These drugs decrease intraglomerular pressure, lower systemic arterial blood pressure, reduce urinary protein excretion, and delay the progression of chronic kidney disease to end-stage renal disease.[8–10] A report from the Lupus in Minorities: Nature versus Nurture cohort suggests that ACE inhibitor use delays the development of renal involvement in SLE.[11] Eighty of 378 patients (21%) in the cohort used ACE inhibitors. The probability of renal-involvement-free survival at 10 years was 88% for ACE inhibitor users and 75% for nonusers ($P = .01$), and by multivariable Cox proportional hazards regression analyses, ACE inhibitors use was associated with a longer time-to-renal involvement occurrence (hazard ratio 0.27; 95% confidence interval [CI] 0.09–0.78). ACE inhibitor use was also associated with a decreased risk of disease activity (hazard ratio 0.56; 95% CI 0.34–0.94).

The RAAS, and its pharmacologic blockade, may play a role in the pathogenesis and prognosis of SLE independent of its effects on systemic blood pressure and glomerular hemodynamics. Several animal studies have highlighted the inflammatory components of the RAAS and the potential benefits of RAAS blockade in reducing or eliminating this inflammation in lupus nephritis.[12] De Albuquerque and colleagues[13] treated lupus-prone mice with captopril and found that captopril treatment delayed the onset of proteinuria when administered to prenephritic mice and slowed disease progression in mice with early and advanced nephritis. These results were not seen in a control group treated with verapamil. The ACE inhibitor–induced improvement in renal disease correlated with reduced transforming growth factor (TGF)-β expression, particularly of the TGF-β1 and TGF-β2 isoforms, in the kidneys. Moreover, in vivo or in vitro exposure to captopril reduced splenic levels of interleukin-4 (IL-4) and IL-10, suggesting an effect of captopril on the immune system of treated animals. In an experiment on the effect of aldosterone blockade on the development and progression of glomerulonephritis in a murine model of lupus, spironolactone significantly reduced the incidence of nephrotic range proteinuria and, on histology, showed far less severe glomerular injuries (no crescents, diminished overall cellularity, and less prominent deposits in the capillary loops and mesangium) compared with controls.[14] The investigators found significant differences in anti–single-stranded DNA and anti–double-stranded DNA antibody levels between control mice and mice treated with spironolactone by 36 weeks of age, again highlighting a potential anti-inflammatory, immune-mediating component of RAAS blockade.

Importantly, lupus nephritis classes are not static entities and may transform from one class to another, both spontaneously and after therapy, and influence treatment decisions. In a review of more than 700 patients with lupus nephritis who underwent repeat biopsies during their disease courses, performed on average at 3.0 years after the initial biopsy, 52.6% of cases demonstrated some form of class switching.[15] This phenomenon of class switching is particularly important for patients whose biopsies show class I or class II lesions and have been maintained on conservative therapy alone. In 9 studies encompassing 519 lupus patients with repeat renal biopsies, the rate of class switching in patients with class I or class II lesions on their initial biopsies was 70% when a repeat biopsy was performed: 54% transforming into a proliferative (ie, class III or IV) lesion, 4% evolving into a pure class V membranous lesion, and 12% manifesting a mixed proliferative and membranous pattern.[15–23] This class switching is crucial to recognize because it may move a patient from a low-risk group that does not require immunosuppressive therapy to a high-risk group that does warrant renal-directed immunosuppression. Therefore, patients with class I or II lesions who manifest increased proteinuria and/or renal dysfunction despite effective use of RAAS blockade should be targeted for repeat biopsies.

LUPUS PODOCYTOPATHY

In 2002, Dube and colleagues[24] and Hertig and colleagues[25] described small series of patients with SLE, nephrotic syndrome, and biopsy findings of MCD or FSGS. Eight of 18 patients in these reports had mesangial deposits, including 7 of 11 with MCD and 1 of 7 with FSGS, consistent with concurrent mesangial lupus nephritis (ie, class I or II lesions). The patients with MCD universally showed rapid remission of nephrotic syndrome with steroid therapy; the response to steroids was inconsistent in patients with FSGS lesions. In 2005, Kraft and colleagues[26] reported 8 additional patients with SLE, nephrotic syndrome, and light microscopic findings of MCD, FSGS, or mesangial proliferative glomerulonephritis. These investigators argued that the development of nephrotic range proteinuria in patients with SLE without subendothelial or subepithelial immune deposits on biopsy is more likely a manifestation of SLE than the coexistence of idiopathic MCD/FSGS and SLE. The term lupus podocytopathy thus arose to describe these lesions as part of the lupus nephritis spectrum.

More recently, Hu and colleagues[27] presented 50 patients classified as having lupus podocytopathy, culled from a 14-year biopsy registry (2000–2013) and representing 1.3% of all lupus nephritis biopsies read at Nanjing University during this time period. Thirteen patients had normal light microscopy findings; 28 showed mesangial proliferative changes, and 9 had FSGS lesions. Forty-seven of the 50 patients had mesangial immune deposits as confirmed by immunofluorescence and electron microscopy. All of the patients had full nephrotic syndrome. This series, the largest cohort of lupus podocytopathy, provided representative data on clinical presentations, treatment responses, and relapse rates in patients with this entity. For example, the remission rate with immunosuppression of 94% was not altogether surprising on the basis of prior series, but the median time to remission of 4 weeks added a new layer of important, clinically relevant information. Response and relapse rates differed among the histologic subtypes: all of the patients with MCD and 27 of the 28 patients with mesangial proliferative changes responded, whereas nonresponders were disproportionately high in the FSGS subgroup. As with podocytopathies not associated with SLE, relapse rates were high (56%) and did not differ by histologic pattern. Therefore, many of these lupus podocytopathy patients will require multiple rounds of immunosuppression for relapses, and the use of steroid-sparing agents, such as mycophenolate mofetil (MMF), calcineurin inhibitors, cyclophosphamide, and rituximab, may need to be used in the same way these agents are used in frequently relapsing forms of steroid-sensitive MCD and FSGS.

A finding that emerged in virtually every case series of lupus podocytopathy is that morphologic findings of FSGS are associated with a distinctly worse prognosis. In the series from Hu and colleagues,[27] patients with FSGS compared with those with MCD or mesangial proliferative changes had higher rates of hypertension and acute kidney injury on clinical presentation and more severe tubulointerstitial involvement on biopsy. In follow-up, not only were the patients with FSGS less likely to respond to therapy, but also, when responses did occur, the remissions happened later, at a median of 8 weeks compared with 4 weeks for the MCD and mesangial proliferative subgroups. These observations raise the question of whether it is appropriate to use the same umbrella term of lupus podocytopathy for all 3 of these patterns of glomerular injury.

The ISN/RPS classification of lupus does not include lupus podocytopathy. A 2016 paper[28] proposed fairly simple criteria to diagnose lupus podocytopathy: (1) clinical presentation of full nephrotic syndrome in a patient with SLE, (2) diffuse and severe foot process effacement, and (3) the absence of subendothelial or subepithelial immune deposits. Mesangial deposits and mesangial proliferation were not part of the criteria. If these findings are present, then the additional diagnosis of mesangial proliferative lupus nephritis (ie, class II) is merited. If mesangial deposits are not accompanied by mesangial proliferation, the diagnosis of minimal mesangial lupus nephritis (class I) is given. In this manner, the classic forms of immune complex–mediated lupus nephritis are separated from lupus podocytopathy, with a willingness to diagnose both in the appropriate situation, and the need for a mesangial proliferative category of lupus podocytopathy is avoided. Lupus podocytopathy was also subdivided into patients who would otherwise meet criteria for MCD or FSGS, including the morphologic subtypes of FSGS (collapsing, tip lesion, and so forth).

CLASS V LUPUS NEPHRITIS

Class V, or membranous, lupus nephritis is defined by subepithelial immune deposits. The membranous alterations may be present alone or on a background of mesangial hypercellularity and mesangial immune deposits. In the past, reports have varied regarding renal survival rates for different populations with membranous LN. These differences were, in part, due to problems with the World Health Organization (WHO) classification of lupus nephritis, which included proliferative lesions superimposed on pure lupus membranous nephropathy (WHO class Vc and Vd) along with those with only predominantly pure membranous features (Va and Vb).[6] With the updated ISN/RPS classification, a distinction was clearly made between pure class V lesions and mixed proliferative and membranous cases (III + V or IV + V lesions). The latter follows a much more aggressive course, and treatment generally should focus on the proliferative component (discussed later). In contrast, patients with pure membranous lupus nephropathy, especially when proteinuria remains in the subnephrotic range, often do extremely well regardless of treatment options and may not require any specific therapy beyond RAAS blockade.

Most treatment regimens studied for pure class V lupus nephritis with nephrotic range proteinuria have been based on successful therapies used for primary membranous nephropathy. For example, Austin and colleagues[29] randomized 42 patients with membranous lupus nephritis to 3 groups: cyclosporine for 11 months (on top of steroids), alternate-month intravenous pulse cyclophosphamide for 6 doses (also on top of steroids), and alternate-day prednisone alone. At 1 year, the cumulative probability of remission was 27% with prednisone, 60% with cyclophosphamide, and 83% with cyclosporine. Remissions occurred more quickly in the cyclosporine group, but there were fewer relapses in the cyclophosphamide group.[30] Similar data are available from small numbers of patients treated with tacrolimus monotherapy.[31–34] Two large trials of MMF versus intravenous cyclophosphamide induction in lupus nephritis,[35,36] conducted primarily in patients with proliferative lesions, included 84 (of total 510) patients with pure membranous lesions. In a pooled analysis of these participants, remissions, relapses, and overall clinical course were similar in the membranous patients treated with oral MMF and intravenous cyclophosphamide induction therapy.[37] Therefore, the 2012 ACR guidelines for Screening, Treatment, and Management of Lupus Nephritis allowed for MMF as first-line immunosuppression for patients with class V lupus nephritis requiring immunosuppression due to nephrotic range proteinuria and/or declining renal function.

The data supporting the use of other immunosuppressive agents are less robust. Rituximab and abatacept have been used off-label for pure class V lesions based on post hoc analyses of studies that included both proliferative and nonproliferative cases of lupus nephritis with higher response rates in patients with nephrotic range proteinuria.[38,39] There has also been renewed interest in calcineurin inhibitor use in patients with class V lupus nephritis based on the early results with the novel calcineurin inhibitor, voclosporin. In a phase 2 study, whose results were presented in abstract form, voclosporin (at low and high doses added on top of background steroids and MMF) yielded complete remission rates at 48 weeks between 40% and 49% compared with a 24% complete remission rate in control group patients treated with steroids and MMF alone. This drug is now being evaluated in a larger phase 3 study with planned enrollment exceeding 300 patients (clinicaltrials.gov identifier NCT 03021499).

MIXED PROLIFERATIVE AND NONPROLIFERATIVE LUPUS NEPHRITIS

Some patients with lupus nephritis will have evidence of endocapillary proliferative disease, fulfilling criteria for either class III or class IV lesions, as well as a membranous nephropathy pattern of glomerular basement membrane thickening due to subepithelial deposits, fulfilling criteria for class V disease. These mixed cases should be classified as III + V or IV + V, and the treatment is usually dictated by the proliferative lesion.

Therefore, first-line therapy will generally be a combination of steroids with cyclophosphamide or MMF for induction therapy, followed by MMF for maintenance therapy.

Another induction treatment strategy studied in small settings is to combine a calcineurin inhibitor with MMF plus corticosteroids. This multitargeted immunosuppressant regimen is akin to those used in protecting kidney transplants. For example, Bao and colleagues[40] randomized 40 patients with diffuse proliferative LN superimposed on membranous LN (ISN class IV + V) to induction therapy with MMF, tacrolimus, and steroids (multitarget therapy) or intravenous cyclophosphamide plus steroids. Intention-to-treat analysis revealed a higher rate of complete remission with multitarget therapy at both 6 and 9 months (50% and 65%, respectively) than with cyclophosphamide (5% and 15%, respectively). Adverse events were lower in the multitarget group, too. In a subsequent report using a much larger patient population drawn from 26 nephrology centers across China, this multitarget therapy at 24 weeks, compared with cyclophosphamide-based induction, showed higher rates of complete (46% vs 26%) and complete plus partial (84% vs 63%) remission. The median time to overall response was shorter in the multitarget group as well.[41]

Recently, these investigators have reported an open-label, multicenter study for 18 months to assess the efficacy and safety of multitarget maintenance therapy in patients who had responded at 24 weeks during the induction phase.[42] Those induced on multitarget therapy (N = 116) remained on low-dose MMF, tacrolimus, and prednisone, whereas those induced with cyclophosphamide (N = 90) were given azathioprine plus prednisone. The multitarget and azathioprine groups had similar cumulative renal relapse rates (6% vs 8%, respectively), and serum creatinine levels remained stable in both groups. The azathioprine group had more adverse events (44% vs 16% for multitarget therapy). The caveats for both the induction and the maintenance phase of these multitarget therapy studies include (a) whether they will be generalizable beyond Asian populations of lupus nephritis and (b) whether the remission rates achieved will be sustained once calcineurin inhibitors are weaned off, given the high rate of proteinuria relapse when calcineurin inhibitors have been stopped in other glomerular diseases.

SUMMARY

The approach to patients with class I, II, and V lesions of lupus nephritis requires an understanding of the unique nature of each of these lesions as well as the possibility that, over the course of disease, class switching may occur. Conservative, nonimmunomodulatory therapy is sufficient for all patients with class I and II lesions and for patients with class V lesions, preserved renal function, and nonnephrotic range proteinuria. For patients who require kidney-targeted immunosuppression, MMF is the current mainstay of therapy, but a variety of other treatment options, ranging from multitargeted therapy to novel agents under investigation, are available for patients whose disease courses stray outside the conventional parameters.

REFERENCES

1. Bomback AS, Appel GB. Updates on the treatment of lupus nephritis. J Am Soc Nephrol 2010;21(12):2028–35.
2. Zhang X, Nagaraja HN, Nadasdy T, et al. A composite urine biomarker reflects interstitial inflammation in lupus nephritis kidney biopsies. Kidney Int 2012; 81(4):401–6.
3. Schwartz N, Rubinstein T, Burkly LC, et al. Urinary TWEAK as a biomarker of lupus nephritis: a multicenter cohort study. Arthritis Res Ther 2009;11(5):R143.

4. Hahn BH, McMahon MA, Wilkinson A, et al. American College of Rheumatology guidelines for screening, treatment, and management of lupus nephritis. Arthritis Care Res (Hoboken) 2012;64(6):797–808.

5. Beck L, Bomback AS, Choi MJ, et al. KDOQI US commentary on the 2012 KDIGO clinical practice guideline for glomerulonephritis. Am J Kidney Dis 2013;62(3): 403–41.

6. Markowitz GS, D'Agati VD. The ISN/RPS 2003 classification of lupus nephritis: an assessment at 3 years. Kidney Int 2007;71(6):491–5.

7. K/DOQI clinical practice guidelines on hypertension and antihypertensive agents in chronic kidney disease. Am J Kidney Dis 2004;43(5 Suppl 1):S1–290.

8. Lewis EJ, Hunsicker LG, Bain RP, et al. The effect of angiotensin-converting-enzyme inhibition on diabetic nephropathy. The Collaborative Study Group. N Engl J Med 1993;329(20):1456–62.

9. Lewis EJ, Hunsicker LG, Clarke WR, et al. Renoprotective effect of the angiotensin-receptor antagonist irbesartan in patients with nephropathy due to type 2 diabetes. N Engl J Med 2001;345(12):851–60.

10. MacKinnon M, Shurraw S, Akbari A, et al. Combination therapy with an angiotensin receptor blocker and an ACE inhibitor in proteinuric renal disease: a systematic review of the efficacy and safety data. Am J Kidney Dis 2006;48(1):8–20.

11. Duran-Barragan S, McGwin G Jr, Vila LM, et al. Angiotensin-converting enzyme inhibitors delay the occurrence of renal involvement and are associated with a decreased risk of disease activity in patients with systemic lupus erythematosus–results from LUMINA (LIX): a multiethnic US cohort. Rheumatology (Oxford) 2008;47(7):1093–6.

12. Teplitsky V, Shoenfeld Y, Tanay A. The renin-angiotensin system in lupus: physiology, genes and practice, in animals and humans. Lupus 2006;15(6):319–25.

13. De Albuquerque DA, Saxena V, Adams DE, et al. An ACE inhibitor reduces Th2 cytokines and TGF-beta1 and TGF-beta2 isoforms in murine lupus nephritis. Kidney Int 2004;65(3):846–59.

14. Monrad SU, Killen PD, Anderson MR, et al. The role of aldosterone blockade in murine lupus nephritis. Arthritis Res Ther 2008;10(1):R5.

15. Narvaez J, Ricse M, Goma M, et al. The value of repeat biopsy in lupus nephritis flares. Medicine (Baltimore) 2017;96(24):e7099.

16. Daleboudt GM, Bajema IM, Goemaere NN, et al. The clinical relevance of a repeat biopsy in lupus nephritis flares. Nephrol Dial Transplant 2009;24(12): 3712–7.

17. Alsuwaida AO. The clinical significance of serial kidney biopsies in lupus nephritis. Mod Rheumatol 2014;24(3):453–6.

18. Bajaj S, Albert L, Gladman DD, et al. Serial renal biopsy in systemic lupus erythematosus. J Rheumatol 2000;27(12):2822–6.

19. Pagni F, Galimberti S, Goffredo P, et al. The value of repeat biopsy in the management of lupus nephritis: an international multicentre study in a large cohort of patients. Nephrol Dial Transpl 2013;28(12):3014–23.

20. Moroni G, Pasquali S, Quaglini S, et al. Clinical and prognostic value of serial renal biopsies in lupus nephritis. Am J Kidney Dis 1999;34(3):530–9.

21. Wang GB, Xu ZJ, Liu HF, et al. Changes in pathological pattern and treatment regimens based on repeat renal biopsy in lupus nephritis. Chin Med J (Engl) 2012;125(16):2890–4.

22. Greloni G, Scolnik M, Marin J, et al. Value of repeat biopsy in lupus nephritis flares. Lupus Sci Med 2014;1(1):e000004.

23. Tannor EK, Bates WD, Moosa MR. The clinical relevance of repeat renal biopsies in the management of lupus nephritis: a South African experience. Lupus 2018; 27(4):525–35.

24. Dube GK, Markowitz GS, Radhakrishnan J, et al. Minimal change disease in systemic lupus erythematosus. Clin Nephrol 2002;57(2):120–6.

25. Hertig A, Droz D, Lesavre P, et al. SLE and idiopathic nephrotic syndrome: coincidence or not? Am J Kidney Dis 2002;40(6):1179–84.

26. Kraft SW, Schwartz MM, Korbet SM, et al. Glomerular podocytopathy in patients with systemic lupus erythematosus. J Am Soc Nephrol 2005;16(1):175–9.

27. Hu W, Chen Y, Wang S, et al. Clinical-morphological features and outcomes of lupus podocytopathy. Clin J Am Soc Nephrol 2016;11(4):585–92.

28. Bomback AS, Markowitz GS. Lupus podocytopathy: a distinct entity. Clin J Am Soc Nephrol 2016;11(4):547–8.

29. Austin HA 3rd, Illei GG, Braun MJ, et al. Randomized, controlled trial of prednisone, cyclophosphamide, and cyclosporine in lupus membranous nephropathy. J Am Soc Nephrol 2009;20(4):901–11.

30. Cattran DC, Alexopoulos E, Heering P, et al. Cyclosporin in idiopathic glomerular disease associated with the nephrotic syndrome : workshop recommendations. Kidney Int 2007;72(12):1429–47.

31. Tse KC, Lam MF, Tang SC, et al. A pilot study on tacrolimus treatment in membranous or quiescent lupus nephritis with proteinuria resistant to angiotensin inhibition or blockade. Lupus 2007;16(1):46–51.

32. Asamiya Y, Uchida K, Otsubo S, et al. Clinical assessment of tacrolimus therapy in lupus nephritis: one-year follow-up study in a single center. Nephron Clin Pract 2009;113(4):c330–6.

33. Miyasaka N, Kawai S, Hashimoto H. Efficacy and safety of tacrolimus for lupus nephritis: a placebo-controlled double-blind multicenter study. Mod Rheumatol 2009;19(6):606–15.

34. Uchino A, Tsukamoto H, Nakashima H, et al. Tacrolimus is effective for lupus nephritis patients with persistent proteinuria. Clin Exp Rheumatol 2010;28(1): 6–12.

35. Ginzler EM, Dooley MA, Aranow C, et al. Mycophenolate mofetil or intravenous cyclophosphamide for lupus nephritis. N Engl J Med 2005;353(21):2219–28.

36. Appel GB, Contreras G, Dooley MA, et al. Mycophenolate mofetil versus cyclophosphamide for induction treatment of lupus nephritis. J Am Soc Nephrol 2009;20(5):1103–12.

37. Radhakrishnan J, Moutzouris DA, Ginzler EM, et al. Mycophenolate mofetil and intravenous cyclophosphamide are similar as induction therapy for class V lupus nephritis. Kidney Int 2010;77(2):152–60.

38. Rovin BH, Furie R, Latinis K, et al. Efficacy and safety of rituximab in patients with active proliferative lupus nephritis: the Lupus Nephritis Assessment with Rituximab study. Arthritis Rheum 2012;64(4):1215–26.

39. Furie R, Nicholls K, Cheng TT, et al. Efficacy and safety of abatacept in lupus nephritis: a twelve-month, randomized, double-blind study. Arthritis Rheumatol 2014;66(2):379–89.

40. Bao H, Liu ZH, Xie HL, et al. Successful treatment of class V+IV lupus nephritis with multitarget therapy. J Am Soc Nephrol 2008;19(10):2001–10.

41. Liu Z, Zhang H, Liu Z, et al. Multitarget therapy for induction treatment of lupus nephritis: a randomized trial. Ann Intern Med 2015;162(1):18–26.

42. Zhang H, Liu Z, Zhou M, et al. Multitarget therapy for maintenance treatment of lupus nephritis. J Am Soc Nephrol 2017;28(12):3671–8.

Renal Manifestations of Rheumatoid Arthritis

Teja Kapoor, MD*, Joan Bathon, MD[1]

KEYWORDS

- Rheumatoid arthritis • RA • Rheumatoid nephropathy • Rheumatoid kidney
- RA glomerulonephritis • Chronic kidney disease in RA • DMARDs in CKD

KEY POINTS

- Renal manifestations in patients with rheumatoid arthritis (RA) have evolved as management of RA has improved.
- Older disease-modifying antirheumatic drugs, uncontrolled systemic inflammation, and chronic nonsteroidal antiinflammatory drug (NSAID) use contributed to kidney disease in the past.
- The increased use of methotrexate and biologic medications, decrease in chronic NSAID use, and a treat-to-target strategy has contributed to a decrease in renal manifestations.
- Chronic kidney disease in patients with RA is now more closely associated with cardiovascular risk factors than with RA disease severity.
- In patients with established chronic kidney disease, medications such as NSAIDs, methotrexate, and tofacitinib may need to be adjusted or avoided to prevent adverse events.

INTRODUCTION

Rheumatoid arthritis (RA) is a systemic autoimmune disease that primarily causes inflammation of the joints. The prevalence of RA is 1%, with a greater predominance in women.[1] Chronic inflammation in RA can result in joint destruction and significant physical disability, as well as premature cardiovascular disease (CVD).[2,3]

Renal manifestations can be seen in RA but have become less prevalent as medical therapies for treating RA evolved. Historically, the primary cause of renal insufficiency in patients with RA was nephrotoxicity of therapies for RA, such as nonsteroidal antiinflammatory drugs (NSAIDs) and disease-modifying antirheumatic drugs (DMARDs),

Disclosures: T. Kapoor, none; J. Bathon: consultant to Regeneron (<$5000).
Department of Medicine, Division of Rheumatology, Columbia University College of Physicians and Surgeons, 630 West 168th Street, New York, NY 10032, USA
[1] Present address: 630 West 168th Street, Physician & Surgeons Building 3rd Floor, Room 450, New York, NY 10032.
* Corresponding author. 161 Fort Washington, Herbert Irving Pavilion, 2nd Floor, Room 205, New York, NY 10032.
E-mail address: Tmk2134@cumc.columbia.edu

Rheum Dis Clin N Am 44 (2018) 571–584
https://doi.org/10.1016/j.rdc.2018.06.008
0889-857X/18/© 2018 Elsevier Inc. All rights reserved.

such as penicillamine, bucillamine, gold, and cyclosporine. Poorly controlled systemic inflammation also led to mesangial proliferative glomerulonephritis (GN) or secondary amyloidosis. The emergence of methotrexate and targeted biologic agents, coupled with treat-to-target therapeutic approaches, marked a revolutionary turning point in the treatment of RA and greatly ameliorated the long-term consequences of chronic systemic inflammation and the need for older, more nephrotoxic DMARDs. In Asian nations, such as Japan and Korea, where older DMARD use is still common, medication-associated renal complications in patients with RA are still reported.

THE PREMETHOTREXATE AND PRE–TARGETED BIOLOGIC ERA
Prevalence of Renal Involvement in Rheumatoid Arthritis

In the era before methotrexate and targeted biologics, chronic kidney disease (CKD) was common in patients with RA, with a prevalence of 37% to 57%.[4,5] In contrast with systemic lupus erythematosus (SLE), clinically significant renal damage directly related to RA is typically not observed, except in the case of patients with poorly controlled disease activity who may develop secondary amyloidosis, which can lead to end-stage renal disease (ESRD).[6]

Most reports of CKD in patients with RA in more recent decades are in Asian populations, which may be attributed to differences in specific DMARD usage. RA medications that continue to be used in Asian nations such as Japan, Korea, and China, but are now rarely used in Western nations, include azathioprine, gold, bucillamine, cyclophosphamide, cyclosporine, and mycophenolate mofetil.[7,8]

Types of Renal Involvement in Rheumatoid Arthritis

Multiple regions of the kidney can be affected by RA and/or by treatment with RA medications. These regions include the glomerulus, vasculature, tubules, and the interstitium (**Box 1**). The level of proteinuria, active urinary sediment, and clinical symptoms do not accurately predict the renal histology in RA. Therefore, if unexplained CKD or proteinuria is detected, a renal biopsy is necessary for diagnosis.[6]

Glomerulonephritis
Autopsy studies in patients with RA describe mesangial proliferative, membranous GN, and crescentic GN, although there was little to no associated compromise in renal function reported.[9] Sub–nephrotic-range proteinuria is common in membranous GN and mesangial GN. Estimated glomerular filtration rate (eGFR), as defined by serum creatinine levels, was normal in most patients with RA who had mesangial and membranous GN.[6]

Mesangial glomerulonephritis The prevalence of mesangial GN ranges from 35% to 78% among patients with RA with known nephropathy.[6] It is usually associated with long-standing RA disease (12.9 ± 10.4 years).[6] However, it typically has a mild course and nephrotic syndrome and renal failure have only rarely been reported.[8] Interleukin (IL)-6, which is at increased levels in the peripheral blood and synovia of patients with RA, may be a growth factor for mesangial cells. In animal models, IL-6 induced proliferation of mesangial cells in the kidneys in a dose-dependent manner. In a small study by Horii and colleagues[10] of patients without RA who had primary mesangial proliferative GN, higher urine IL-6 levels were observed compared with patients with primary minimal change disease, primary membranous GN, and normal healthy controls. Whether chronically high levels of IL-6 cause mesangial GN in RA remains unclear.

Membranous glomerulonephritis Immune-complex deposition can occur in the glomerular basement membrane and lead to membranous GN. Immune-complex

---

Box 1
Types of renal involvement in patients with rheumatoid arthritis glomerulonephritis

Glomerulonephritis
- Mesangial GN
- Immunoglobulin A mesangial GN
- Membranous GN
  - Medication induced
  - Non–medication induced
- Minimal change disease
- Focal segmental glomerulosclerosis

Interstitial nephritis
- NSAIDs

Papillary necrosis
- Medication

Rheumatoid vasculitis

Renal amyloidosis

CKD caused by CVD
- Elderly age
- Hypertension
- Diabetes

---

deposition can occur in a segmental or diffuse pattern.[6,8] Most cases of membranous GN in patients with RA have been associated with DMARDs, including gold, bucillamine, and penicillamine, and has only rarely been described in patients with RA not taking these medications (**Table 1**).[6,8] Nephrotic-range proteinuria is a common presentation in membranous GN.[7] In contrast with mesangial GN, membranous GN was associated with a shorter RA disease duration (3.8 ± 2.9 years).[6] The primary treatment of drug-induced membranous GN is discontinuation of the offending medication. The use of immunosuppressants and prednisone does not significantly influence the time to remission.[6,11–16]

Other types of glomerulonephritis and renal vasculitis in patients with rheumatoid arthritis Immunoglobulin (Ig) A GN is one of the most common primary glomerular

Table 1
Medication-induced nephropathy in rheumatoid arthritis medication

Medication	Renal Manifestation
Bucillamine[6,14–16]	Membranous GN
Penicillamine[6,14–16]	Membranous GN
Gold[6,14–16]	Membranous GN Minimal change disease
Auranofin[6,14–16]	Membranous GN Minimal change disease
Phenacetin[22,80]	Renal papillary necrosis
Cyclosporine[12]	Obliterative vasculopathy of the afferent arteriole Tubulointerstitial fibrosis
NSAIDs	Acute kidney injury (via endothelial injury and/or tubular injury) Interstitial nephritis Type 4 renal tubular acidosis (hyperkalemia)

diseases in the general population.[17] The frequency of IgA GN in patients with RA is similar to that seen in the general population,[18] with a prevalence as high as 12% among patients with RA.[8] IgA GN is histologically indistinguishable between patients with and without RA.[6,8,9] Treatment of idiopathic IgA nephropathy has primarily consisted of angiotensin-converting enzyme inhibitors. Severe cases with progressively worsening renal function have been treated with glucocorticoids.[19]

Other nephropathies, such as minimal change disease and focal segmental glomerulosclerosis, are rare and have been reported only in a handful of patients with RA, with literature limited primarily to case reports.[8,20] Several cases of severe necrotizing renal vasculitis with microscopic hematuria, proteinuria, and renal insufficiency have been described in patients with severe seropositive erosive RA.[6,9,21] Some of these cases were also associated with cutaneous and pulmonary involvement.[6] However, early literature did not differentiate rheumatoid vasculitis from polyarteritis nodosa or antineutrophil cytoplasmic antibody (ANCA)–associated vasculitis.[22] Patients were primarily treated with high-dose glucocorticoids and immunosuppressants such as rituximab and cyclophosphamide.[6,9,21]

Secondary amyloidosis

Renal deposition of amyloid A protein was once a common cause of nephrotic syndrome in patients with RA with poorly controlled disease. The acute-phase reactant precursor protein, serum amyloid A (SAA), is synthesized by hepatocytes in response to proinflammatory cytokines such as tumor necrosis factor (TNF), IL-1, and IL-6.[23] Chronically increased levels of SAA can lead to secondary amyloidosis, particularly in genetically susceptible patients who have the SAA allele.[23] Amyloid may deposit in the glomeruli, blood vessels, peritubules, and interstitium of the kidney.[6] Patients classically present with proteinuria and increased serum creatinine level and develop progressive renal failure.[6] Secondary amyloidosis was associated with longer RA disease duration (17.2 ± 7.3 years) compared with patients with RA with membranous nephropathy (3.8 ± 2.9 years) or mesangial nephropathy (12.9 ± 10.4 years).[6]

Before the 1970s, and well before the advent of both methotrexate and targeted biologic agents, the prevalence of secondary amyloidosis was noted to be 16% to 19% of patients with RA[22,24] and was a major cause of ESRD and death in patients with RA compared with controls.[1] In a recent report from the Japan Renal Biopsy Registry, the prevalence of secondary renal amyloidosis remains high at 21% among patients with RA, likely because of the continued use of older pre–biologic era DMARDs.[7] Treatment of secondary amyloidosis is primarily focused on control of the underlying disease and supportive care.[23]

Secondary amyloidosis results from defective metabolism of the inflammatory acute-phase reactant precursor protein SAA, whose concentration strongly correlates with inflammatory disease activity. Accordingly, treating the underlying disease is the conventional approach in amyloid A (AA) amyloidosis, because no specific treatment exists. Despite the poor prognosis of amyloid renal involvement, the outcome of AA amyloidosis might be improved by suppressing the acute inflammatory response.

The postmethotrexate and postbiologic era

The American College of Rheumatology updated its recommendations in 2015 to include a treat-to-target strategy to treat RA to a state of low disease activity or remission, predefined by one of the American College of Rheumatology recommended disease active measures. Follow-up every 1 to 3 months is recommended during active disease with escalation of therapy with the goal to reach the target in 3 to 6 months.[25] Randomized controlled trials have shown superiority of the treat-to-target strategy compared with usual clinical care.[25,26]

In addition to the treat-to-target strategy, the advent of methotrexate, an oral synthetic DMARD, and the development of targeted biologic DMARDs such as TNF inhibitors, significantly affected the outcomes of patients with RA. Use of these agents as monotherapy, or in combination therapy, dramatically reduces the systemic and articular burden of inflammation and prevents or slows joint damage.

The incidence of renal amyloidosis in RA has significantly decreased over the years, because RA is treated more effectively and aggressively, and some have suggested that TNF inhibitors in particular may prevent amyloidosis.[6,9,27] Whether TNF inhibitors are effective at treating AA amyloidosis once it is already established is controversial. Some studies suggest improvement, whereas others suggest that, despite TNF inhibitor therapy, many patients progress to ESRD.[28]

Note that there have been paradoxic reports of lupuslike events (LLEs) and vasculitislike events (VLEs) occurring in patients treated with TNF inhibitors.[29] Reports surfaced of patients with RA treated with TNF inhibitors who developed new antinuclear antibodies, double-stranded DNA antibodies, and biopsy-proven lupus GN. Some cases of LLEs resolved with discontinuation of the anti-TNF agent, whereas others have required the addition of glucocorticoids and SLE immunosuppressants. Rare cases of ANCA vasculitis with biopsy-proven pauci-immune necrotizing GN, myeloperoxidase antibodies, and pulmonary involvement were also reported in patients receiving treatment with TNF inhibitors. However, the absolute risk of these events in patients treated with TNF inhibitors is low. The British Society for Rheumatology Biologics Registry, a national registry of patients with RA receiving targeted biologic therapy, prospectively followed 12,937 patients who were treated with TNF inhibitors and a comparison group of 3673 patients treated with nonbiologic DMARDs. The study showed that the absolute risk of LLE and VLE was low in the TNF inhibitor cohort (LLE 10 per 10,000 patient-years; VLE 15 per 10,000 patient-years) and, after adjusting for baseline patient differences, there were no differences in the risks of LLE (hazard ratio [HR], 1.86; 95% confidence interval [CI], 0.52–6.58) or VLEs (HR, 1.27; 95% CI, 0.40–4.04) for patients treated with TNF inhibitors compared with those treated with nonbiologic DMARDs.[30]

Chronic kidney disease and cardiovascular disease in rheumatoid arthritis

In recent years, CKD in patients with RA seems to be increasingly linked to CVD and cardiovascular risk factors, as in the general population (**Fig. 1**). In a cross-sectional study of 1908 Japanese patients with RA, those with CKD (defined as eGFR<60 mL/min) had a greater prevalence of diabetes mellitus (17.2% vs 8.6%; $P<.001$), hypertension (60.1% vs 26.3%; odds ratio [OR] 3.05; $P<.001$), and advanced age (73.1 years vs 61.0 years; OR 5.19 $P<.001$) compared with patients without CKD. There was no significant difference in NSAID use between the two groups.[31] In a cross-sectional analysis by Daoussis and colleagues[32] of 400 patients with RA in the United Kingdom, traditional cardiovascular risk factors such as hyperlipidemia, hypertension, and insulin resistance were associated with CKD, whereas RA disease activity, severity, and duration were not. Patients with RA have an increased risk for CVD and have a higher prevalence of some conventional CVD risk factors, such as hypertension, compared with the general population.[2,3] This excess CVD risk is thought to be caused by the chronically enhanced levels of inflammation that characterize RA. In

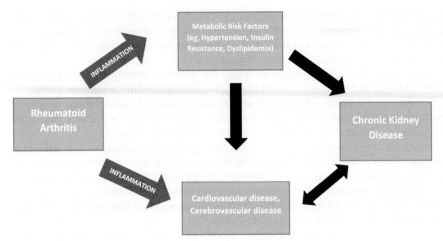

Fig. 1. CKD, CVD, and RA.

turn, acute CVD events that lead to heart failure may further promote decline of renal function.

The presence of CKD further worsens the CVD mortality risk in patients with RA. Sihvonen and Korpela[33] showed a 2 to 4 times greater mortality in patients with RA who had CKD compared with those without CKD (HR, 2.77–4.45). In another nationwide longitudinal cohort study of 12,579 patients with RA in Taiwan, those with CKD had a significantly greater risk for ischemic heart disease (adjusted HR, 1.57; CI, 1.38–1.79; $P<.001$) and stroke (adjusted HR, 1.24; CI, 1.06–1.43; $P<.05$) compared with patients with RA who did not have CKD, after adjusting for gender, age, and other CVD risk factors such as diabetes, hypertension, and hyperlipidemia.[34] Aggressive management of conventional CVD and CKD risk factors is recommended to reduce morbidity and mortality in patients with RA.

MANAGEMENT OF RHEUMATOID ARTHRITIS IN PATIENTS WITH CHRONIC KIDNEY DISEASE AND END-STAGE RENAL DISEASE

Management of RA may have to be modulated in patients with CKD. Some medications are excreted through the kidneys and a reduction in dose may be required in patients with compromised renal function to prevent drug toxicity. **Table 2** summarizes the medication dose adjustments for patients with RA who have CKD or ESRD and are on dialysis.

Nonsteroidal Antiinflammatory Drugs

In the premethotrexate and prebiologic era, NSAIDs were considered one of the first-line treatments for RA. Over time, NSAIDs have taken more of an adjunctive role to DMARD therapy as awareness of their adverse renal, gastrointestinal, and cardiovascular effects has increased. Thus, use is limited to on-demand use in many patients with arthritis.

The antiinflammatory mechanism of NSAIDs is mediated by the inhibition of cyclooxygenase (COX) enzymes, with consequent reduction in levels of inflammatory and vasodilatory prostaglandins.[35] Prostaglandins are synthesized in many regions of the kidney, including the glomeruli, vascular endothelial cells, renal tubules, and medullary interstitial cells.[36] In the setting of reduced renal perfusion,

Table 2
Dose adjustments of therapies for rheumatoid arthritis in patients with chronic kidney disease and end-stage renal disease medication

Medication	Dosing Adjustments
NSAIDs	CrCl 30–59 mL/min: use with caution. Evaluate risks vs benefits of use CrCl ≤30 mL/min: contraindicated In hemodialysis: avoid use. Evaluate risks vs benefits of use
Methotrexate	CrCl >50 mL/min: no adjustments in dosing needed CrCl 31–50 mL/min: reduce dose by 50% CrCl ≤30 mL/min: contraindicated In hemodialysis or peritoneal dialysis: contraindicated
Leflunomide	CrCl<60 mL/min: no adjustments in dosing needed In hemodialysis or peritoneal dialysis: no adjustments in dosing needed
Sulfasalazine	CrCl<60 mL/min: no adjustments in dosing needed In hemodialysis or peritoneal dialysis: no adjustments in dosing needed
Hydroxychloroquine	CrCl<60 mL/min: no adjustments in dosing needed In hemodialysis or peritoneal dialysis: no adjustments in dosing needed
Tofacitinib	CrCl>50 mL/min: no adjustments in dosing needed CrCl ≤50 mL/min: decrease dose to 5 mg once a day In hemodialysis or peritoneal dialysis: decrease dose to 5 mg once a day. No supplement necessary
TNF inhibitors (91–150 kDa)	No adjustments in dosing needed
Rituximab (144kDa)	No adjustments in dosing needed
Abatacept (92 kDa)	No adjustments in dosing needed
Tocilizumab (148 kDa)	No adjustments in dosing needed
Sarilumab (144 kDa)	No adjustments in dosing needed

Abbreviation: CrCl, creatinine clearance.

prostaglandin synthesis promotes vasodilation and leads to increased renin secretion. In patients with prolonged renal vasoconstriction, such as in patients with CKD, elderly patients, or patients with chronic heart failure, prostaglandins act to protect glomerular filtration. NSAID-induced inhibition of COX enzymes and the decrease in prostaglandin synthesis lead to reversible renal ischemia by inhibiting afferent vasodilation, decreasing the glomerular filtration by decreasing peritubular blood flow, increasing tubular ischemia and injury, and therefore leading to kidney injury.[37,38] Decreased prostaglandin synthesis in other regions of the kidney by NSAIDs may also lead to tubulointerstitial nephritis, type 4 renal tubular acidosis with hyperkalemia, and renal papillary necrosis.[37,39] NSAIDs may also cause an allergic hypersensitivity reaction, leading to acute interstitial nephritis. Continued long-term NSAID use in these patients may lead to chronic interstitial nephritis with interstitial fibrosis and CKD.[40] Treatment involves discontinuation of the NSAID or addition of glucocorticoids in more severe cases of biopsy-proven acute interstitial nephritis.

Metabolism of NSAIDs occurs by the liver and excretion occurs by the kidneys. The American College of Rheumatology recommends caution with NSAID use in patients with a creatinine clearance of 30 to 59 mL/min and avoidance of NSAIDs in patients with a creatinine clearance of less than 30 mL/min[41] In a case-control study of patients on hemodialysis, Jankovic and colleagues[42] showed that NSAID use was associated with increased gastrointestinal bleeding, after adjusting for age, sex, medications, and comorbidities (OR adjusted, 5.8; 95% CI, 1.3–26.9; P = .024) compared with non–NSAID users on hemodialysis. Thus it is recommended that NSAIDs be avoided in patients with ESRD.

Oral Nonbiologic Disease-Modifying Antirheumatic Drugs

Methotrexate

Methotrexate is a folic acid antagonist that binds to dihydrofolate reductase and inhibits DNA, RNA, and protein synthesis.[43] Methotrexate is excreted primarily through the kidneys via both glomerular filtration and active tubular secretion. The half-life of methotrexate can range from 4.5 hours to 10 hours. However, the elimination half-life of methotrexate increases with the degree of renal impairment.[44] According to American College of Physicians, a dose reduction of 50% is recommended in patients with creatinine clearance of less than or equal to 50 mL/min[44–46] The 2008 American College of Rheumatology guidelines recommend against the use of methotrexate in patients with creatinine clearance less than or equal to 30 mL/min[45] In dialysis patients, guidelines recommend against use of methotrexate because of the risk of bone marrow toxicity.[47,48]

Leflunomide

Leflunomide was first approved by the US Food and Drug Administration in 1998 for RA. After oral absorption, nearly 95% of leflunomide is converted to its active metabolite, teriflunomide, within the intestinal wall and liver. The primary effect of teriflunomide is through noncompetitive inhibition of dihydroorotate dehydrogenase, an enzyme required for the de novo production of pyrimidine in lymphocytes. Therefore, there is a reduction in T-cell and B-cell activation and proliferation.[49]

The elimination half-life of leflunomide is 14 to 18 days[50] with excretion through the urine (43%) and feces (48%).[49] More than 99% of teriflunomide is bound to plasma albumin with a low volume of distribution (0.14 L/kg). In patients with RA, the steady-state concentration of teriflunomide is fairly stable even in the setting of renal disease, thus dose adjustments are not needed in patients with CKD. In ESRD, plasma concentrations of teriflunomide did not significantly change with dialysis.[51,52] These findings are consistent with the notion that hemodialysis is less likely to affect highly protein-bound medications.[53]

Sulfasalazine

Sulfasalazine is metabolized into sulfapyridine and 5-aminosalicylic acid (5-ASA), which are primarily responsible for the disease-modifying effects in RA.[54–62] Rare cases of interstitial nephritis have been reported in patients with inflammatory bowel disease with continued long-term use of 5-ASA, via inhibition of cyclooxygenase or because of analgesic hypersensitivity, similar to NSAIDs. Treatment involves discontinuation of the medication, which may reverse the interstitial nephritis.[63] Only 10% to 30% of the parent drug sulfasalazine is absorbed in the small intestine. In the large intestine, sulfasalazine is metabolized by intestinal bacteria into sulfapyridine and mesalazine. Approximately 60% of sulfapyridine is further absorbed in the large intestine, whereas mesalazine largely remains unmetabolized. 5-ASA has a 10% to 30% bioavailability. Absorbed 5-ASA and sulfapyridine are eliminated through the urine. The renal clearance of sulfasalazine was estimated to be 37%, whereas the remainder is eliminated through the feces.[54] Studies with sulfasalazine report safety in patients with CKD and ESRD and dose adjustments are not necessary.[63,64]

Hydroxychloroquine

Hydroxychloroquine is an antimalarial medication widely used as an immunomodulatory DMARD. By increasing the acidic pH of intracellular lysosomes, hydroxychloroquine interferes with the antigen-processing cascade in macrophages and antigen-presenting cells and ultimately downregulates the CD4 T-cell immune response to autoantigenic peptides.[65,66] Additional effects of hydroxychloroquine include inhibiting toll-like receptors, which activate the innate immune system,[67] and decreasing the production of cytokines, including TNF-α.[68–73]

The oral bioavailability of hydroxychloroquine is approximately 74%, with a large variability of 30% to 100% among patients with RA. The medication is metabolized by the liver. Approximately 16% to 30% is excreted by the kidneys, 25% is excreted in the feces, and the remainder is stored long term in tissues. Renal excretion does not correlate with creatinine clearance, because of the long half-life of the medication and extensive tissue uptake. The terminal half-life is approximately 40 to 50 days and is attributed to the widespread distribution of hydroxychloroquine in the bone marrow, liver, kidneys, lungs, adrenal gland, pituitary gland, and the choroid and ciliary body of the eye. Urine concentrations of hydroxychloroquine can still be detectable several months after single doses. Because renal clearance of hydroxychloroquine does not correlate with creatinine clearance, dosage adjustments are not required or clearly specified in patients with CKD or ESRD.[74]

Tofacitinib

Tofacitinib is an oral janus kinase (JAK) inhibitor that inhibits JAK1, JAK2, and JAK3. Inhibition of JAK1 and JAK3 leads to a decrease in IL-2, IL-4, IL-7, IL-9, IL-15, and IL-21, which are crucial for lymphocyte activation, function, and proliferation.[75]

Tofacitinib is primarily metabolized by the liver. The medication is 70% eliminated by the liver and 30% by the kidney.[75] Patients with mild renal dysfunction (Cockcroft-Gault creatinine clearance >50 mL/min) do not require dose adjustments. Patients with moderate (Cockcroft-Gault creatinine clearance >30 and ≤50 mL/min) to severe (Cockcroft-Gault creatinine clearance ≤30 mL/min) renal impairment had higher serum tofacitinib levels compared with those with normal renal function. Thus, a reduced daily dose of tofacitinib 5 mg once a day is recommended for patients with RA with moderate to severe CKD. In patients with ESRD, plasma concentrations decreased because of both increased hepatic metabolism of tofacitinib as well as clearance from dialysis; 5 mg/d dosing is suggested and supplemental doses after dialysis are not necessary in patients with ESRD.[75]

Targeted Biologic Disease-Modifying Antirheumatic Drugs

The renal glomerulus is generally only able to filter molecules smaller than 60 kDa[76] Most biologic medications are larger than this filtration cutoff, with the exception of the IL-1 inhibitor anakinra, which has a molecular weight of 17.3 kDa. Therefore, large proteins, such as monoclonal antibodies and the soluble TNF receptor etanercept, are not affected by glomerular filtration rate and thus do not seem to be affected by the degree of CKD.[76,77] In a pharmacokinetics study in patients with psoriasis, Don and colleagues[77] showed that steady-state levels of etanercept were comparable between patients on hemodialysis and patients with normal renal function. Findings by Hueber and colleagues[78] and Sumida and colleagues[79] showed that TNF inhibitors were safe and well tolerated in patients with RA with renal insufficiency and on hemodialysis. There was no effect on renal function in patients with CKD.

SUMMARY

Renal manifestations in patients with RA can be divided into sequelae of RA (including secondary amyloidosis, mesangial GN, and increased CVD risk) and medication nephrotoxicity. The prevalence of these renal manifestations has evolved over the years in parallel with the improved management of RA, leading to less secondary amyloidosis and less medication toxicity. Older DMARDs, such as penicillamine, bucillamine, gold, and cyclosporine, contributed to renal toxicity in patients with RA; however, these are very rarely used in the current era. The establishment of methotrexate as a first-line DMARD, decrease in chronic NSAID use, emergence of biologic medications, and a treat-to-target strategy not only improved the treatment of RA but also decreased the likelihood of renal manifestations caused by chronic inflammation as well as from drug-related nephrotoxicity in patients with RA. In more recent years, CKD in patients with RA seems to be predominantly associated with cardiovascular metabolic risk factors such as hypertension and insulin resistance, rather than with RA disease severity. Importantly, the presence of CKD significantly worsens the mortality risk from CVD in patients with RA.

In patients with established CKD, medications such as NSAIDs, methotrexate, and tofacitinib may need to be adjusted or avoided to prevent adverse events. Leflunomide, sulfasalazine, hydroxychloroquine, and biologic medications are safe and effective in patients with CKD and ESRD without the need for dose adjustments.

REFERENCES

1. Mutru O, Laakso M, Isomaki H, et al. Ten year mortality and causes of death in patients with rheumatoid arthritis. Br Med J 1985;290:1797–9.
2. Avina-Zubieta JA, Choi HK, Sadatsafavi M, et al. Risk of cardiovascular mortality in patients with rheumatoid arthritis: a meta-analysis of observational studies. Arthritis Rheum 2008;59:1690–7.
3. Meune C, Touzé E, Trinquart L, et al. Trends in cardiovascular mortality in patients with rheumatoid arthritis over 50 years: a systematic review and meta-analysis of cohort studies. Rheumatology (Oxford) 2009;48:1309–13.
4. Kanevskaia M, Varshavskii V. The problem of rheumatoid nephropathy. Ter Arkh 2003;75(5):24–9.
5. Krel O, Varshavskii V, Kanevskaia M, et al. Kidney involvement in patients with rheumatoid arthritis. Ter Arkh 1990;62(6):104–13.
6. Helin H, Korpela M, Mustonen J, et al. Renal biopsy findings and clinicopathologic correlations in rheumatoid arthritis. Arthritis Rheum 1995;38(2):242–7.
7. Ichikawa K, Konta T, Sato H, et al. The clinical and pathological characteristics of nephropathies in connective tissue diseases in the Japan Renal Biopsy Registry (J-RBR). Clin Exp Nephrol 2017;21(6):1024–9.
8. Makino H, Yoshinaga Y, Yamasaki Y, et al. Renal involvement in rheumatoid arthritis: analysis of renal biopsy specimens from 100 patients. Mod Rheumatol 2002;12(2):148–54.
9. Horak P, Smrzova A, Krejci K, et al. Renal manifestations of rheumatic diseases. A review. Biomed Pap Med Fac Univ Palacky Olomouc Czech Repub 2013;157(2):98–104.
10. Horii Y, Muraguchi A, Iwano M, et al. Involvement of IL-6 in mesangial proliferative glomerulonephritis. J Immunol 1989;143(12):3949–55.
11. Hoshino J, Ubara Y, Hara S, et al. Outcome and treatment of bucillamine-induced nephropathy. Nephron Clin Pract 2006;104(1):c15–9.

12. Busauschina A, Schnuelle P, van der Woude FJ. Cyclosporine nephrotoxicity. Transplant Proc 2004;36(2 Suppl):229S–33S.
13. Hall C. Gold nephropathy. Nephron 1988;50:265–72.
14. Isozaki T, Kimura M, Ikegaya N, et al. Bucillamine (a new therapeutic agent for rheumatoid arthritis) induced nephrotic syndrome: a report of two cases and review of the literature. Clin Investig 1992;70(11):1036–42.
15. Nagahama K, Matsushita H, Hara M, et al. Bucillamine induces membranous glomerulonephritis. Am J Kidney Dis 2002;39(4):706–12.
16. Yoshida A, Morozumi K, Suganuma T, et al. Clinicopathological findings of bucillamine-induced nephrotic syndrome in patients with rheumatoid arthritis. Am J Nephrol 1991;11(4):284–8.
17. Nakano M, Ueno M, Nishi S, et al. Determination of IgA- and IgM-rheumatoid factors in patients with rheumatoid arthritis with and without nephropathy. Ann Rheum Dis 1996;55(8):520–4.
18. Korpela M, Mustonen J, Helin H, et al. Immunological comparison of patients with rheumatoid arthritis with and without nephropathy. Ann Rheum Dis 1990;49(4):214–8.
19. Lv J, Xu D, Perkovic V, et al. TESTING study group. corticosteroid therapy in IgA nephropathy. J Am Soc Nephrol 2012;23(6):1108.
20. Mirzaei A, Ataeipoor Y, Asgari M, et al. Seropositivity of rheumatoid arthritis specific tests in a patient with nephrotic syndrome: successful treatment with rituximab. Iran J Kidney Dis 2017;11(6):467–8.
21. Karie S, Gandjbakhch F, Janus N, et al. Kidney disease in RA patients: prevalence and implication on RA-related drugs management: the MATRIX study. Rheumatology (Oxford) 2008;47(3):350–4.
22. Lawson A, Maclean N. Renal disease and drug therapy in rheumatoid arthritis. Ann Rheum Dis 1966;25(5):441–9.
23. Real de Asúa D, Costa R, Galván JM, et al. Systemic AA amyloidosis: epidemiology, diagnosis, and management. Clin Epidemiol 2014;6:369–77.
24. Pollak V, Pirani C, Steck I, et al. The kidney in rheumatoid arthritis: studies by renal biopsy. Arthritis Rheum 1962;5:1–9.
25. Singh JA, Saag GK, Bridges LB Jr, et al. American College of Rheumatology 2015 recommendations for the treatment of rheumatoid arthritis. Arthritis Care Res 2016;68(1):1–25.
26. Solomon DH, Bitton A, Katz JN, et al. Treat to target in rheumatoid arthritis: fact, fiction or hypothesis? Arthritis Rheumatol 2014;66(4):775–82.
27. Karstila K, Korpela M, Sihvonen S, et al. Prognosis of clinical renal disease and incidence of new renal findings in patients with rheumatoid arthritis: follow-up of a population-based study. Clin Rheumatol 2007;26(12):2089–95.
28. Esatoglu S, Hatemi G, Ugurlu S, et al. Long-term follow-up of secondary amyloidosis patients treated with tumor necrosis factor inhibitor therapy: a STROBE-compliant observational study. Medicine (Baltimore) 2017;96(34):e7859.
29. Stokes MB, Foster K, Markowitz GS, et al. Development of glomerulonephritis during anti-TNF-alpha therapy for rheumatoid arthritis. Nephrol Dial Transplant 2005;20:1400–6.
30. Jani M, Dixon W, Chinoy H. Drug safety and immunogenicity of tumour necrosis factor inhibitors: the story so far. Rheumatology (Oxford) 2018. https://doi.org/10.1093/rheumatology/kex434.
31. Mori S, Yoshitama T, Hirakata N, et al. Prevalence of and factors associated with renal dysfunction in rheumatoid arthritis patients: a cross-sectional study in community hospitals. Clin Rheumatol 2017;36(12):2673–82.

32. Daoussis D, Panoulas VF, Antonopoulos I, et al. Cardiovascular risk factors and not disease activity, severity or therapy associate with renal dysfunction in patients with rheumatoid arthritis. Ann Rheum Dis 2010;69:517–21.

33. Sihvonen S, Korpela M, Mustonen J, et al. Renal disease as a predictor of increased mortality among patients with RA. Nephron Clin Pract 2004;96(4): c107–14.

34. Chiu H-Y, Huang H-L, Li C-H, et al. Increased risk of chronic kidney disease in rheumatoid arthritis associated with cardiovascular complications – a national population-based cohort study. PLoS One 2015;10(9):e0136508.

35. Vane JR. Inhibition of prostaglandin synthesis as a mechanism of action for aspirin-like drugs. Nat New Biol 1971;231:232–5.

36. Bonvalet JP, Pradelles P, Farman N. Segmental synthesis and actions of prostaglandins along the nephron. Am J Physiol 1987;253:F377.

37. Whelton A. Nephrotoxicity of nonsteroidal anti-inflammatory drugs: physiologic foundations and clinical implications. Am J Med 1999;106(5):13S–24S.

38. Zhang X, Donnan PT, Bell S, et al. Non-steroidal anti-inflammatory drug induced acute kidney injury in the community dwelling general population and people with chronic kidney disease: systematic review and meta-analysis. BMC Nephrol 2017;18:256.

39. Clive DM, Stoff JS. Renal syndromes associated with nonsteroidal antiinflammatory drugs. N Engl J Med 1984;310:563.

40. Hörl WH. Nonsteroidal anti-inflammatory drugs and the kidney. Pharmaceuticals (Basel) 2010;3(7):2291–321.

41. Hochberg MC, Altman RD, April KT, et al. American College of Rheumatology 2012 recommendations for the use of nonpharmacologic and pharmacologic therapies in osteoarthritis of the hand, hip, and knee. Arthritis Care Res 2012; 64(4):465–74.

42. Jankovic S, Aleksic J, Rakovic S, et al. Nonsteroidal antiinflammatory drugs and risk of gastrointestinal bleeding among patients on hemodialysis. J Nephrol 2009; 22(4):502–7.

43. Lopez-Olivo M, Siddhanamatha H, Shea B, et al. Methotrexate for treating rheumatoid arthritis. Cochrane Database Syst Rev 2014;(6):CD000957.

44. Brown P, Pratt A, Isaacs J. Mechanism of action of methotrexate in rheumatoid arthritis, and the search for biomarkers. Nat Rev Rheumatol 2016;12(12):731–42.

45. Aronoff G, Bennett W, Berns J, et al. Drug prescribing in renal failure: dosing guidelines for adults and children. 5th edition. Philadelphia: American College of Physicians; 2007. p. 97–177.

46. Bressolle F, Bologna C, Kinowski JM, et al. Effects of moderate renal insufficiency on pharmacokinetics of methotrexate in rheumatoid arthritis patients. Ann Rheum Dis 1998;57:110–3.

47. Saag KG, Teng GG, Patkar NM, et al. American College of Rheumatology 2008 recommendations for the use of nonbiologic and biologic disease-modifying antirheumatic drugs in rheumatoid arthritis. Arthritis Rheum 2008;59(6):762–84.

48. Yang C, Kuo M, Guh J, et al. Pancytopenia after low dose methotrexate therapy in a hemodialysis patient: case report and review of the literature. Ren Fail 2006;28: 95–7.

49. Aly L, Hemmer B, Korn T. From leflunomide to teriflunomide: drug development and immuno-suppressive oral drugs in the treatment of multiple sclerosis. Curr Neuropharmacol 2017;15(6):874–91.

50. Rozman B. Clinical pharmacokinetics of leflunomide. Clin Pharmacokinet 2002; 41:421.

51. Russo P, Wiese M, Smith M, et al. Leflunomide for inflammatory arthritis in end-stage renal disease on peritoneal dialysis: a pharmacokinetic and pharmacogenetic study. Ann Pharmacother 2013;47:3.

52. Beaman J, Hackett L, Luxton G, et al. Effect of hemodialysis on leflunomide plasma concentrations. Ann Pharmacother 2002;36:75–7.

53. Lam Y, Banerji S, Hatfield C, et al. Principles of drug administration in renal insufficiency. Clin Pharmacokinet 1997;32:30–57.

54. Plosker G, Croom K. Sulfasalazine: a review of its use in the management of rheumatoid arthritis. Drugs 2005;65:1825–49.

55. Smedegard G, Bjork J. Sulphasalazine: mechanism of action in rheumatoid arthritis. Br J Rheumatol 1995;34(Suppl. 2):7–15.

56. Fujiwara M, Mitsui K, Yamamoto I. Inhibition of proliferative responses and interleukin 2 productions by salazosulfapyridine and its metabolites. Jpn J Pharmacol 1990;54(2):121–31.

57. Hashimoto J, Sato K, Higaki M, et al. The effects of antirheumatic drugs on the production of, and the responsiveness to cytokines (IL-1 and IL-6). J Drug Eval 1991;11(3):279–86.

58. Kang B, Chung S, Im S, et al. Sulfasalazine prevents T- helper 1 immune response by suppressing interleukin-12 production in macrophages. Immunology 1999;98(1):98–103.

59. Rodenburg R, Ganga A, van Lent P, et al. The anti-inflammatory drug sulfasalazine inhibits tumor necrosis factor alpha expression in macrophages by inducing apoptosis. Arthritis Rheum 2000;43(9):1941–50.

60. Hirohata S, Ohshima N, Yanagida T, et al. Regulation of human B cell function by sulfasalazine and its metabolites. Int Immunopharmacol 2002;2(5):631–40.

61. Comer S, Jasin H. In vitro immunomodulatory effects of sulfasalazine and its metabolites. J Rheumatol 1988;15(4):580–6.

62. Imai F, Suzuki T, Ishibashi T, et al. Effect of sulfasalazine on B cell hyperactivity in patients with rheumatoid arthritis. J Rheumatol 1994;21(4):612–5.

63. Patel H, Barr A, Jeejeebhoy KN. Renal effects of long-term treatment of 5-aminosalicylic acid. Can J Gastroenterol 2009;23(3):170–6.

64. Akiyama Y, Sakurai Y, Kato Y, et al. Retrospective study of salazosulfapyridine in eight patients with rheumatoid arthritis on hemodialysis. Mod Rheumatol 2014;24: 285–90.

65. Paudyal S, Yang F, Rice C, et al. End-stage renal disease in patients with rheumatoid arthritis. Semin Arthritis Rheum 2017;46:418–22.

66. Fox R. Mechanism of action of hydroxychloroquine as an antirheumatic drug. Semin Arthritis Rheum 1993;23(2 Suppl 1):82–91.

67. Kalia S, Kutz J. New concepts in antimalarial use and mode of action in dermatology. Dermatol Ther 2007;20:160–74.

68. Van Den Borne B, Dijkmans B, De Rooij H, et al. Chloroquine and hydroxychloroquine equally affect tumor necrosis factor-alpha, interleukin 6, and interferon-gamma production by peripheral blood mononuclear cells. J Rheumatol 1997; 24:55–60.

69. Karres I, Kremer J, Dietl I, et al. Chloroquine inhibits proinflammatory cytokine release into human whole blood. Am J Physiol 1998;274:R1058–64.

70. Landewe R, Miltenburg A, Breedveld F, et al. Cyclosporine and chloroquine synergistically inhibit the interferon-gamma production by CD4-positive and CD8-positive synovial T-cell clones derived from a patient with rheumatoid arthritis. J Rheumatol 1992;19:1353–7.

71. Sperber K, Quraishi H, Kalb T, et al. Selective regulation of cytokine secretion by hydroxychloroquine. Inhibition of interleukin 1 alpha (IL-1-alpha) and IL-6 in human monocytes and T cells. J Rheumatol 1993;20:803–8.
72. Wozniacka A, Lesiak A, Narbutt J, et al. Chloroquine treatment influences proinflammatory cytokine levels in systemic lupus erythematosus patients. Lupus 2006;15:268.
73. Weber S, Levitz S. Chloroquine interferes with lipopolysaccharide-induced TNF-alpha gene expression by a nonlysosomotropic mechanism. J Immunol 2000;165:1534–40.
74. Hydroxychloroquine. 2018. Physician's desk reference. Available at: http://www.pdr.net/drug-summary/Plaquenil-hydroxychloroquine-sulfate-1911.7193. Accessed April 18, 2018.
75. Krishnaswami S, Chow V, Boy M, et al. Pharmacokinetics of tofacitinib, a janus kinase inhibitor, in patients with impaired renal function and end-stage renal disease. J Clin Pharmacol 2013;54(1):46–52.
76. Meibohm B, Zhou H. Characterizing the impact of renal impairment on the clinical pharmacology of biologics. J Clin Pharmacol 2012;52(1 Suppl):54S–62S.
77. Don BR, Spin G, Nestorov I, et al. The pharmacokinetics of etanercept in patients with end-stage renal disease on haemodialysis. J Pharm Pharmacol 2005;57(11):1407–13.
78. Hueber AJ, Tunc A, Schett G, et al. Anti-tumour necrosis factor α therapy in patients with impaired renal function. Ann Rheum Dis 2007;66(7):981–2.
79. Sumida K, Ubara Y, Suwabe T, et al. Adalimumab treatment in patients with rheumatoid arthritis with renal insufficiency. Arthritis Care Res (Hoboken) 2013;65(3):471–5.
80. Schourup K. Necrosis of the renal papillae; post-mortem series. Acta Pathol Microbiol Scand 1957;41(6):462–78.

Secondary, AA, Amyloidosis

Riccardo Papa, MD[a,*], Helen J. Lachmann, MD, FRCP, FRCPath[b]

KEYWORDS

- Systemic amyloidosis • AA amyloidosis • Serum amyloid A • SAA1 gene
- Congo red staining • SAP scintigraphy • Rheumatoid arthritis
- Autoinflammatory syndrome

KEY POINTS

- Secondary, AA, amyloidosis can complicate any long-term inflammatory disorder.
- Extracellular deposition of serum amyloid A (SAA) protein as amyloid primarily affects kidney function, with proteinuria as first clinical manifestation.
- Biopsy is the diagnostic gold standard and serum amyloid P component scintigraphy can help to define amyloid type and distribution.
- Targeted anti-inflammatory treatment promotes normalization of circulating SAA levels, preventing further amyloid deposition and renal damage.
- Clearance of existing amyloid deposits may be an effective treatment approach in the near future.

INTRODUCTION

Secondary, AA, amyloidosis is a rare systemic complication that can develop in any long-term inflammatory disorder, characterized by the pathogenic extracellular deposition of misfolded protein in a confirmation rich in beta pleated sheet. In AA amyloid, the fibrils are derived from serum amyloid A (SAA) protein, an acute-phase reactant synthetized largely by hepatocytes under the transcriptional regulation of proinflammatory cytokines. In Western countries, the low incidence of chronic infections and improving treatments for autoimmune diseases have resulted in a falling incidence of AA amyloidosis, which is now less common than primary, amyloid light-chain (AL), or wild-type transthyretin (previously known as senile) amyloidosis.

The kidney is the major involved organ, with proteinuria as first clinical manifestation. The extent of renal damage defines the patient prognosis, and renal biopsy is the commonest diagnostic investigation. Targeted anti-inflammatory treatment aimed

Disclosure Statement: The authors have nothing to disclosure.
[a] Autoinflammatory Diseases and Immunodeficiencies Centre, Pediatric and Rheumatology Clinic, Giannina Gaslini Institute, University of Genoa, Via Gerolamo Gaslini 5, Genova 16147, Italy; [b] National Amyloidosis Centre, Royal Free Campus, University College Medical School, Rowland Hill Street, London NW3 2PF, UK
* Corresponding author.
E-mail address: papariccardo86@gmail.com

at promoting a sustained and complete normalization of circulating SAA levels prevents progressive amyloid deposition and protects renal function, avoiding the need for renal replacement therapy. Novel therapies aimed at promoting clearance of existing amyloid deposits may be an effective treatment approach in the near future.

PATHOGENESIS
Formation of AA Amyloid

Amyloid is an amorphous and insoluble proteolytic resistant material derived from the spontaneous aggregation of fibrils composed of twisted protofilaments.[1–3] Protofilaments derive from misfolded proteins, called amyloid precursors, and share a common X-ray diffraction fingerprint of a β-sheet structure in cross-β conformation.[4] At least 30 different proteins can be deposited as amyloid in humans. In addition to the fibrillary protein a number of other proteins are also present in all types of amyloid, including serum amyloid P component, ApoE, ApoA4, and glycosaminoglycans.

In AA amyloidosis, the amyloid precursor is SAA, a soluble apolipoprotein mostly encoded by the *SAA1* gene, although *SAA2*-derived amyloid is also recognized.[5] *SAA1* has 5 polymorphic coding alleles that are defined by single nucleotide polymorphisms located on exon 3, varying by only a few amino acids at positions 52, 57, 60, and 72 of the mature protein. SAA isoforms show different capability to interact with the SAA receptors and homozygosity for SAA1.1 is a recognized risk factor for the formation of AA amyloidosis in Europeans.[6]

Like C-reactive protein (CRP), SAA is an acute-phase reactant synthesized by hepatocytes but also other cells, including macrophages, endothelial cells, and smooth muscle cells, under the transcriptional regulation of proinflammatory cytokines, particularly tumor necrosis factor (TNF) alpha, interleukin-1 (IL-1) beta and IL-6.[5] In fact, hepatocyte-specific mutations in some transcriptional regulators markedly reduced the expression of SAA.[7] The median plasma concentration of SAA in health is 3 mg/L and can increase to more than 1 mg/mL during an acute-phase response, making it a highly sensitive disease activity marker.[8]

There is evidence for a role for SAA in the regulation of inflammation and immunity, inducing expression of proinflammatory cytokines/chemokines and activation of immune cells at the site of inflammation.[9–14] Antibodies against SAA contribute to control of inflammation in patients treated with intravenous immunoglobulin.[15] SAA also inhibits dendritic cell differentiation from the bone marrow, limiting the inflammatory response.[16] SAA acts as opsonin, promoting bacteria uptake by neutrophils,[17] and as retinol-binding protein, limiting bacterial burden in the intestine starting from the neonatal period.[18–20] The capability of SAA to induce the expression of matrix metalloproteinase and angiogenesis promotes tumor metastasis in carcinoma[21,22] and joint destruction in inflammatory arthritis.[23] The direct impact of SAA on high-density lipoprotein (HDL) levels and apoA1 clearance may be lower than previously expected,[24] but, at least in mice, there is evidence that SAA contributes to maintenance of normal body weight and protects from hepatic steatosis.[25] Dissociation of SAA from HDL facilitates the formation of AA amyloid[26] and impairs the antioxidative functionality of HDL.[27]

Normally folded SAA is taken up by macrophages, transported to the lysosomal compartment and completely degraded. In patients with amyloidosis, intermediate SAA products have a propensity to aggregate into protofilaments. Glycosaminoglycans, serum amyloid P component (SAP), and lipid components associate with these accumulated intermediates in the extracellular space and are thought to contribute to formation of mature fibrils and confer resistance to proteolysis.[28,29] Although matrix metalloproteinases are able to degrade both SAA and amyloid A fibrils in vitro and display varying capacity regarding the SAA1 isoforms, there is little evidence in humans that polymorphisms in these proteases contribute to the risk of amyloid formation.[30]

Risk Factors

Virtually any persistent inflammatory disorders can be complicated by AA amyloidosis (**Box 1**), but chronic infections and inflammatory arthritis are the commonest causes in the developing and developed world, respectively. In rheumatoid arthritis, longer disease activity seems to be more relevant then severity.[31] Immunodeficiency usually underlays atypical chronic infections in the developed world, and treatment delay is the leading risk factor for the development of AA amyloidosis in these patients.[32–35] Obesity and aging may be susceptibility factors in patients with AA amyloidosis from undefined cause.[36] However, only a minority of patients with long-lasting inflammation develop this complication, and it seems highly likely that other undetermined environmental and genetic factors are involved.[37]

The SAA1 gene alleles alter the propensity of SAA to autoaggregate as amyloid fibrils and their susceptibility to degradation by matrix metalloproteinases, independent of the underlying disease.[38,39] In particular, in the White population, a strong positive association with AA amyloidosis has been established with SAA1.1 allele in patients affected by juvenile idiopathic arthritis, familial Mediterranean fever (FMF), and Behçet disease.[40–42] Conversely, Japanese patients with homozygous SAA1.3 allele and rheumatoid arthritis are at higher risk of developing AA amyloidosis, with a shorter latency period before disease onset, whereas SAA1.1 appears to be protective.[43–45] These contrary results suggest that homozygosity for the SAA1 allele may be more important in predisposing the development of AA amyloidosis than the specific allele itself.

The monogenic periodic fever syndromes, such as FMF and TNF Receptor associated periodic syndrome (TRAPS), carry very high risks of AA amyloidosis.[46] However, to date the only statistically significant correlations identified have been homozygous M694V variants in FMF[41] and country of recruitment.[47,48] Whether the country of origin reflects genetic factors associated with ethnicity or environmental factors is not yet clear.

DIAGNOSIS
Epidemiology

AA amyloidosis has almost certainly been underdiagnosed; the estimated incidence varies from 1 to 2 cases per million person-years, but is now clearly decreasing.[49–54] Prevalence in chronic inflammatory diseases is 5% to 10% or substantially higher if asymptomatic patients are considered.[31,55–57] A recently reported rise in the median age of diagnosis, from 50 to 70 years, probably reflects changes in the underlying diseases and improved access to effective therapies.[58] As with all types of amyloidosis, women appear to be slightly less affected, accounting for 44% of the largest series.[59] Although it is very uncommon, AA type is the most frequent cause of amyloidosis in children.[60] Only 0.9% of patients starting renal replacement therapy are affected by AA amyloidosis.

Clinical Features

Proteinuria is the first clinical manifestation in almost 95% of patients with AA amyloidosis, whereas 50% present with nephrotic syndrome. In a large cohort of 374 patients,

Box 1
Causes of secondary, AA, amyloidosis

Chronic Infections

Tuberculosis

Leprosy

Whipple Disease

Osteomyelitis

Chronic pyelonephritis

Subacute bacterial endocarditis

Chronic cutaneous ulcers

Conditions Predisposing to Chronic Infections

Cystic fibrosis

Bronchiectasis

Kartagener syndrome

Epidermolysis bullosa

Injected drug abuse

Jejuno-ileal bypass

Paraplegia

Sickle cell anemia

Immunodeficiency

Common variable immunodeficiency

Cyclic neutropenia

Hyperimmunoglobulin M syndrome

Hypogammaglobulinemia

Sex-linked agammaglobulinemia

Human immunodeficiency virus/AIDS

Neoplasia

Adenocarcinoma

Basal cell carcinoma

Carcinoid tumor

Castleman disease

Gastrointestinal stromal tumor

Hairy cell leukemia

Hepatic adenoma

Hodgkin disease

Mesothelioma

Renal cell carcinoma

Sarcoma

Inflammatory Arthritis

Adult-onset Still disease

Ankylosing spondylitis

Juvenile idiopathic arthritis

Psoriatic arthropathy

Reiter syndrome

Rheumatoid arthritis

Gout

Systemic Vasculitis

Antineutrophil cytoplasmic antibody–associated vasculitis

Behçet disease

Giant cell arteritis

Polyarteritis nodosa

Polymyalgia rheumatica

Systemic lupus erythematosus

Takayasu arteritis

Periodic Fevers

Cryopyrin-associated periodic fever syndrome

Familial Mediterranean fever

Mevalonate kinase deficiency

Tumor necrosis factor receptor associated periodic syndrome

Inflammatory Bowel Disease

Ulcerative colitis

Crohn diseases

Others

Atrial myxoma

Inflammatory abdominal aortic aneurism

Retroperitoneal fibrosis

SAPHO (synovitis, acne, pustulosis, hyperostosis, and osteitis) syndrome

Sarcoidosis

Sinus histiocytosis with massive lymphadenopathy

the median 24-hour urine protein leak was 3.9 g, with 12% of patients losing more than 10 g per day. End-stage renal disease (ESRD) has been reported in 10% of patients at presentation.[59]

Acute manifestations are extremely rare but can be dramatic. Amyloid deposits in spleen and liver can present as atraumatic organ rupture requiring emergency surgery.[61–64] Amyloid deposits in the gastrointestinal wall can predispose acute obstruction or bleeding, which can be massive.[65–67] Other symptoms of gut involvement are recurrent abdominal pain and malabsorption with chronic diarrhea.[68–70] Cardiac and neuropathic involvement are both extremely rare but cardiac failure has been reported.[59] Lung amyloid and thyroid enlargement can occur.[71]

Although only 10% of patients have detectable hepatomegaly on clinical examination,[59] liver amyloid deposits are visualized on SAP scintigraphy in 23% of patients. No data about functional hyposplenism have been reported in AA amyloidosis, but 24% of patients with primary AL amyloidosis are hyposplenic at presentation and this may contribute to septic complications.[72] Clearly there are other risk factors for infections in these patients, including nephrotic syndrome, use of immunosuppressive medications, or the underlying disease process itself.

Imaging

Imaging is a noninvasive method to provide information on the distribution and extent of amyloid deposits.

Total body SAP component scintigraphy was discovered by Mark Pepys, and later developed for clinical use by Philip Hawkins in London.[73,74] The diagnostic sensitivity is almost 90% and the dose of radioactivity is small, 80 to 90 MBq for a 6-hour scan, and 120 to 190 MBq for a 24-hour scan, so serial scans can be safely used for monitoring amyloid deposition during follow-up.[75,76] The radiolabeled SAP reversibly binds to all types of amyloid and localizes in proportion to the quantity of amyloid present, enabling deposits to be visualized in a semiquantitative manner (**Fig. 1**). SAP is a plasma glycoprotein of the pentraxin family, highly concentrated within amyloid deposits where it accounts for up to 15% of the total mass as a nonfibrillar constituent, and can also act as a calcium-dependent ligand-binding protein. After intravenous injection, ^{123}I-SAP rapidly equilibrates between the relatively small pool of endogenous SAP within the circulation and much larger pool of SAP within the extravascular amyloid deposits. Unfortunately, there is limited correlation between the quantity of amyloid and the severity of organ dysfunction and the imaging resolution is not sufficient to identify deposits in hollow, diffuse, or small structures, such as the gastrointestinal tract, skin, and nerves. It is also unable to evaluate deposits in the heart and lungs due to movement and blood pool content. However, SAP scintigraphy has shown that the distribution of amyloid can be patchy, justifying false-negative biopsy results, and varies between different forms of amyloidosis. It also has demonstrated the dynamic nature of amyloid deposition. SAP scintigraphy is limited to a few clinical centers in Europe and is not commercially available. New non-nuclear imaging techniques, such as positron emission computed tomography and single-photon emission computed tomography, already used to detect other types of amyloid, are now being developed in the United States.[77–79]

Imaging techniques to evaluate cardiac amyloidosis have been developed because electrocardiography may be normal until advanced disease. A left ventricular wall thickness of greater than 12 mm in the absence of hypertension or other causes of left ventricular hypertrophy fulfill consensus criteria for cardiac involvement in patients with amyloidosis. By 2-dimensional Doppler echocardiography, the evidence of thickening of valves or a predominantly diastolic restrictive dysfunction has been also reported. Cardiac magnetic resonance (CMR) demonstrates the characteristic late gadolinium enhancement in the sub-endocardium or more diffusely.[80] However, cardiac involvement in AA amyloidosis is rarely seen and staging systems using cardiac imaging or biomarkers (eg, troponin T or N-terminal-pro brain natriuretic protein) have not been validated. Furthermore, uremic cardiomyopathy can often be difficult to distinguish from cardiac amyloid, and CMR has been relatively contraindicated in patients with advanced renal disease, making it challenging to confidently diagnose cardiac involvement in this subset of patients.

Elastography has been experimentally used to measure liver stiffness induced by amyloid deposition around hepatic stellate cells.[81]

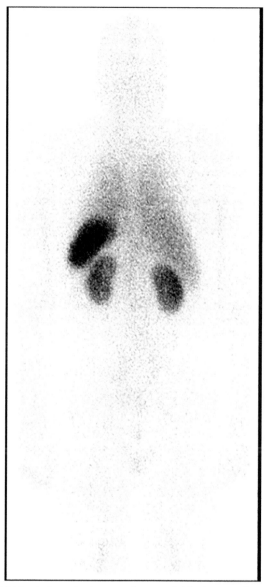

Fig. 1. I^{123} labeled SAP scintigraphy in secondary amyloidosis. Posterior whole-body image showing amyloid deposition in liver, spleen, and kidney of a patient affected by rheumatoid arthritis complicated by AA amyloidosis.

Histology

Positive histology is required for the diagnosis of amyloidosis, but a negative result does not exclude the presence of amyloidosis. In general, histology is a very poor method to establish the extent or distribution of amyloid, as deposits can be patchy.

The current diagnostic gold standard is the presence of apple green birefringence when a tissue biopsy stained with Congo red is viewed under cross-polarized light

(**Fig. 2**). Adequate experience and sufficient amyloid are required. For optimal results, the tissue sections need to be cut thicker than usual. The apple green optical effect is produced by alignment of the dye molecules along the amyloid fibrils. Thioflavin T fluorescence correlates linearly with amyloid concentration, but the binding capability is less specific.[82]

Using electron microscopy, amyloid fibrils are 10 to 15 nm in diameter, straight, rigid, nonbranching, of indeterminate length, and composed of twisted protofilaments.[3]

Immunohistochemistry is usually sufficient to determine the fibril protein type in AA amyloid, as there are excellent commercially available antibodies, but tandem mass spectrometry can be useful in nondiagnostic or un-interpretable cases.[83–87]

Renal biopsy can be performed without increased incidence of bleeding[88]; this is a concern with biopsy of other organs, probably due to increased fragility of blood vessels and reduced elasticity of the parenchyma. Renal glomeruli are the most common site of deposition.[89,90] The percentage of patients with AA amyloidosis diagnosed from a renal biopsy varies from 7% to more than 40%.[91–94] Less invasive procedures, such as fine-needle aspiration of subcutaneous fat or rectal biopsy, are useful but of lower sensitivity.[95]

Outcomes

AA amyloidosis is a potentially fatal disease complication with median survival of 6 to 9 years.[59,96] Adverse prognostic factors include higher level of serum creatinine and proteinuria, ESRD, cardiac involvement, evidence of amyloid deposits in the liver,

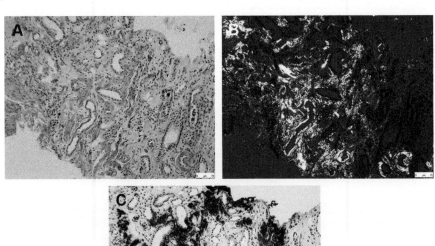

Fig. 2. Renal biopsy showing characteristic histologic appearance of amorphous deposits stained with Congo red (*A*, original magnification × 10) demonstrating apple green birefringence under cross-polarized light (*B*). Immunohistochemical staining of the same section with antibodies to AA (*C*, original magnification × 10).

underlying Crohn disease or chronic sepsis, and older age at the time of diagnosis. Positive prognostic factors are an underlying periodic fever syndrome and the regression of amyloid deposits on the SAP scintigraphy, which is related to sustained reduction in SAA synthesis.[97]

MANAGEMENT
General Management

Widespread availability of effective agents to control chronic inflammatory conditions, such as antibiotics and biologics, are likely to continue to reduce the incidence of AA amyloidosis in the future (**Table 1**).[98–102] Once AA amyloid is present, long-term suppression of the circulating SAA level is pivotal to improving patient and renal outcomes,[59,96,103,104] and must be achieved by aggressively treating the underlying disease with the aim of persistent normalization of the hepatic acute-phase response. The choice of treatment regimen depends entirely on the underlying cause of chronic inflammation, but the aim is always to suppress production of SAA to within the normal range. Long-term inflammatory control can be accompanied by gradual regression of amyloid deposits and improvement in renal function (**Fig. 3**). If SAA assays are unavailable, serial CRP level, measures of organ function, and symptoms related to the inflammatory condition can be used as indicators of treatment efficacy. It must be recognized that in some patients there is a discrepancy between CRP and SAA level and the relationship should be established in each patient by several concurrent measurements before electing to follow a patient with only CRP measurements.

The kidney is the major affected organ in AA amyloidosis and maintenance of organ function is a primary treatment goal. Potential renal insults, such as hypoperfusion, hypertension, infections, nephrotoxic drugs, and surgery, should be avoided if possible. In the nephrotic syndrome, patients should be advised to limit their liquid and sodium intake to reduce edema.[105] There was no evidence for supporting antibiotic prophylaxis, but vaccinations are recommended.[106–109] Diuretics are often required, especially high doses of loop diuretics in combination with either thiazide or potassium-sparing diuretics. Angiotensin-converting enzyme inhibitors reduce the risk of progression to ESRD and proteinuria, but whether these confer any long-term benefit in AA amyloidosis specifically is unknown.[110,111] When renal replacement therapy is needed, peritoneal dialysis had a higher total incidence of infections then hemodialysis, although this has improved during the past decade.[112] During the interdialytic period, weight gains and hypotensive episodes also may occur. Severe nephrotic syndrome can be very difficult to manage and renal artery embolization has been reportedly successful in some case reports.[113–115] Quality of life is usually improved by renal transplantation, although the survival of patients has been reported to be significantly worse than in other causes of ESRD, with 5-year and 10-year survival reportedly 82.5% and 61.7%, respectively.[116,117] Furthermore, amyloid recurrence in the renal transplant can occur if inflammation is not controlled, with reported onset of proteinuria after a median of 118 months. Sepsis should be treated early and aggressively. Infectious complications have been reportedly high following renal transplantation, but there is no significant increased risk of infections in patients who had received higher cumulative doses of immunosuppressant agents, and patients whose underlying disease was due to infection did not exhibit worsening of their initial disease after transplant immunosuppression. Cardiovascular complications have been reported as a common cause of death in patients with AA amyloidosis after transplantation.[118]

Adrenal insufficiency is rare, even though amyloid deposition in the adrenal glands is common. Because blood pressure abnormalities are usually related to kidney

Table 1
Examples of treatments for the commonest disorders underlying AA amyloidosis

Underlying Disorder	Treatment	Examples
Inflammatory arthritis	Conventional disease-modifying agents	Gold Hydroxychloroquine sulfasalazine Azathioprine Methotrexate
	Other immunosuppressant agents	Cyclosporine Cyclophosphamide Mycophenolate Leflunomide
	Biologic agents	Infliximab Etanercept Adalimumab Tocilizumab Rituximab
Periodic fevers	On-demand agents	Nonsteroidal anti-inflammatory drugs Prednisone
	Colchicine[a]	
	Biologic agents	Anakinra Canakinumab
Inflammatory bowel disease	Conventional disease-modifying agents	Sulfasalazine Mesalazine Azathioprine Methotrexate
	Biologic agents	Infliximab Adalimumab
	Antibiotics	Metronidazole Ciprofloxacin Azithromycin
	Surgery	
Systemic vasculitis	Conventional disease-modifying agents	Azathioprine Methotrexate
	Other immunosuppressant agents	Cyclophosphamide Mycophenolate
	Biologic agents	Rituximab
	Plasma exchange	
Immunodeficiency	Immunoglobulins	
	Antibiotics	Cotrimoxazole Miconazole
Chronic infections	Antibiotics and surgery	
	Physiotherapy[b]	
Neoplasia	Chemotherapy and surgery	
	Biologic agents[c]	Tocilizumab

[a] Familial Mediterranean fever.
[b] Bronchiectasis.
[c] Castleman disease.

involvement, Addisonian symptoms may be difficult to determine and investigation for adrenal insufficiency may be required.[119,120]

Amyloid deposition in vessels can increase the risk of bleeding and case reports of spontaneous organ rupture have been reported. Conversely, very heavy proteinuria

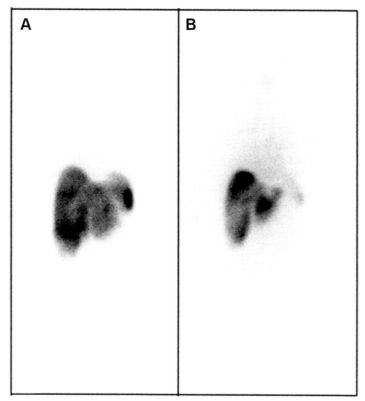

Fig. 3. Regression of hepatic AA amyloid deposits demonstrated on whole body anterior I[123] labeled SAP scintigraphy before (*A*) and 1 year after (*B*) anti-interleukin 1 treatment in a patient with an underlying periodic fever syndrome.

increases the risk of thrombosis and the decision to anticoagulate must be made on an individual patient basis.

Chronic diarrhea and protein-losing enteropathy due to gastrointestinal amyloid can be treated with long-acting somatostatin analogs or octreotide,[121,122] but promotility agents are usually not successful and total parenteral nutrition may be needed. Dimethylsulfoxide has not achieved any improvement in AA amyloidosis.[123]

Targeted Therapy

In patients with AA amyloidosis whose underlying condition is refractory to treatment, development of targeted therapies to inhibit amyloid formation or enhance the clearance of existing deposits is crucial.

Eprodisate (1, 3-propanedisulfonate) is a negatively charged, sulfonated molecule of low molecular weight that has structural similarities to heparan sulfate. It binds to the binding site on SAA to prevent its interaction with glycosaminoglycans. Highly sulfated glycosaminoglycans, particularly heparan and dermatan sulfate proteoglycans, are a universal constituent of amyloid deposits and are thought to promote fibril assembly and aid in maintenance of the conformational changes associated with amyloidogenesis. In vivo studies have shown that eprodisate inhibits the development of amyloid deposits in mouse models and has been tested in a phase II/III multicenter, placebo-controlled, double-blinded study in AA amyloidosis.[124] Unfortunately, the study failed to demonstrate a significant benefit from active therapy on progression to ESRD or risk of death, although there was a trend to benefit. In particular, the mean rate of decline in creatinine clearance was significantly slower in the eprodisate group than placebo: 10.9 compared with 15.6 mL per minute per 1.73 m^2 of body surface area per year (P = .02). A second clinical study also failed to reach its primary end points, although results have not been published yet.[125]

An alternative approach has been to target other components of amyloid deposits to destabilize fibrils and promote amyloid clearance by macrophages.[126] SAP protein is a universal constituent of amyloid deposits and the R-1-(6-[R-2-carboxy-pyrrolidin-1-yl]-6-oxo-hexanoyl) pyrrolidine-2-carboxylic acid (CPHPC) was developed to inhibit the binding of SAP to amyloid.[127] A preliminary clinical study confirmed that regular administration of CPHPC produced sustained and profound depletion of SAP from the blood, with no adverse effects.[128] Administration of repeated doses of anti-SAP antibodies has been demonstrated to trigger the clearance of amyloid deposits.[129,130] This approach may improve management and outcome for patients with AA amyloidosis whose underlying condition is refractory to treatment.

SUMMARY

AA amyloidosis can complicate any chronic inflammatory disorders. Despite its rarity, physicians from many specialities may encounter affected patients due to variety of possible underlying causes. Proteinuria is the typical presentation and progression to renal insufficiency occurs if the diagnosis is missed. A routine urine dipstick in patients with inflammatory conditions is an inexpensive screening test. Histology is required for the final diagnosis and positive immunohistochemistry for AA deposits is usually straightforward with commercial antibodies. SAP scintigraphy may be useful for characterization of disease extent and monitoring deposits. Suppression of SAA levels remains the primary goal of treatment, but supportive care is needed. New approaches are being developed for patients with AA amyloidosis whose underlying disease is resistant to targeted treatments.

REFERENCES

1. Pepys MB. Amyloidosis. Annu Rev Med 2006;57:223–41.
2. Schmidt A, Annamalai K, Schmidt M, et al. Cryo-EM reveals the steric zipper structure of a light chain-derived amyloid fibril. Proc Natl Acad Sci U S A 2016;113:6200–5.
3. Close W, Neumann M, Schmidt A, et al. Physical basis of amyloid fibril polymorphism. Nat Commun 2018;9:699.
4. Perutz MF, Finch JT, Berriman J, et al. Amyloid fibers are water-filled nanotubes. Proc Natl Acad Sci U S A 2002;99:5591–5.
5. Sun L, Ye RD. Serum amyloid A1: structure, function and gene polymorphism. Gene 2016;583:48–57.
6. Chen M, Zhou H, Cheng N, et al. Serum amyloid A1 isoforms display different efficacy at Toll-like receptor 2 and formyl peptide receptor 2. Immunobiology 2014;219:916–23.
7. Quinton LJ, Blahna MT, Jones MR, et al. Hepatocyte-specific mutation of both NF-κB RelA and STAT3 abrogates the acute phase response in mice. J Clin Invest 2012;122:1758–63.
8. Hijmans W, Sipe JD. Levels of the serum amyloid A protein (SAA) in normal persons of different age groups. Clin Exp Immunol 1979;35:96–100.

9. Ji YR, Kim HJ, Bae KB, et al. Hepatic serum amyloid A1 aggravates T cell-mediated hepatitis by inducing chemokines via toll-like receptor 2 in mice. J Biol Chem 2015;290:12804–11.

10. De Buck M, Gouwy M, Wang JM, et al. The cytokine-serum amyloid A-chemokine network. Cytokine Growth Factor Rev 2016;30:55–69.

11. Sano T, Huang W, Hall JA, et al. An IL-23R/IL-22 circuit regulates epithelial serum amyloid A to promote local effector Th17 responses. Cell 2015;163:381–93.

12. Hershkoviz R, Preciado-Patt L, Lider O, et al. Extracellular matrix-anchored serum amyloid A preferentially induces mast cell adhesion. Am J Physiol 1997;273:C179–87.

13. Niemi K, Teirilä L, Lappalainen J, et al. Serum amyloid A activates the NLRP3 inflammasome via P2X7 receptor and a cathepsin B-sensitive pathway. J Immunol 2011;186:6119–28.

14. O'Neill L, Rooney P, Molloy D, et al. Regulation of inflammation and angiogenesis in giant cell arteritis by acute-phase serum amyloid A. Arthritis Rheumatol 2015;67:2447–56.

15. Kuret T, Lakota K, Mali P, et al. Naturally occurring antibodies against serum amyloid A reduce IL-6 release from peripheral blood mononuclear cells. PLoS One 2018;13:e0195346.

16. Kim JC, Jung YS, Lee HY, et al. Serum amyloid A inhibits dendritic cell differentiation by suppressing GM-CSF receptor expression and signaling. Exp Mol Med 2017;49:e369.

17. Shah C, Hari-Dass R, Raynes JG. Serum amyloid A is an innate immune opsonin for gram-negative bacteria. Blood 2006;108:1751–7.

18. Derebe MG, Zlatkov CM, Gattu S, et al. Serum amyloid A is a retinol binding protein that transports retinol during bacterial infection. Elife 2014;3:e03206.

19. Esterházy D, Mucida D. Serum Amyloid A proteins take retinol for a ride. Trends Immunol 2018;35:505–6.

20. Sack GH Jr, Zachara N, Rosenblum N, et al. Serum amyloid A1 (SAA1) protein in human colostrum. FEBS Open Bio 2018;8:435–41.

21. Hansen MT, Forst B, Cremers N, et al. A link between inflammation and metastasis: serum amyloid A1 and A3 induce metastasis, and are targets of metastasis-inducing S100A4. Oncogene 2014;34:424.

22. Lung HL, Man OY, Yeung MC, et al. SAA1 polymorphisms are associated with variation in antiangiogenic and tumor-suppressive activities in nasopharyngeal carcinoma. Oncogene 2014;34:878.

23. Connolly M, Mullan RH, McCormick J, et al. Acute-phase serum amyloid A regulates tumor necrosis factor α and matrix turnover and predicts disease progression in patients with inflammatory arthritis before and after biologic therapy. Arthritis Rheum 2012;64:1035–45.

24. de Beer MC, Wroblewski JM, Noffsinger VP, et al. The impairment of macrophage-to-feces reverse cholesterol transport during inflammation does not depend on serum amyloid A. J Lipids 2013;2013:283486.

25. Ather JL, Poynter ME. Serum amyloid A3 is required for normal weight and immunometabolic function in mice. PLoS One 2018;13:e0192352.

26. Lu J, Yu Y, Zhu I, et al. Structural mechanism of serum amyloid A-mediated inflammatory amyloidosis. Proc Natl Acad Sci U S A 2014;111:5189–94.

27. Dullaart RP, de Boer JF, Annema W, et al. The inverse relation of HDL antioxidative functionality with serum amyloid a is lost in metabolic syndrome subjects. Obesity (Silver Spring) 2013;21:361–6.

28. Kisilevsky R, Raimondi S, Bellotti V. Historical and current concepts of fibrillogenesis and in vivo amyloidogenesis: implications of amyloid tissue targeting. Front Mol Biosci 2016;3:17.

29. Jayaraman S, Gantz DL, Haupt C, et al. Serum amyloid A forms stable oligomers that disrupt vesicles at lysosomal pH and contribute to the pathogenesis of reactive amyloidosis. Proc Natl Acad Sci U S A 2017;114:E6507–15.

30. Stix B, Kähne T, Sletten K, et al. Proteolysis of AA amyloid fibril proteins by matrix metalloproteinases-1, -2, and -3. Am J Pathol 2001;159:561–70.

31. Koivuniemi R, Paimela L, Suomalainen R, et al. Amyloidosis is frequently undetected in patients with rheumatoid arthritis. Amyloid 2008;15:262–8.

32. Esenboga S, Çagdas Ayvaz D, Saglam Ayhan A, et al. CVID associated with systemic amyloidosis. Case Rep Immunol 2015;2015:879179.

33. Arslan S, Ucar R, Yavsan DM, et al. Common variable immunodeficiency and pulmonary amyloidosis: a case report. J Clin Immunol 2015;35:344–7.

34. Darougar S, Rashid Farokhi F, Tajik S, et al. Amyloidosis as a renal complication of chronic granulomatous disease. Iran J Kidney Dis 2016;10(4):228–32.

35. Gupta K, Rawat A, Agrawal P, et al. Infectious and non-infectious complications in primary immunodeficiency disorders: an autopsy study from North India. J Clin Pathol 2018;71(5):425–35.

36. Blank N, Hegenbart U, Dietrich S, et al. Obesity is a significant susceptibility factor for idiopathic AA amyloidosis. Amyloid 2018;25:37–45.

37. Obici L, Raimondi S, Lavatelli F, et al. Susceptibility to AA amyloidosis in rheumatic diseases: a critical overview. Arthritis Rheum 2009;61:1435–40.

38. van der Hilst JCH, Yamada T, Op den Camp HJ, et al. Increased susceptibility of serum amyloid A 1.1 to degradation by MMP-1: potential explanation for higher risk of type AA amyloidosis. Rheumatology (Oxford) 2008;47:1651–4.

39. Srinivasan S, Patke S, Wang Y, et al. Pathogenic serum amyloid A 1.1 shows a long Oligomer-rich fibrillation lag phase contrary to the highly amyloidogenic non-pathogenic SAA2.2. J Biol Chem 2013;288:2744–55.

40. Booth DR, Booth SE, Gillmore JD, et al. SAA1 alleles as risk factors in reactive systemic AA amyloidosis. Amyloid 1998;5:262–5.

41. Gershoni-Baruch R, Brik R, Zacks N, et al. The contribution of genotypes at the MEFV and SAA1 loci to amyloidosis and disease severity in patients with familial Mediterranean fever. Arthritis Rheum 2003;48:1149–55.

42. Utku U, Dilek M, Akpolat I, et al. SAA1 α/α alleles in Behçet's disease related amyloidosis. Clin Rheumatol 2007;26:927–9.

43. Moriguchi M, Terai C, Koseki Y, et al. Influence of genotypes at SAA1 and SAA2 loci on the development and the length of latent period of secondary AA-amyloidosis in patients with rheumatoid arthritis. Hum Genet 1999;105:360–6.

44. Nakamura T, Higashi S, Tomoda K, et al. Significance of SAA1.3 allele genotype in Japanese patients with amyloidosis secondary to rheumatoid arthritis. Rheumatology 2006;45:43–9.

45. Yamada T, Okuda Y, Takasugi K, et al. Relative serum amyloid A (SAA) values: the influence of SAA1 genotypes and corticosteroid treatment in Japanese patients with rheumatoid arthritis. Ann Rheum Dis 2001;60:124–7.

46. Papa R, Doglio M, Lachmann HJ, et al. A web-based collection of genotype-phenotype associations in hereditary recurrent fevers from the Eurofever registry. Orphanet J Rare Dis 2017;12:167.

47. Touitou I, Sarkisian T, Medlej-Hashim M, et al. Country as the primary risk factor for renal amyloidosis in familial Mediterranean fever. Arthritis Rheum 2007;56:1706–12.

48. Resul Y, Samet O, Huseyin O, et al. Familial Mediterranean fever gene mutations in the inner northern region of Turkey and genotype–phenotype correlation in children. J Paediatr Child Health 2009;45:641–5.
49. Kyle RA, Linos A, Beard CM, et al. Incidence and natural history of primary systemic amyloidosis in Olmsted County, Minnesota, 1950 through 1989 [see comments]. Blood 1992;79:1817–22.
50. Pinney JH, Smith CJ, Taube JB, et al. Systemic amyloidosis in England: an epidemiological study. Br J Haematol 2013;161:525–32.
51. Hemminki K, Li X, Försti A, et al. Incidence and survival in non-hereditary amyloidosis in Sweden. BMC Public Health 2012;12:974.
52. Aguirre MA, Boietti BR, Nucifora E, et al. Incidence rate of amyloidosis in patients from a medical care program in Buenos Aires, Argentina: a prospective cohort. Amyloid 2016;23:184–7.
53. Magy-Bertrand N, Dupond JL, Mauny F, et al. Incidence of amyloidosis over 3 years: the AMYPRO study. Clin Exp Rheumatol 2008;26:1074–8.
54. Immonen K, Finne P, Grönhagen-Riska C, et al. A marked decline in the incidence of renal replacement therapy for amyloidosis associated with inflammatory rheumatic diseases–data from nationwide registries in Finland. Amyloid 2011;18:25–8.
55. Alishiri GH, Salimzadeh A, Owlia MB, et al. Prevalence of amyloid deposition in long standing rheumatoid arthritis in Iranian patients by abdominal subcutaneous fat biopsy and assessment of clinical and laboratory characteristics. BMC Musculoskelet Disord 2006;7:43.
56. Ozen S, Demirkaya E, Amaryan G. Results from a multicentre international registry of familial Mediterranean fever: impact of environment on the expression of a monogenic disease in children. Ann Rheum Dis 2014;73:662–7.
57. Barile L, Ariza R, Muci H, et al. Tru-cut needle biopsy of subcutaneous fat in the diagnosis of secondary amyloidosis in rheumatoid arthritis. Arch Med Res 1993; 24:189–92.
58. Costa R. Systemic AA amyloidosis: epidemiology, diagnosis, and management. Clin Epidemiol 2014;6:369–77.
59. Lachmann HJ, Goodman HJ, Gilbertson JA, et al. Natural history and outcome in systemic AA amyloidosis. N Engl J Med 2007;356:2361–71.
60. Bilginer Y, Akpolat T, Ozen S. Renal amyloidosis in children. Pediatr Nephrol 2011;26:1215–27.
61. Renzulli P, Hostettler A, Schoepfer AM, et al. Systematic review of atraumatic splenic rupture. Br J Surg 2009;96:1114–21.
62. Renzulli P, Schoepfer A, Mueller E, et al. Atraumatic splenic rupture in amyloidosis. Amyloid 2009;16:47–53.
63. Shobeiri H, Einakchi M, Khajeh M, et al. Spontaneous rupture of the spleen secondary to amyloidosis. J Coll Physicians Surg Pak 2013;23:427–9.
64. Sandberg-Gertzén H, Ericzon BG, Blomberg B. Primary amyloidosis with spontaneous splenic rupture, cholestasis, and liver failure treated with emergency liver transplantation. Am J Gastroenterol 1998;93:2254.
65. Satapathy SK, Kurtz LE, Sheikh-Fayyaz S, et al. Gastric amyloidosis presenting as massive upper gastrointestinal bleeding. Am J Gastroenterol 2009;104:2113.
66. Ebert EC, Nagar M. Gastrointestinal manifestations of amyloidosis. Am J Gastroenterol 2008;103:776.
67. Kim SH, Kim JH, Gu MJ. Secondary intestinal amyloidosis presenting intractable hematochezia: a case report and literature review. Int J Clin Exp Pathol 2014;7: 1805–8.

68. Rowe K, Pankow J, Nehme F, et al. Gastrointestinal amyloidosis: review of the literature. Cureus 2017;9:e1228.
69. Sattianayagam PT, Hawkins PN, Gillmore JD. Systemic amyloidosis and the gastrointestinal tract. Nat Rev Gastroenterol Hepatol 2009;6:608.
70. Park SW, Jee SR, Kim JH, et al. Duodenal amyloidosis secondary to ulcerative colitis. Intest Res 2018;16:151–4.
71. Calatayud J, Candelas G, Gómez A, et al. Nodular pulmonary amyloidosis in a patient with rheumatoid arthritis. Clin Rheumatol 2007;26:1797–8.
72. Gertz MA, Kyle RA, Greipp PR. Hyposplenism in primary systemic amyloidosis. Ann Intern Med 1983;98:475–7.
73. Hawkins PN, Lavender JP, Pepys MB. Evaluation of systemic amyloidosis by scintigraphy with 123i-labeled serum amyloid P component. N Engl J Med 1990;323:508–13.
74. Hawkins PN, Lavender JP, Myers MJ, et al. Diagnostic radionuclide imaging of amyloid: biological targeting by circulating human serum amyloid P component. Lancet 2018;331:1413–8.
75. Hawkins PN. Serum amyloid P component scintigraphy for diagnosis and monitoring amyloidosis. Curr Opin Nephrol Hypertens 2002;11:649–55.
76. Hazenberg BP, van Rijswijk MH, Piers DA, et al. Diagnostic performance of ^{123}I-labeled serum amyloid P component scintigraphy in patients with amyloidosis. Am J Med 2018;119:355.e15-24.
77. Martin EB, Williams A, Richey T, et al. Comparative evaluation of p5+14 with SAP and peptide p5 by dual-energy SPECT imaging of mice with AA amyloidosis. Sci Rep 2016;6:22695.
78. Wall JS, Kennel SJ, Martin EB. Dual-energy SPECT and the development of peptide p5+14 for imaging amyloidosis. Mol Imaging 2017;16. 1536012117708705.
79. Herholz K, Ebmeier K. Clinical amyloid imaging in Alzheimer's disease. Lancet Neurol 2018;10:667–70.
80. Fontana M, Martinez-Naharro A, Hawkins PN. Staging cardiac amyloidosis with CMR. JACC Cardiovasc Imaging 2016;9:1278–9.
81. Trifanov DS, Dhyani M, Bledsoe JR, et al. Amyloidosis of the liver on shear wave elastography: case report and review of literature. Abdom Imaging 2015;40: 3078–83.
82. Xue C, Lin TY, Chang D, et al. Thioflavin T as an amyloid dye: fibril quantification, optimal concentration and effect on aggregation. R Soc Open Sci 2017;4: 160696.
83. Sethi S, Vrana JA, Theis JD, et al. Laser microdissection and mass spectrometry-based proteomics aids the diagnosis and typing of renal amyloidosis. Kidney Int 2018;82:226–34.
84. Vrana JA, Gamez JD, Madden BJ, et al. Classification of amyloidosis by laser microdissection and mass spectrometry-based proteomic analysis in clinical biopsy specimens. Blood 2009;114:4957–9.
85. Mollee P, Boros S, Loo D, et al. Implementation and evaluation of amyloidosis subtyping by laser-capture microdissection and tandem mass spectrometry. Clin Proteomics 2016;13:30.
86. Larsen BT, Mereuta OM, Dasari S, et al. Correlation of histomorphological pattern of cardiac amyloid deposition with amyloid type: a histological and proteomic analysis of 108 cases. Histopathology 2016;68:648–56.
87. Vrana JA, Theis JD, Dasari S, et al. Clinical diagnosis and typing of systemic amyloidosis in subcutaneous fat aspirates by mass spectrometry-based proteomics. Haematologica 2014;99:1239–47.

88. Fish R, Pinney J, Jain P, et al. The incidence of major hemorrhagic complications after renal biopsies in patients with monoclonal gammopathies. Clin J Am Soc Nephrol 2010;5:1977–80.

89. Khalighi MA, Dean Wallace W, Palma-Diaz MF. Amyloid nephropathy. Clin Kidney J 2014;7:97–106.

90. Hopfer H, Wiech T, Mihatsch MJ. Renal amyloidosis revisited: amyloid distribution, dynamics and biochemical type. Nephrol Dial Transplant 2011;26:2877–84.

91. Said SM, Sethi S, Valeri AM, et al. Renal amyloidosis: origin and clinicopathologic correlations of 474 recent cases. Clin J Am Soc Nephrol 2013;8:1515–23.

92. von Hutten H, Mihatsch M, Lobeck H, et al. Prevalence and origin of amyloid in kidney biopsies. Am J Surg Pathol 2009;33:1198–205.

93. da Fonseca EO, Filho PJ, da Silva LE, et al. Epidemiological, clinical and laboratorial profile of renal amyloidosis: a 12-year retrospective study of 37 cases. J Nephropathol 2015;4:7–12.

94. Potysová Z, Merta M, Tesar V, et al. Renal AA amyloidosis: survey of epidemiologic and laboratory data from one nephrology centre. Int Urol Nephrol 2009;41:941.

95. Hazenberg BPC, Bijzet J, Limburg PC, et al. Diagnostic performance of amyloid A protein quantification in fat tissue of patients with clinical AA amyloidosis. Amyloid 2007;14:133–40.

96. Bergesio F, Ciciani AM, Manganaro M, et al. Renal involvement in systemic amyloidosis: an Italian collaborative study on survival and renal outcome. Nephrol Dial Transplant 2008;23:941–51.

97. Gillmore JD, Lovat LB, Persey MR, et al. Amyloid load and clinical outcome in AA amyloidosis in relation to circulating concentration of serum amyloid A protein. Lancet 2018;358:24–9.

98. ter Haar NM, Oswald M, Jeyaratnam J, et al. Recommendations for the management of autoinflammatory diseases. Ann Rheum Dis 2015;74:1636–44.

99. Lane T, Gillmore JD, Wechalekar AD, et al. Therapeutic blockade of interleukin-6 by tocilizumab In the management of AA amyloidosis and chronic inflammatory disorders: a case series and review of the literature. Clin Exp Rheumatol 2015;33(6 Suppl 94):S46–53.

100. Gattorno M, Obici L, Cattalini M, et al. Canakinumab treatment for patients with active recurrent or chronic TNF receptor-associated periodic syndrome (TRAPS): an open-label, phase II study. Ann Rheum Dis 2017;76:173–8.

101. De Benedetti F, Miettunen P, Kallinich T, et al. Genetic phenotypes impacting E cacy and safety of canakinumab in patients with colchicine-resistant FMF, TRAPS and Hids/Mkd: results from cluster study. Arthritis Rheumatol 2017;69(suppl 10).

102. Prakken B, Martini A. Digging deeper for greater precision and more impact in JIA. Nat Rev Rheumatol 2015;11:70.

103. Lachmann HJ, Gillmore JD. Renal amyloidosis. Br J Hosp Med 2010;71:83–6.

104. Bollée G, Guery B, Joly D, et al. Presentation and outcome of patients with systemic amyloidosis undergoing dialysis. Clin J Am Soc Nephrol 2008;3:375–81.

105. McCaffrey J, Lennon R, Webb NJA. The non-immunosuppressive management of childhood nephrotic syndrome. Pediatr Nephrol 2016;31:1383–402.

106. Mantan M, Pandharikar N, Yadav S, et al. Seroprotection for hepatitis B in children with nephrotic syndrome. Pediatr Nephrol 2013;28:2125–30.

107. Vandecasteele SJ, Ombelet S, Blumental S, et al. The ABC of pneumococcal infections and vaccination in patients with chronic kidney disease. Clin Kidney J 2015;8:318–24.

108. Wu HM, Tang J-L, Cao L, et al. Interventions for preventing infection in nephrotic syndrome. Cochrane Database Syst Rev 2012. https://doi.org/10.1002/14651858.CD003964.pub3.

109. Kamei K, Miyairi I, Ishikura K, et al. Prospective study of live attenuated vaccines for patients with nephrotic syndrome receiving immunosuppressive agents. J Pediatr 2018;196:217–22.e1.

110. Odabas AR, Cetinkaya R, Selcuk Y, et al. Effect of losartan treatment on the proteinuria in normotensive patients having proteinuria due to secondary amyloidosis. Ups J Med Sci 2001;106:183–8.

111. Dilek K, Usta M, Ersoy A, et al. Long-term effects of losartan on proteinuria and renal function in patients with renal amyloidosis. Scand J Urol Nephrol 2002;36:443–6.

112. Mehrotra R, Devuyst O, Davies SJ, et al. The current state of peritoneal dialysis. J Am Soc Nephrol 2016;27:3238–52.

113. Solak Y, Polat I, Atalay H, et al. When urine is no longer beneficial: renal artery embolisation in severe nephrotic syndrome secondary to amyloidosis. Amyloid 2010;17:24–6.

114. Turgut F, Kanbay M, Kaya A, et al. Bilateral renal artery embolization in a case with severe proteinuria secondary to amyloidosis in a hemodialysis patient. Amyloid 2007;14:157–8.

115. Yeh CT, Tseng HS, Liu WS, et al. Severe proteinuria secondary to amyloidosis requiring bilateral renal artery embolization. Case Rep Nephrol Dial 2012;2:78–82.

116. Kofman T, Grimbert P, Canouï-Poitrine F, et al. Renal transplantation in patients with AA amyloidosis nephropathy: results from a French multicenter study. Am J Transplant 2011;11:2423–31.

117. Gursu M, Yelken B, Caliskan Y, et al. Outcome of patients with amyloidosis after renal transplantation: a single-center experience. Int J Artif Organs 2012;35:444–9.

118. Haq A, Hussain S, Meskat B, et al. Complications of renal transplantation in patients with amyloidosis. Transplant Proc 2018;39:120–4.

119. Emeksiz H, Bakkaloglu S, Camurdan O, et al. Acute adrenal crisis mimicking familial Mediterranean fever attack in a renal transplant FMF patient with amyloid goiter. Rheumatol Int 2010;30:1647–9.

120. Gharabaghi MA, Behdadnia A, Gharabaghi MA, et al. Hypoadrenal syndrome in a patient with amyloidosis secondary to familial Mediterranean fever. BMJ Case Rep 2013;2013 [pii:bcr2012007991].

121. Fushimi T, Takahashi Y, Kashima Y, et al. Severe protein losing enteropathy with intractable diarrhea due to systemic AA amyloidosis, successfully treated with corticosteroid and octreotide. Amyloid 2005;12:48–53.

122. Shin JK, Jung YH, Bae MN, et al. Successful treatment of protein-losing enteropathy due to AA amyloidosis with octreotide in a patient with rheumatoid arthritis. Mod Rheumatol 2013;23(2):406–11.

123. Amemori S, Iwakiri R, Endo H, et al. Oral dimethyl sulfoxide for systemic amyloid A amyloidosis complication in chronic inflammatory disease: a retrospective patient chart review. J Gastroenterol 2006;41:444–9.

124. Dember LM, Hawkins PN, Hazenberg BP, et al. Eprodisate for the treatment of renal disease in AA amyloidosis. N Engl J Med 2007;356:2349–60.

125. Rumjon A, Coats T, Javaid MM. Review of eprodisate for the treatment of renal disease in AA amyloidosis. Int J Nephrol Renovasc Dis 2012;5:37–43.

126. Bodin K, Ellmerich S, Kahan MC, et al. Antibodies to human serum amyloid P component eliminate visceral amyloid deposits. Nature 2010;468:93.
127. Pepys MB, Herbert J, Hutchinson WL, et al. Targeted pharmacological depletion of serum amyloid P component for treatment of human amyloidosis. Nature 2002;417:254.
128. Gillmore JD, Tennent GA, Hutchinson WL, et al. Sustained pharmacological depletion of serum amyloid P component in patients with systemic amyloidosis. Br J Haematol 2010;148:760–7.
129. Richards DB, Cookson LM, Berges AC, et al. Therapeutic clearance of amyloid by antibodies to serum amyloid P component. N Engl J Med 2015;373:1106–14.
130. Richards DB, Cookson LM, Barton SV, et al. Repeat doses of antibody to serum amyloid P component clear amyloid deposits in patients with systemic amyloidosis. Sci Transl Med 2018;10 [pii:eaan3128].

Nephrotoxicity of Select Rheumatologic Drugs

Tyler Woodell, MD, Rupali S. Avasare, MD*

KEYWORDS

- Drug-induced nephrotoxicity • Drug-induced electrolyte disorders
- Drug dosing in chronic kidney disease • Drug dosing in hemodialysis

KEY POINTS

- Close monitoring of kidney function, blood pressure, and electrolytes is required when using nephrotoxic agents, such as nonsteroidal antiinflammatory drugs and calcineurin inhibitors in high-risk patients (elderly; concomitant use of renin-angiotensin-aldosterone blockade and/or diuretics; comorbid conditions, such as congestive heart failure, cirrhosis, and/or chronic kidney disease).
- Drug dosing may need to be adjusted for decreased glomerular filtration rate to prevent systemic side effects.
- If drug-induced kidney injury is suspected, then the offending agent should be stopped and patients closely monitored for renal recovery. Evaluation by a nephrologist and consideration of kidney biopsy should take place if the kidney function does not return to baseline after drug discontinuation.

INTRODUCTION

Several drugs commonly used in the management of rheumatic diseases may lead to nephrotoxicity, electrolyte disturbances, and hypertension. Here the authors discuss the adverse kidney effects, risk factors for toxicity, and optimal dosing in chronic kidney disease (CKD), including end-stage kidney disease on dialysis (**Table 1**).

NONSTEROIDAL ANTIINFLAMMATORY DRUGS

Nonsteroidal antiinflammatory drugs (NSAIDs) nonspecifically block the cyclooxygenase enzymes responsible for prostaglandin, prostacyclin, and thromboxane synthesis and thereby reduce inflammation. Because prostaglandins are important in the regulation of renal hemodynamics, NSAIDs may interfere with normal kidney homeostatic function.[1] NSAIDs exert a variety of effects on the kidney. The most common is

Disclosures: None.

Division of Nephrology and Hypertension, Department of Medicine, Oregon Health & Science University, Oregon Health & Science University, 3181 Southwest Sam Jackson Road, Portland, OR 97239, USA

* Corresponding author.

E-mail address: avasare@ohsu.edu

Rheum Dis Clin N Am 44 (2018) 605–617

https://doi.org/10.1016/j.rdc.2018.06.005

0889-857X/18/© 2018 Elsevier Inc. All rights reserved.

rheumatic.theclinics.com

Table 1
Drug dosing table for patients with kidney disease

Drug	CKD 3–5 Dosing	ESRD Dosing	Comments
Allopurinol[17,18]	Start at 50 mg daily when eGFR <30 mL/min; no dose reduction needed if already on therapy	Start at 50 mg daily for HD and PD	Increase by 50–100 mg every 2–5 wk until target uric acid reached;
Azathioprine	No dose adjustment recommended	No dose adjustment recommended	—
Biologics			
B-cell depleting agents	No dose adjustment recommended	No dose adjustment recommended	—
Costimulation blockers	No dose adjustment recommended	No dose adjustment recommended	—
Cytokine inhibitors	No dose adjustment recommended	No dose adjustment recommended	—
Calcineurin inhibitors	Consider dose reduction or drug discontinuation if eGFR decreases to <45–60 mL/min during therapy	No dose adjustment recommended	Avoid use in patients with moderate to severe interstitial fibrosis on kidney biopsy
Colchicine[7]	*Gout prevention:* reduce dose to 0.3 mg/d when eGFR <30 mL/min *Gout treatment:* Do not repeat treatment course more frequently than every 14 d when eGFR <30 mL/min; consider dose reduction	*Gout prevention:* Reduce dose to 0.3 mg twice weekly *Gout treatment:* 0.6 mg in single dose; do not redose more frequently than every 14 d	Reduce dose or frequency when prescribing other medications known to interact, including calcineurin inhibitors, macrolide antibiotics, and statins
Cyclophosphamide	No dose adjustment required; some experts suggest dose reduction by 25% for eGFR <10 mL/min	For HD, dose after HD session, 25-50% dose reduction For PD, 25% dose reduction	Avoid IV hypotonic fluids because of risk of hyponatremia
Glucocorticoids	No dose adjustment recommended	No dose adjustment recommended	—
IVIG[53,54]	Consider avoiding sucrase-stabilized IVIG and infusing at reduced rate	No dose adjustment recommended	—
Leflunomide	No dose adjustment recommended	No dose adjustment recommended	FDA recommends using with caution in patients with renal impairment
Methotrexate[40]	Reduce dose when eGFR <50–60 mL/min; contraindicated when eGFR <30 mL/min	Reduce dose for HD; contraindicated in PD	—

(continued on next page)

Table 1 (continued)			
Drug	CKD 3–5 Dosing	ESRD Dosing	Comments
Mycophenolate mofetil	No dose adjustment recommended	No dose adjustment recommended	—
NSAIDs	Use sparingly in patients when eGFR 30–60 mL/min; relatively contraindicated when eGFR <30 mL/min	Avoid in dialysis patients who make considerable daily volumes of urine (>250–500 mL); okay to use in oliguric patients	Avoid in combination with ACEi/ARB therapy or calcineurin inhibitors

Abbreviations: ACEi, angiotensin-converting enzyme inhibitor; ARB, angiotensin receptor blocker; eGFR, estimated glomerular filtration rate; ESRD, end-stage renal disease; FDA, Food and Drug Administration; HD, hemodialysis; IV, intravenous; IVIG, intravenous immunoglobulin; NSAIDs, nonsteroidal antiinflammatory drugs; PD, peritoneal dialysis.

sodium retention leading to clinically apparent edema in 3% to 5% of patients and hypertension.[2] Other effects include decreased potassium secretion and hyperkalemia, renal ischemia and acute tubular necrosis, acute tubulointerstitial nephritis due to hypersensitivity, nephrotic syndromes (minimal change disease and less commonly membranous nephropathy), hyponatremia, and papillary necrosis.[2–5]

NSAIDs are so commonly used in the management of many rheumatic diseases that the prevalence of NSAID-induced nephrotoxicity is high, though the individual patient risk of nephrotoxicity is low. Those at highest risk of hemodynamically mediated kidney injury are the elderly and those with CKD stage 3 or greater, effective volume depletion (ie, congestive heart failure and cirrhosis, gastrointestinal [GI] fluid losses), and/or hypercalcemia.[3,6] Risk of NSAID-induced kidney injury also increases with concomitant use of drugs that block the renin-angiotensin-aldosterone system. NSAID-induced acute kidney injury may be reversible after NSAID cessation and restoration of euvolemia in volume-depleted patients. The best chance of reversibility is in those who received a short (vs long) course of therapy. If kidney injury does not resolve within 1 week of medication discontinuation, then further workup and evaluation by a nephrologist is required.

The authors suggest avoiding NSAIDs in patients who are high risk for developing kidney injury and in dialysis patients with residual kidney function. If NSAIDs must be used, then a short course of therapy with close monitoring of kidney function, electrolytes, and volume status is advised.

ALLOPURINOL

Allopurinol, a xanthine oxidase inhibitor that decreases urate production, is the most widely used therapy in gout.[7] Nearly 75% of patients with gout have CKD.[8] Ultimately, the risk of serious nephrotoxicity is rare and can be minimized with a *start low, go slow* approach.

Nephrotoxicity from allopurinol can occur in combination with any number of abnormalities, including rash, liver injury, and eosinophilia, that are collectively called the allopurinol hypersensitivity syndrome (AHS), which is a form of drug reaction with eosinophilia and systemic symptoms.[9] Kidney biopsies performed in patients with AHS classically reveal interstitial nephritis, although cases of immune-complex glomerulonephritis have also been reported.[10–12] Regardless of underlying pathologic condition, nephrotoxicity in AHS is often severe enough to require hemodialysis. Although the exact mechanism of AHS remains to be elucidated, it is increasingly recognized that oxypurinol, the active metabolite of allopurinol, induces T-cell activation in a dose-dependent manner.[13,14] This immune response is thought to be further influenced by previous infection with herpes viruses as well as HLA-B*58:01 status.[15]

AHS is rare, estimated to occur in just 0.1% of patients receiving allopurinol.[9] The most important risk factor is the presence of the HLA-B*58:01 allele, which binds to oxypurinol with higher affinity than other alleles; 99% of individuals with AHS undergoing genetic testing in one systematic review carried the HLA-B*58:01 allele.[16] The presence of CKD is another risk factor for AHS, with a mean estimated creatinine clearance of 31 mL/min (based on the CKD-Epidemiology equation) among patients with AHS. This finding may reflect the high prevalence of CKD among patients with gout, rather than a mechanistic link between the two conditions.

Allopurinol can be used safely in patients with CKD, including those on hemodialysis or peritoneal dialysis. The American College of Rheumatology recommends a starting dosage of 50 mg daily when creatinine clearance is less than 30 mL/min.[17,18] Importantly, the peak allopurinol dose has *not* been associated with the development of AHS, and studies have consistently demonstrated improved effectiveness with equivalent safety using daily doses beyond the previously recommended 300 mg for patients with CKD.[7,19] Thus, allopurinol should be increased by 50 to 100 mg every 2 to 5 weeks in patients with CKD until the serum uric acid goals are achieved. Patients of Korean descent who have stage 3 to 5 CKD should undergo genetic testing for the HLA-B*58:01 allele given its high prevalence in this population; if present, an alternative therapy should be selected.[18]

COLCHICINE

Colchicine is an alkaloid derivative that is commonly used for prevention and/or treatment of acute gout flares as well as prevention of amyloidosis in familial Mediterranean fever.[20] Colchicine binds to intracellular tubulin proteins to prevent elongation of microtubule polymers, the most important effect of which is to interrupt cell division. When administered in high doses, however, this therapeutic effect becomes toxic by preferentially affecting systems with high turnover, such as the bone marrow and GI tract.[21,22] There are 3 clinical phases of colchicine toxicity: (1) the gastrointestinal phase, (2) multiorgan failure phase, and, if patients survive, (3) the recovery phase.[23] In the first phase, kidney injury may result from vomiting and diarrhea with resultant volume depletion leading to prerenal azotemia or acute tubular necrosis. In the second phase, which is characterized by shock, arrhythmias, and infectious or hematologic complications, dialysis-dependent acute kidney injury ensues and is presumably due to acute tubular necrosis.[24,25] Neuromyopathy may also occur, characterized by elevations in creatinine kinase activity and potential rhabdomyolysis, which may itself cause acute kidney injury.[26] Colchicine nephrotoxicity is not organ specific but instead reflects the impact of systemic toxicity on the kidneys. Reduced kidney function is a major risk factor for systemic toxicity, and appropriate use of colchicine requires careful dosing with serial monitoring of renal function. Additionally, comprehensive patient education on drug-drug interactions and early signs of toxicity are important strategies that can prevent potentially fatal complications.

Treatment of colchicine toxicity is supportive; efforts, thus, center on prevention. Although it is estimated that only 10% to 20% of colchicine is cleared by the kidneys,[20] dose reduction is needed when creatinine clearance is impaired. The American College of Rheumatology does not recommend a specific creatinine clearance threshold at which dosing should be reduced, but the Food and Drug Administration (FDA) recommends a dose or frequency reduction for gout prevention or treatment, respectively, when creatinine clearance decreases to less than 30 mL/min.[7,18] Colchicine may be used in patients on hemodialysis or peritoneal dialysis at reduced dosing and frequency, which is supported by pharmacokinetic studies.[27] Further dose reduction should be considered when patients are prescribed medications known to increase serum concentrations of colchicine by inhibiting CYP3A4 activity, such as statins, macrolides, and calcineurin inhibitors (CNIs).[23]

5-AMINOSALICYLIC ACID

Sulfasalazine is used for the treatment of rheumatoid arthritis and inflammatory bowel disease. It is metabolized to sulfapyridine and mesalamine (5-aminosalicylic acid), which has antiinflammatory properties. Adverse renal effects are exceedingly rare and include interstitial nephritis, minimal change disease, papillary necrosis (at doses several folds higher than treatment dosage), and kidney stones.[28–30] Nephrotoxicity may occur at any point during treatment but most often presents within the first 12 months of therapy.[31] If acute kidney injury occurs, the drug should be discontinued. Kidney biopsy may be considered if renal insufficiency persists after drug discontinuation.

The FDA recommends caution when using these agents in patients with kidney disease. Kidney function should be checked before initiating therapy and periodically during therapy. These agents are safe to use in hemodialysis patients, and gradual dose titration is advised.[32]

METHOTREXATE

Methotrexate is the first-line therapy for rheumatoid arthritis and is additionally used off-label for rheumatic diseases, including lupus, dermatomyositis, and polymyositis. Methotrexate nephrotoxicity occurs primarily through the formation of crystals in renal tubules, which causes tubular toxicity and obstruction.[33] Because crystal formation only occurs when the solubility of methotrexate is saturated, much of the current understanding of nephrotoxicity applies to high-dose methotrexate (>500 mg/m^2) administered for some cancers; methotrexate nephrotoxicity in rheumatic diseases is less well studied. Nevertheless, evidence exists that even at low doses, methotrexate is associated with, and may contribute to, nephrotoxicity.[34] According to one study, approximately 40% of individuals receiving up to 30 mg/wk of methotrexate had worsened renal function (defined as an increase in creatinine $\geq$20 μmol/L or 0.23 mg/dL) after 2 years of therapy.[35] It is important to note that most patients also received NSAIDs, and one-fifth of patients started CNIs after study entry. To better understand the direct impact of methotrexate on renal function, creatinine clearance has been directly measured using radioisotopes (ethylenediaminetetraacetic acid–labeled with chromium-51) in patients receiving low-dose methotrexate alone for rheumatoid arthritis.[36] Within weeks of initiating methotrexate, creatinine clearance decreased by an average of 11 mL/min. Importantly, when aspirin (2 g daily) was added to these patients' treatment, their creatinine clearance decreased further, again by an average of 11 mL/min; this second decrease was completely reversed after discontinuing aspirin. These findings suggest there are separate, but additive, effects of methotrexate and other medications used for rheumatic diseases, such as NSAIDs.

The mechanism by which low-dose methotrexate nephrotoxicity occurs has not been definitively identified in humans. Animal studies suggest that methotrexate is directly toxic to renal tubules, potentially by inducing oxidative stress.[37] In contrast to crystal-induced nephrotoxicity from high-dose methotrexate, there are no established risk factors for nephrotoxicity with low-dose methotrexate; clinical suspicion must, therefore, be maintained for all patients. Methotrexate nephrotoxicity should be considered in patients found to have an elevated creatinine in the absence of hematuria or proteinuria. Despite its tubular toxicity, methotrexate has not been reported to cause tubulopathies, such as Fanconi syndrome or renal tubular acidosis.

Methotrexate is almost entirely cleared by the kidneys; reduced kidney function is, therefore, the major risk factor for systemic methotrexate toxicity.[38,39] Therefore, close monitoring of serum creatinine before initiating and throughout treatment with methotrexate is advised. The American College of Rheumatology recommends that serum creatinine be measured every 2 to 4 weeks during the first 3 months of therapy with methotrexate and every 8 to 12 weeks thereafter.[40] If not discontinued, methotrexate dosing should be reduced when creatinine clearance decreases to less than 50 to 60 mL/min; the use of methotrexate is contraindicated when creatinine clearance is less than 30 mL/min. However, patients with end-stage renal disease who are on hemodialysis can resume methotrexate at reduced doses following hemodialysis sessions. There are no data regarding the safety of low-dose methotrexate in peritoneal dialysis, but the use of peritoneal dialysis for high-dose methotrexate toxicity has been described to inefficiently clear methotrexate.[41] Although hemodialysis provides significantly more effective methotrexate clearance, intensive peritoneal dialysis may be considered if vascular access for hemodialysis is untenable.

INTRAVENOUS IMMUNOGLOBULIN

Intravenous immunoglobulin (IVIG) is used off-label in several rheumatic conditions, including lupus, dermatomyositis, and polymyositis.[42] With just a few hundred reported cases to date, nephrotoxicity is a rare adverse event of IVIG not widely recognized until the 1990s.[43–45] The risk of nephrotoxicity relates not to IVIG itself but to the solution in which it is prepared. To prevent immunoglobulins from dimerizing or polymerizing (a process that may cause fever, chills, and joint pain), IVIG is stabilized by adding macromolecules (including carbohydrates or amino acids) to the solution.[46] Importantly, these macromolecules are taken up in the proximal tubular cells of the kidney where they cannot be efficiently digested, if at all.[47] The resultant accumulation of macromolecules in proximal tubular cell lysosomes causes cell swelling and, if severe, tubular obstruction with subsequent kidney injury. Different macromolecules are taken up and digested to varying degrees, but sucrose-stabilized IVIG confers the greatest risk of nephrotoxicity given the complete absence of sucrase in proximal tubular cells; up to 90% of reported cases of IVIG nephrotoxicity occur with sucrose-stabilized solutions.[44] Although lysosomal accumulation of sucrose is the primary mechanism by which IVIG nephrotoxicity occurs, it should be noted that Coombs-positive hemolysis is another known adverse event of IVIG use, more commonly associated with proline- or glycine-stabilized solutions, that can cause pigment nephropathy if hemolysis is severe.[48,49]

Onset of IVIG nephrotoxicity typically occurs within a few days of IVIG administration and is often characterized by oliguria; kidney biopsy reveals cytoplasmic vacuolization with degeneration of the proximal tubular cells and narrowing or complete obstruction of the tubular lumina.[43,50] Treatment is supportive, with up to 40% requiring dialysis temporarily and most patients developing renal recovery within weeks of stopping IVIG therapy.[44] In addition to the use of sucrose-stabilized solutions, proposed risk factors for the development of IVIG nephrotoxicity include CKD (in some studies defined as a serum creatinine >1.5 mg/dL), age greater than 65 years, comorbid diabetes, and concurrent use of other potentially nephrotoxic agents, including intravenous (IV) contrast dye.[43,47,51,52]

Although there are no specific recommendations proposed by the FDA or drug manufacturers for patients with CKD, some experts suggest that sucrose-stabilized solutions be avoided and slower infusion rates be considered in such patients.[53,54] IVIG is considered safe in patients on hemodialysis; a controlled clinical trial among hemodialysis patients demonstrated no difference in side effects or adverse events between IVIG and placebo.[55] The safety of IVIG in peritoneal dialysis is unknown, though case reports of toxicity among patients on peritoneal dialysis do not exist.

CYCLOPHOSPHAMIDE

Cyclophosphamide is an alkylating agent with antineoplastic and immunosuppressant properties used to manage lupus, scleroderma, myopathies, and antineutrophil cytoplasmic antibody (ANCA)–associated vasculitis. The dose used for rheumatic diseases is lower than that used for neoplasms. Notably, the toxic effects of cyclophosphamide, such as hemorrhagic cystitis and bladder malignancy, are related to dose and duration of therapy.

Electrolyte abnormalities, specifically hyponatremia, may occur in patients treated with IV cyclophosphamide. In one retrospective analysis, up to 14% of patients developed hyponatremia with low-dose pulse IV cyclophosphamide, especially when given alongside hypotonic IV fluids.[56] Thus, if forced diuresis is desired and patients are not hypervolemic, IV isotonic solutions are preferable to hypotonic solutions.

Clearance of the cyclophosphamide parent drug and some metabolites may be decreased in renal insufficiency, but there is no consensus guideline about dose reduction.[57] In dialysis patients, cyclophosphamide should be administered after a hemodialysis session at 75% of the standard dose, based on expert opinion.[58]

CALCINEURIN INHIBITORS

CNIs are frequently used as adjunctive therapy in the management of proliferative lupus nephritis with or without class V lesions. The two most studied CNIs are cyclosporine and tacrolimus. Although they are structurally distinct, they both bind to immunophilins, which inhibit calcineurin, and thereby lead to T-cell suppression.[59]

Use of cyclosporine in systemic lupus erythematosus was first reported in 1981[60] at a high dosage of 10 mg/kg/d. All patients (n = 5) eventually stopped therapy because of side effects, including nephrotoxicity and angioedema. Since then, CNIs have been used safely at lower doses with close monitoring of trough levels and kidney function.

Several mechanisms for nephrotoxicity have been identified, including renal vasoconstriction, tubular toxicity that can lead to an acute and/or chronic nephropathy, thrombotic microangiopathy, and focal sclerosis. CNIs also lead to hyperkalemia and hypertension by promoting salt retention and decreasing kaliuresis.[61,62] Other electrolyte derangements include hypomagnesemia, hyperuricemia, and metabolic acidosis. Furthermore, CNIs (in particular, tacrolimus) are associated with the development of diabetes that may be due to their effect on B-cell function.[63]

Risk factors for CNI toxicity include older age, NSAID use, volume depletion, and genetic factors.[64] There are no clear guidelines for dosing in patients with CKD, but in clinical practice these agents are avoided in CKD stage 3 and greater. If the medication is necessary, such as in transplant recipients, then the lowest acceptable trough level is targeted. CNIs are probably not dialyzable because they are highly protein bound; trough levels should guide dosing in the dialysis population.

NEPHROTOXICITY OF BIOLOGICAL AGENTS

Biological therapies for rheumatic conditions have emerged as an attractive treatment option for patients with CKD, both because most agents do not require dose adjustment and because there has yet to be any mechanistic link identified between their use and nephrotoxicity. In fact, evidence suggests that the use of biologics is associated with reduced incidence of CKD (compared with not receiving biologics) as well as slowed kidney disease progression after initiating biological therapy.[65] Nevertheless, idiosyncratic cases of nephrotoxicity associated with certain biologics deserve mention here. Clinicians should maintain suspicion for biological nephrotoxicity in any patient found to have new-onset kidney disease and consult with a nephrologist.

Cytokine Inhibitors

Much of what is known about nephrotoxicity in cytokine inhibitors relates to tumor necrosis factor α (TNFα) inhibitors commonly used to treat rheumatoid arthritis, spondyloarthropathies, and inflammatory bowel disease. Although relatively rare, there is a growing recognition of nephrotoxicity in association with TNFα inhibitors. Most cases reported involve the use of infliximab or etanercept, though cases involving adalimumab are also described.[66] Although all cases are characterized by some combination of increasing creatinine, hematuria, and proteinuria, histopathologic features are heterogeneous and may reveal glomerular or tubulointerstitial disease. The most common finding reported to date in association with etanercept and infliximab is drug-induced lupus nephritis,[66–68] though cases of renal sarcoidosis, ANCA-associated vasculitis, and Henoch-Schönlein purpura temporally related to the initiation of TNFα inhibitors are also described.[69–72] Case reports also exist describing membranous nephropathy and minimal change disease; spontaneous resolution of the renal disorder following cessation of TNFα inhibitors suggests a causal role of the biological agents rather than chance association.[73–75]

Treatment of TNFα inhibitor nephrotoxicity includes cessation of the culprit drug and, in some instances, immunosuppression that is tailored to the underlying renal pathology after consulting with a nephrologist. TNFα inhibitors are generally considered safe for use in patients with CKD, including those on hemodialysis; TNFα inhibitors do not require dose adjustment for CKD or dialysis dependence.[76,77]

Costimulation Blockers

Abatacept is approved for use in the management of rheumatoid and psoriatic arthritis. Although its use has not been studied in patients with advanced CKD or those on dialysis, a systematic review did not identify nephrotoxicity as a potential adverse event of the drug; there are no case reports to the authors' knowledge of nephrotoxicity associated with abatacept.[78]

B-Cell Depleting Agents

Belimumab and rituximab are B-cell depleting agents used in the management of extrarenal lupus and a variety of rheumatic conditions, respectively. As with abatacept, neither belimumab nor rituximab has been linked to nephrotoxicity in systematic reviews or case reports.[79,80] Indeed, rituximab has emerged as a promising therapy for many autoimmune renal disorders, including membranous nephropathy and frequently relapsing minimal change disease.[81–84] No dose adjustment is needed for patients with advanced CKD or dialysis dependence, and the presence of existing CKD has not been identified as a risk factor for extrarenal adverse events to date.

LEFLUNOMIDE

Leflunomide is a pyrimidine synthesis inhibitor whose active metabolite, teriflunomide, is used for the treatment of rheumatoid arthritis. There are no reports of nephrotoxicity attributed to leflunomide when used for rheumatoid arthritis. However, approximately 1% of patients receiving teriflunomide in placebo-controlled trials for multiple sclerosis had acute kidney injury (defined as a doubling of serum creatinine) and, separately, hyperkalemia greater than 6.5 mEq/L.[85,86] The generalizability of these findings to patients with rheumatoid arthritis receiving leflunomide cannot be determined. The FDA advises caution when prescribing leflunomide in the setting of kidney disease (no specific estimated glomerular filtration rate defined) because of a lack of pharmacokinetic studies in patients with CKD, but dose adjustment is not advised. Pharmacokinetic studies confirm that no dose adjustment is needed for patients on dialysis.[87]

RHEUMATIC DRUGS WITHOUT KNOWN NEPHROTOXICITY

Glucocorticoids are among the most common agents used to treat a broad range of rheumatic conditions. Although glucocorticoids can increase blood pressure or worsen preexisting hypertension, which is itself a risk factor for CKD, there is no direct nephrotoxicity attributed to their use.[88] Dose adjustments are not required for patients with CKD, including those on dialysis.

Mycophenolate mofetil is a purine synthesis inhibitor commonly used in the management of lupus and scleroderma. Its use has not been associated with nephrotoxicity; dose adjustment is not necessary for patients with CKD, including those on dialysis.

REFERENCES

1. Yared A, Kon V, Ichikawa I. Mechanism of preservation of glomerular perfusion and filtration during acute extracellular fluid volume depletion. Importance of intrarenal vasopressin-prostaglandin interaction for protecting kidneys from constrictor action of vasopressin. J Clin Invest 1985;75(5):1477–87.
2. Whelton A, Hamilton CW. Nonsteroidal anti-inflammatory drugs: effects on kidney function. J Clin Pharmacol 1991;31(7):588–98.
3. Gooch K, Culleton BF, Manns BJ, et al. NSAID use and progression of chronic kidney disease. Am J Med 2007;120(3):280.e1-7.
4. Wharam PC, Speedy DB, Noakes TD, et al. NSAID use increases the risk of developing hyponatremia during an Ironman triathlon. Med Sci Sports Exerc 2006;38(4):618–22.
5. Braden GL, O'Shea MH, Mulhern JG, et al. Acute renal failure and hyperkalaemia associated with cyclooxygenase-2 inhibitors. Nephrol Dial Transplant 2004;19(5): 1149–53.
6. Whelton A, Stout RI, Spilman PS, et al. Renal effects of ibuprofen, piroxicam, and sulindac in patients with asymptomatic renal failure. A prospective, randomized, crossover comparison. Ann Intern Med 1990;112(8):568–76.
7. Vargas-Santos AB, Neogi T. Management of gout and hyperuricemia in CKD. Am J Kidney Dis 2017;70(3):422–39.
8. Dalbeth N, Merriman TR, Stamp LK. Gout. Lancet 2016;388(10055):2039–52.
9. Singer JZ, Wallace SL. The allopurinol hypersensitivity syndrome. Unnecessary morbidity and mortality. Arthritis Rheum 1986;29(1):82–7.

10. Gelbart DR, Weinstein AB, Fajardo LF. Allopurinol-induced interstitial nephritis. Ann Intern Med 1977;86(2):196–8.
11. Grussendorf M, Andrassy K, Waldherr R, et al. Systemic hypersensitivity to allopurinol with acute interstitial nephritis. Am J Nephrol 1981;1(2):105–9.
12. Kantor GL. Toxic epidermal necrolysis, azotemia, and death after allopurinol therapy. JAMA 1970;212(3):478–9.
13. Yun J, Mattsson J, Schnyder K, et al. Allopurinol hypersensitivity is primarily mediated by dose-dependent oxypurinol-specific T cell response. Clin Exp Allergy 2013;43(11):1246–55.
14. Yun J, Marcaida MJ, Eriksson KK, et al. Oxypurinol directly and immediately activates the drug-specific T cells via the preferential use of HLA-B*58:01. J Immunol 2014;192(7):2984–93.
15. Stamp LK, Day RO, Yun J. Allopurinol hypersensitivity: investigating the cause and minimizing the risk. Nat Rev Rheumatol 2016;12(4):235–42.
16. Ramasamy SN, Korb-Wells CS, Kannangara DR, et al. Allopurinol hypersensitivity: a systematic review of all published cases, 1950-2012. Drug Saf 2013;36(10): 953–80.
17. Khanna D, Fitzgerald JD, Khanna PP, et al. 2012 American College of Rheumatology guidelines for management of gout. Part 1: systematic nonpharmacologic and pharmacologic therapeutic approaches to hyperuricemia. Arthritis Care Res (Hoboken) 2012;64(10):1431–46.
18. Khanna D, Khanna PP, Fitzgerald JD, et al. 2012 American College of Rheumatology guidelines for management of gout. Part 2: therapy and antiinflammatory prophylaxis of acute gouty arthritis. Arthritis Care Res (Hoboken) 2012;64(10): 1447–61.
19. Stamp LK, O'Donnell JL, Zhang M, et al. Using allopurinol above the dose based on creatinine clearance is effective and safe in patients with chronic gout, including those with renal impairment. Arthritis Rheum 2011;63(2):412–21.
20. Terkeltaub RA. Colchicine update: 2008. Semin Arthritis Rheum 2009;38(6): 411–9.
21. Hood RL. Colchicine poisoning. J Emerg Med 1994;12(2):171–7.
22. Folpini A, Furfori P. Colchicine toxicity–clinical features and treatment. Massive overdose case report. J Toxicol Clin Toxicol 1995;33(1):71–7.
23. Finkelstein Y, Aks SE, Hutson JR, et al. Colchicine poisoning: the dark side of an ancient drug. Clin Toxicol (Phila) 2010;48(5):407–14.
24. Stapczynski JS, Rothstein RJ, Gaye WA, et al. Colchicine overdose: report of two cases and review of the literature. Ann Emerg Med 1981;10(7):364–9.
25. Putterman C, Ben-Chetrit E, Caraco Y, et al. Colchicine intoxication: clinical pharmacology, risk factors, features, and management. Semin Arthritis Rheum 1991; 21(3):143–55.
26. Kuncl RW, Duncan G, Watson D, et al. Colchicine myopathy and neuropathy. N Engl J Med 1987;316(25):1562–8.
27. Wason S, Mount D, Faulkner R. Single-dose, open-label study of the differences in pharmacokinetics of colchicine in subjects with renal impairment, including end-stage renal disease. Clin Drug Investig 2014;34(12):845–55.
28. World MJ, Stevens PE, Ashton MA, et al. Mesalazine-associated interstitial nephritis. Nephrol Dial Transplant 1996;11(4):614–21.
29. Novis BH, Korzets Z, Chen P, et al. Nephrotic syndrome after treatment with 5-aminosalicylic acid. Br Med J 1988;296(6634):1442.
30. Durando M, Tiu H, Kim JS. Sulfasalazine-induced crystalluria causing severe acute kidney injury. Am J Kidney Dis 2017;70(6):869–73.

31. Gisbert JP, Gonzalez-Lama Y, Mate J. 5-Aminosalicylates and renal function in inflammatory bowel disease: a systematic review. Inflamm Bowel Dis 2007;13(5): 629–38.

32. Akiyama Y, Sakurai Y, Kato Y, et al. Retrospective study of salazosulfapyridine in eight patients with rheumatoid arthritis on hemodialysis. Mod Rheumatol 2014; 24(2):285–90.

33. Howard SC, McCormick J, Pui CH, et al. Preventing and managing toxicities of high-dose methotrexate. Oncologist 2016;21(12):1471–82.

34. Kremer JM, Petrillo GF, Hamilton RA. Pharmacokinetics and renal function in patients with rheumatoid arthritis receiving a standard dose of oral weekly methotrexate: association with significant decreases in creatinine clearance and renal clearance of the drug after 6 months of therapy. J Rheumatol 1995;22(1):38–40.

35. Verstappen SM, Bakker MF, Heurkens AH, et al. Adverse events and factors associated with toxicity in patients with early rheumatoid arthritis treated with methotrexate tight control therapy: the CAMERA study. Ann Rheum Dis 2010; 69(6):1044–8.

36. Seideman P, Muller-Suur R. Renal effects of aspirin and low dose methotrexate in rheumatoid arthritis. Ann Rheum Dis 1993;52(8):613–5.

37. Kolli VK, Abraham P, Isaac B, et al. Neutrophil infiltration and oxidative stress may play a critical role in methotrexate-induced renal damage. Chemotherapy 2009; 55(2):83–90.

38. Takeuchi A, Masuda S, Saito H, et al. Role of kidney-specific organic anion transporters in the urinary excretion of methotrexate. Kidney Int 2001;60(3):1058–68.

39. The effect of age and renal function on the efficacy and toxicity of methotrexate in rheumatoid arthritis. Rheumatoid Arthritis Clinical Trial Archive Group. J Rheumatol 1995;22(2):218–23.

40. Saag KG, Teng GG, Patkar NM, et al. American College of Rheumatology 2008 recommendations for the use of nonbiologic and biologic disease-modifying antirheumatic drugs in rheumatoid arthritis. Arthritis Rheum 2008;59(6):762–84.

41. Murashima M, Adamski J, Milone MC, et al. Methotrexate clearance by high-flux hemodialysis and peritoneal dialysis: a case report. Am J Kidney Dis 2009;53(5): 871–4.

42. Leong H, Stachnik J, Bonk ME, et al. Unlabeled uses of intravenous immune globulin. Am J Health Syst Pharm 2008;65(19):1815–24.

43. Cayco AV, Perazella MA, Hayslett JP. Renal insufficiency after intravenous immune globulin therapy: a report of two cases and an analysis of the literature. J Am Soc Nephrol 1997;8(11):1788–94.

44. Centers for Disease Control and Prevention. Renal insufficiency and failure associated with immune globulin intravenous therapy–United States, 1985-1998. MMWR Morb Mortal Wkly Rep 1999;48(24):518–21.

45. Dantal J. Intravenous immunoglobulins: in-depth review of excipients and acute kidney injury risk. Am J Nephrol 2013;38(4):275–84.

46. Duhem C, Dicato MA, Ries F. Side-effects of intravenous immune globulins. Clin Exp Immunol 1994;97(Suppl 1):79–83.

47. Dickenmann M, Oettl T, Mihatsch MJ. Osmotic nephrosis: acute kidney injury with accumulation of proximal tubular lysosomes due to administration of exogenous solutes. Am J Kidney Dis 2008;51(3):491–503.

48. Daw Z, Padmore R, Neurath D, et al. Hemolytic transfusion reactions after administration of intravenous immune (gamma) globulin: a case series analysis. Transfusion 2008;48(8):1598–601.

49. Welles CC, Tambra S, Lafayette RA. Hemoglobinuria and acute kidney injury requiring hemodialysis following intravenous immunoglobulin infusion. Am J Kidney Dis 2010;55(1):148–51.

50. Cantu TG, Hoehn-Saric EW, Burgess KM, et al. Acute renal failure associated with immunoglobulin therapy. Am J Kidney Dis 1995;25(2):228–34.

51. Chacko B, John GT, Balakrishnan N, et al. Osmotic nephropathy resulting from maltose-based intravenous immunoglobulin therapy. Ren Fail 2006; 28(2):193–5.

52. Cheng MJ, Christmas C. Special considerations with the use of intravenous immunoglobulin in older persons. Drugs Aging 2011;28(9):729–36.

53. Vo AA, Cam V, Toyoda M, et al. Safety and adverse events profiles of intravenous gammaglobulin products used for immunomodulation: a single-center experience. Clin J Am Soc Nephrol 2006;1(4):844–52.

54. Katz U, Achiron A, Sherer Y, et al. Safety of intravenous immunoglobulin (IVIG) therapy. Autoimmun Rev 2007;6(4):257–9.

55. Jordan SC, Tyan D, Stablein D, et al. Evaluation of intravenous immunoglobulin as an agent to lower allosensitization and improve transplantation in highly sensitized adult patients with end-stage renal disease: report of the NIH IG02 trial. J Am Soc Nephrol 2004;15(12):3256–62.

56. Lee YC, Park JS, Lee CH, et al. Hyponatraemia induced by low-dose intravenous pulse cyclophosphamide. Nephrol Dial Transplant 2010;25(5):1520–4.

57. Haubitz M, Bohnenstengel F, Brunkhorst R, et al. Cyclophosphamide pharmacokinetics and dose requirements in patients with renal insufficiency. Kidney Int 2002;61(4):1495–501.

58. Janus N, Thariat J, Boulanger H, et al. Proposal for dosage adjustment and timing of chemotherapy in hemodialyzed patients. Ann Oncol 2010;21(7):1395–403.

59. Kapturczak MH, Meier-Kriesche HU, Kaplan B. Pharmacology of calcineurin antagonists. Transplant Proc 2004;36(2 Suppl):25S–32S.

60. Isenberg DA, Snaith ML, Morrow WJW, et al. Cyclosporin a for the treatment of systemic lupus erythematosus. Int J Immunopharmacol 1981;3(2):163–9.

61. Hoorn EJ, Walsh SB, McCormick JA, et al. The calcineurin inhibitor tacrolimus activates the renal sodium chloride cotransporter to cause hypertension. Nat Med 2011;17(10):1304–9.

62. Shoda W, Nomura N, Ando F, et al. Calcineurin inhibitors block sodium-chloride cotransporter dephosphorylation in response to high potassium intake. Kidney Int 2017;91(2):402–11.

63. Heit JJ, Apelqvist AA, Gu X, et al. Calcineurin/NFAT signalling regulates pancreatic beta-cell growth and function. Nature 2006;443(7109):345–9.

64. Naesens M, Kuypers DR, Sarwal M. Calcineurin inhibitor nephrotoxicity. Clin J Am Soc Nephrol 2009;4(2):481–508.

65. Sumida K, Molnar MZ, Potukuchi PK, et al. Treatment of rheumatoid arthritis with biologic agents lowers the risk of incident chronic kidney disease. Kidney Int 2018;93(5):1207–16.

66. Oikonomou KA, Kapsoritakis AN, Stefanidis I, et al. Drug-induced nephrotoxicity in inflammatory bowel disease. Nephron Clin Pract 2011;119(2):c89–94 [discussion: c96].

67. Neradova A, Stam F, van den Berg JG, et al. Etanercept-associated SLE with lupus nephritis. Lupus 2009;18(7):667–8.

68. Saint Marcoux B, De Bandt M, CRI (Club Rhumatismes et Inflammation). Vasculitides induced by TNFalpha antagonists: a study in 39 patients in France. Joint Bone Spine 2006;73(6):710–3.

69. Ortiz-Sierra MC, Echeverri AF, Tobon GJ, et al. Developing of granulomatosis with polyangiitis during etanercept therapy. Case Rep Rheumatol 2014;2014:210108.
70. Akiyama M, Kaneko Y, Hanaoka H, et al. Acute kidney injury due to renal sarcoidosis during etanercept therapy: a case report and literature review. Intern Med 2015;54(9):1131–4.
71. Rolle AS, Zimmermann B, Poon SH. Etanercept-induced Henoch-Schonlein purpura in a patient with ankylosing spondylitis. J Clin Rheumatol 2013;19(2):90–3.
72. Hirohama D, Hoshino J, Hasegawa E, et al. Development of myeloperoxidase-antineutrophil cytoplasmic antibody-associated renal vasculitis in a patient receiving treatment with anti-tumor necrosis factor-alpha. Mod Rheumatol 2010; 20(6):602–5.
73. Koya M, Pichler R, Jefferson JA. Minimal-change disease secondary to etanercept. Clin Kidney J 2012;5(5):420–3.
74. Kaushik P, Rahmani M, Ellison W. Membranous glomerulonephritis with the use of etanercept in ankylosing spondylitis. Ann Pharmacother 2011;45(12):e62.
75. Chin G, Luxton G, Harvey JM. Infliximab and nephrotic syndrome. Nephrol Dial Transpl 2005;20(12):2824–6.
76. Don BR, Spin G, Nestorov I, et al. The pharmacokinetics of etanercept in patients with end-stage renal disease on haemodialysis. J Pharm Pharmacol 2005;57(11): 1407–13.
77. Cho SK, Sung YK, Park S, et al. Etanercept treatment in rheumatoid arthritis patients with chronic kidney failure on predialysis. Rheumatol Int 2010;30(11): 1519–22.
78. Maxwell L, Singh JA. Abatacept for rheumatoid arthritis. Cochrane Database Syst Rev 2009;(4):CD007277.
79. Lopez-Olivo MA, Amezaga Urruela M, McGahan L, et al. Rituximab for rheumatoid arthritis. Cochrane Database Syst Rev 2015;(1):CD007356.
80. Blair HA, Duggan ST. Belimumab: a review in systemic lupus erythematosus. Drugs 2018;78(3):355–66.
81. De Vita S, Quartuccio L, Isola M, et al. A randomized controlled trial of rituximab for the treatment of severe cryoglobulinemic vasculitis. Arthritis Rheum 2012; 64(3):843–53.
82. Ruggenenti P, Cravedi P, Chianca A, et al. Rituximab in idiopathic membranous nephropathy. J Am Soc Nephrol 2012;23(8):1416–25.
83. Guitard J, Hebral AL, Fakhouri F, et al. Rituximab for minimal-change nephrotic syndrome in adulthood: predictive factors for response, long-term outcomes and tolerance. Nephrol Dial Transpl 2014;29(11):2084–91.
84. Specks U, Merkel PA, Seo P, et al. Efficacy of remission-induction regimens for ANCA-associated vasculitis. N Engl J Med 2013;369(5):417–27.
85. O'Connor PW, Li D, Freedman MS, et al. A phase II study of the safety and efficacy of teriflunomide in multiple sclerosis with relapses. Neurology 2006;66(6): 894–900.
86. O'Connor P, Wolinsky JS, Confavreux C, et al. Randomized trial of oral teriflunomide for relapsing multiple sclerosis. N Engl J Med 2011;365(14):1293–303.
87. Bergner R, Peters L, Schmitt V, et al. Leflunomide in dialysis patients with rheumatoid arthritis–a pharmacokinetic study. Clin Rheumatol 2013;32(2):267–70.
88. Whelton PK, Carey RM, Aronow WS, et al. 2017 ACC/AHA/AAPA/ABC/ACPM/ AGS/APhA/ASH/ASPC/NMA/PCNA guideline for the prevention, detection, evaluation, and management of high blood pressure in adults: a report of the American College of Cardiology/American Heart Association Task Force on Clinical Practice Guidelines. Hypertension 2018;71(6):e13–115.

Acute and Chronic Tubulointerstitial Nephritis of Rheumatic Causes

Nestor Oliva-Damaso, MD[a],*, Elena Oliva-Damaso, MD, PhD[b],
Juan Payan, MD[a]

KEYWORDS

- Tubulointerstitial nephritis • Acute interstitial nephritis • Chronic interstitial nephritis
- Systemic lupus erythematous • Sjögren syndrome • Sarcoidosis • Scleroderma
- TINU syndrome

KEY POINTS

- Rheumatic diseases represent 10% to 20% of all cases of tubulointerstitial nephritis (TIN), and the rest are drug-induced or infectious-related forms.
- TIN may be a complication of sarcoidosis, Sjögren syndrome, TIN with uveitis syndrome, immunoglobulin G4–related disease, systemic lupus erythematous, scleroderma, and vasculitis.
- TIN should be suspected in the decline of kidney function with tubular proteinuria (usually less than 1 g/d), leukocyturia, and extrarenal symptoms.
- Kidney biopsy is generally required to make a definitive diagnosis.
- Corticosteroids represent the first therapeutic approach whereby relapses are frequent in systemic diseases.

INTRODUCTION

Tubulointerstitial nephritis (TIN) is a renal histologic lesion characterized by the presence of inflammatory infiltrates and edema within the tubulo-interstitial compartment, usually not affecting the glomerular and vascular compartments (**Fig. 1**).[1,2] This lesion was first described by Biermer[3] in 1860 and defined as an entity in 1898 by Councilman.[4] Depending on the clinical course, TIN is divided into acute interstitial nephritis (AIN) or chronic interstitial nephritis (CIN). AIN is a frequent cause of acute kidney injury

Conflict of Interest: The authors declare no competing interest.
[a] Department of Medicine, Division of Nephrology, Hospital Costa del Sol, A-7, Km 187, 29305 Marbella, Malaga, Spain; [b] Department of Medicine, Division of Nephrology, Hospital Doctor Negrin, Barranco de la Ballena, 35010 Las Palmas de Gran Canaria, Spain
* Corresponding author. Division of Nephrology, Department of Medicine, Hospital Costa del Sol, A-7, Km 187, 29305, Marbella, Malaga, Spain.
E-mail address: nestorod@hotmail.com

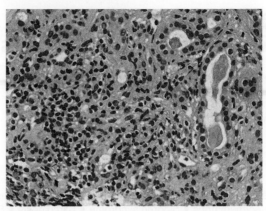

Fig. 1. Kidney biopsy specimen. Light microscopy (hematoxylin-eosin stain, original magnification ×400) demonstrates acute interstitial nephritis with an interstitial lymphoplasmacytic infiltrate with eosinophils and associated interstitial edema.

(AKI) that can lead to chronic kidney disease (CKD).[5] Although AIN is reversible (particularly if an offending medication is discontinued), the disease may progress and cause fibrosis and CIN. The likelihood of chronicity increases with systemic inflammatory or rheumatologic diseases and delayed removal of the causative medication in drug-induced TIN.[6] AIN is divided by cause into the following categories: allergic/drug-induced (antibiotics, nonsteroidal antiinflammatory drugs [NSAIDs], proton pump inhibitors, others); infection-related (including bacteria, fungi, and viruses); auto-immune/systemic; and idiopathic forms of disease.[6] Drug-induced AIN accounts for most cases (71%), of which antibiotics represent the most common responsible class of drug followed by proton-pump inhibitors and NSAIDs.[7] Rheumatic/autoimmune diseases are the second most frequent cause of TIN, accounting for approximately 10% to 20% of all cases; of these, sarcoidosis is the most common cause.[7] The other rheumatic diseases that can cause TIN include systemic lupus erythematous (SLE), Sjögren syndrome, scleroderma, TIN with uveitis (TINU) syndrome, immunoglobulin G4 (IgG4)–related disease, and vasculitis.

The prevalence of biopsy-proven AIN seems to be between 0.5% and 2.6% of all renal biopsies.[8] However, in patients with AKI, AIN represents 18% to 27% of biopsied cases.[8–10] Altogether AIN represents the second leading cause of intrinsic AKI after acute tubular necrosis.[11] The true incidence and prevalence of TIN might be underestimated, as a significant number of patients do not undergo renal biopsy and are treated empirically or because the vagueness of clinical symptoms can be attributed to other causes of renal injury.[11] In recent years, the prevalence of AIN has increased (from 3.6% to 10.5% of total kidney biopsies), which is more marked among elderly patients[12] possibly because of an increased use of certain medications[8] or an increased detection.[13] In adults with TIN the median percentage of interstitial kidney fibrosis was 30% and median glomerulosclerosis was 8% indicating chronic changes.[14] In children, TIN (both acute and chronic) accounts for 1% to 7% of the histologic diagnoses in renal biopsies.[15,16]

Autoimmune and systemic diseases causing AIN are rare in the elderly (65 years of age and older) whereby most cases are drug-related AIN; rheumatic causes are mostly seen in younger patients.[17] AIN is associated with an immune-mediated infiltration of the kidney interstitium by inflammatory cells that can progress to interstitial fibrosis and, therefore, transform into chronic interstitial nephritis.[5] Rheumatic disease and chronic damage induced by drugs (analgesic CIN) are related by chronicity.[18] The causes of AIN and CIN are numerous (summarized in **Table 1**), and the authors focus in this review on acute and chronic TIN related to rheumatic diseases.

CLINICAL FEATURES AND DIAGNOSIS

TIN is a histologic diagnosis due to many conditions (see **Table 1**). Patients with AIN usually present with low-grade proteinuria (about 1 g/24 h or less), decline in glomerular filtration rate (100% of AINs have AKI), leukocyturia (82% of the cases), and microhematuria (67% of cases) as shown in **Table 2**.[11,14,19] In AIN, the classic triad of fever, rash, and eosinophilia is uncommonly seen (more typical of drug-induced AIN) and represents only about 10% of the cases.[7] Interestingly, arthralgia is common in the clinical presentation in AIN (in almost half of all the cases, 45%) and is not exclusive of a rheumatic cause of TIN.[11] Clinical suspicion of AIN in patients with AKI usually relies on the presence of general symptoms (malaise, anorexia, arthralgia), hypersensitivity manifestations (low-grade fever, skin rash, eosinophilia), and urinalysis findings.[6,8,11] A firm final diagnosis requires a confirmatory kidney biopsy. Kidneys are structurally normal by ultrasound but may be enlarged[7]; small kidneys could indicate CKD. CIN usually has a slow and less expressive clinical manifestation, with symptoms usually more related to the causative systemic disease. Tubulointerstitial dysfunction can manifest as Fanconi syndrome. Patients may present with electrolyte disorders, such as hypokalemia (due to salt wasting and secondary hyperaldosteronism), hyperkalemia (due to impaired distal secretion), or metabolic acidosis. Elevated fractional excretion of sodium, glycosuria, and aminoaciduria typical of a proximal tubular dysfunction can also be seen.[6,20] CIN with CKD can also present with nocturia, polyuria, and polydipsia due to nephrogenic diabetes insipidus caused by drugs (eg, lithium), hypercalcemia (sarcoidosis), or immune diseases (Sjögren syndrome).[20] Eosinophiluria defined by eosinophils that account for more than 1% of urinary white cells[21,22] has been associated with AIN.[23] However, urinary eosinophils are not specific to AIN and can be found in other kidney diseases,[24] necessitating a kidney biopsy for diagnosis.[25,26] The only clinical manifestation common to all TIN cases is an acute or subacute kidney injury often resulting in CKD and its signs and symptoms.[27,28] The continued offending AIN cause or a severe episode of AKI that does not respond quickly to the withdrawal or treatment may result in CIN. AIN is histologically characterized by light microscopy with tubulointerstitial edema and infiltration of inflammatory cells (mononuclear, lymphocytes, plasma cells, eosinophils, histiocytes, and neutrophils) with glomerular and vascular structures generally preserved (**Fig. 1**).[11] CIN is characterized by renal interstitial fibrosis with tubular atrophy, a variable extent of inflammation in the fibrotic areas, and frequently inflammation in the atrophied tubules.[29] The degree of kidney function and the likelihood of kidney function recovery are closely linked to the extension of tubulointerstitial fibrosis in kidney histology.[30,31]

Drug-induced AIN follows exposure to a culprit drug and improves on stopping the medication, in which case the kidney biopsy can be unnecessary.[6] Interestingly, patients who are misdiagnosed with drug-induced AIN can develop uveitis, systemic symptoms, or autoantibodies in follow-up, highlighting that AIN can be the first clinical manifestation of an autoimmune disease.[32] Patients who have AIN not related to drugs may have symptoms related to an associated infection, systemic condition, or rheumatic diseases (like SLE, sarcoidosis, scleroderma, TINU, IgG4-related disease, Sjögren syndrome). In these diseases, which can present with different types of renal glomerular involvement (with nephrotic or nephritic syndrome), urinary findings of leukocyturia and white blood cell casts (with no urinary infection, so-called sterile pyuria)

Table 1
Causes of acute and chronic tubulointerstitial disease

	Medications/Toxins	Infection	Autoimmune Diseases	Systemic Diseases	Metabolic Disorders
Acute TIN	B-Lactam antibiotics, sulfonamides, rifampicin, quinine, NSAIDs, PPIs, H2-antagonist, anticonvulsants, allopurinol, diuretics, acute radiation nephritis; any medication can potentially produce AIN	Viruses, bacteria, fungi, parasites, spirochetes, others	Sjögren syndrome, sarcoidosis, IgG4-related disease, SLE, TINU, vasculitis	Dysproteinemias, lymphoproliferative diseases, inflammatory bowel disease, atheroembolic disease, DRESS	Oxalate nephropathy, uric acid nephropathy, nephrocalcinosis
Chronic TIN	NSAIDs, analgesic, lithium, PPIs, calcineurin inhibitors, chemotherapeutic agents, lead, cadmium, aristolochic acid, chronic radiation	Chronic pyelonephritis, malakoplakia, xanthogranulomatous pyelonephritis	Sjögren syndrome, sarcoidosis, SLE, TINU, IgG4-related disease, scleroderma, vasculitis	Dysproteinemias, lymphoproliferative diseases, sickle cell disease, inflammatory bowel disease, cystinosis, Dent disease, atheroembolic disease, DRESS	Oxalate nephropathy, uric acid nephropathy, nephrocalcinosis, hypokalemic nephropathy

Abbreviations: DRESS, drug-related eosinophilia systemic syndrome; PPIs, proton pump inhibitors.
Adapted from Perazella MA. Clinical approach to diagnosing acute and chronic tubulointerstitial disease. Adv Chronic Kidney Dis 2017;24:59; with permission.

Table 2
Clinical and laboratory features at presentation in acute interstitial nephritis

Clinical Features	%
Acute kidney injury	100
Non-nephrotic proteinuria	93
Leukocyturia	82
Microhematuria	67
Arthralgias	45
Dialysis required	40
Fever	36
Eosinophilia	35
Skin rash	22
Macrohematuria	5
Nephrotic-range proteinuria	2

Table shows clinical and laboratory features at presentation in 2 series[14,19] with AIN that included 121 cases. Most (91%) of the cases were drug-induced AIN; all had an acute worsening of kidney function and, in a significant proportion of cases, required dialysis.

are characteristics of TIN. Leukocyturia with low-grade proteinuria is not usually seen in other forms of renal disorders (shown in **Table 3**).[33] Specific clinical features of each rheumatic disease are described in each section.

SARCOID-RELATED TUBULOINTERSTITIAL NEPHRITIS

Sarcoidosis is the most frequent rheumatologic cause of TIN.[7] Sarcoidosis is a multi-system granulomatous disease of unknown cause characterized by the presence of noncaseating granulomas. It may affect any organ, including the kidneys. Granulomatous interstitial nephritis is the most typical histologic renal manifestation of sarcoidosis[34,35] and is usually identified as the initial presentation of the disease.[35] Apart from clinical features of TIN, the presence of pulmonary involvement (hilar adenopathies, pulmonary infiltrates), hypercalcemia, elevated serum levels of angiotensin-converting enzyme, and elevated 1,25 $(OH)_2$ vitamin D levels are typically seen.[8] Although granulomatous TIN is more frequent, interstitial nephritis without granulomas can be present in 20% of the cases.[36] Patients with hypercalcemia and fever with a

Table 3
Classic urinary findings in various kidney disorders

Urine Dipstick/Urine Microscopy	Interstitial Nephritis	Nephritic Syndrome	Nephrotic Syndrome	Tubular Necrosis
Protein	0/+	++	++++	0/+
Blood/RBCs	0/+	++++	0	0
Leukocyte/WBCs	+++	0/+	0	0
RBC casts	0	++	0	0
WBC casts	+++	0	0	0
RTE cell casts, granular casts	+	+	0	++++

Abbreviations: RBCs, red blood cells; RTE, renal tubular epithelial; WBCs, white blood cells.
   Adapted from Perazella MA. Clinical approach to diagnosing acute and chronic tubulointerstitial disease. Adv Chronic Kidney Dis 2017;24:57–63.

decline of glomerular filtration rate (in the absence of significant proteinuria and active urine sediment) should raise clinical suspicion for renal sarcoidosis.[36] Most patients with renal sarcoidosis have evidence of diffuse active sarcoidosis,[36–39] such as thoracic involvement (90%) or systemic symptoms, such as weight loss, fatigue, or fever (42%).[36] The diagnosis of sarcoid-related TIN is made by renal biopsy revealing interstitial infiltration of mononuclear cells, noncaseating granulomas in interstitium, tubular injury, and normal glomeruli. Differential diagnosis on patients with suspected sarcoidosis and TIN includes tuberculosis, mycobacterium infections, granulomatosis with polyangiitis (Wegener), brucellosis, histoplasmosis, TINU syndrome, Crohn disease, and drug-induced TIN.[40–42]

Treatment of sarcoid-related TIN is glucocorticoids as the first-line therapy. Most patients manifest a rapid improvement with 0.5 to 1.0 mg/kg/d of prednisone with the dose tapered down starting at 4 weeks.[8] Another regimen, based on the largest study of sarcoid-related TIN, is 1 mg/kg/d of oral prednisone for 6 to 12 weeks followed by a slow taper to a maintenance dose of 10 to 20 mg for an additional 6 to 9 months.[36] Short intravenous pulses of methylprednisolone have also been used.[36] Although corticosteroids are effective, the renal function recovery is often incomplete because of long-standing disease with irreversible fibrosis and CIN.[36,37,43,44] Relapses can occur and are related with responders whose steroids are tapered too rapidly. Some patients need prolonged treatment or become corticosteroid dependent. In these patients, the adverse effects of prolong corticosteroid use can be significant. Therefore, second-line steroid-sparing therapies have been sought for renal sarcoidosis and can include therapies that are effective in pulmonary sarcoidosis, such as methotrexate, chloroquine, azathioprine,[34] or mycophenolate mofetil.[45] Infliximab has been used as a last resort.[34,46]

TUBULOINTERSTITIAL NEPHRITIS AND UVEITIS (TUBULOINTERSTITIAL NEPHRITIS WITH UVEITIS SYNDROME)

TINU syndrome is defined as an anterior bilateral uveitis associated with AIN.[47] This entity was first described in 1975.[48] The pathogenesis of TINU syndrome is unknown but thought to be immune mediated. Autoantigen modified C-reactive protein is common to both the uvea and renal tubular cells.[49,50] T lymphocytes and interleukin-2 with delayed-type hypersensitivity has also been implicated.[51,52] Most patients are young women (with a median age of 15 years),[53] although it has been reported in adults.[49] The kidney manifestation usually precedes the ophthalmic symptoms,[49] but the two entities may present in any order.[54] The renal manifestations include typical AKI, tubular proteinuria, leukocyturia, microhematuria, and commonly tubular dysfunction. The symptoms of anterior uveitis are usually bilateral eye pain or redness, photophobia, dry eyes, and decreased visual acuity.[55] TINU syndrome may present with systemic manifestations, including arthralgias, myalgias, fever, weight loss, asthenia, anorexia, abdominal pain, polyuria, and nocturia. The diagnosis is made by the combination of ophthalmic findings and a kidney biopsy consistent with AIN in which interstitial granulomas can be seen.[44] Differential diagnosis can be challenging with other systemic diseases, such as Sjögren syndrome, sarcoidosis, SLE, Behçet syndrome, Wegener granulomatosis, and infection (tuberculosis, brucellosis, toxoplasmosis, and histoplasmosis). Corticosteroids are commonly used as a treatment in TINU syndrome; most patients recover kidney function, although relapses can occur.[56] Patients with progressive renal insufficiency can be treated with prednisone at 1 mg/kg/d for 3 to 6 months depending on the response (and then slowly tapered). This regimen is usually more prolonged than in other types of AIN, and even patients who require dialysis initially can recover kidney functionality.[57] Uveitis management requires early referral to an ophthalmologist. In steroid-resistant or relapsing cases, mycophenolate mofetil can be a therapeutic option.[58]

TUBULOINTERSTITIAL NEPHRITIS IN SJÖGREN SYNDROME

Sjögren syndrome is an autoimmune disease associated with lymphocytic and plasmacytic infiltration of exocrine organs (salival, parotid, lacrimal) producing a sicca syndrome. Nonexocrine organs, such as the kidneys, can also be affected. CIN is the most common manifestation; rarely, some patients with Sjögren syndrome develop glomerular disease.[59,60] Sjögren syndrome histologically presents as a renal interstitial infiltrate (as with other forms of TIN) with chronic features of tubular atrophy and interstitial fibrosis (CIN).[61,62] It may present with granuloma formation and uveitis; therefore, differentiating sarcoidosis and TINU syndrome is necessary.[59,63] As renal histologic findings are not specific, ocular tests and a biopsy of salivary glands are performed. These studies can be supported by positive autoantibodies, anti-Ro (anti-Sjögren-syndrome–related antigen A [SSA]) and anti-La (anti-Sjögren-syndrome–related type B antigen [SSB]), that are relatively specific to Sjögren syndrome and can be helpful for diagnosis.[8] Clinical manifestations include systemic sicca syndrome and CIN features. These features include mild deterioration of kidney function with a relatively benign urinalysis (low-grade proteinuria, leukocyturia, and microhematuria) and tubular dysfunction.[62] Abnormalities in tubular function associated with Sjögren syndrome include Fanconi syndrome, distal tubular acidosis, nephrogenic diabetes insipidus, and hypokalemia.[62] Patients can have metabolic acidosis with low plasma bicarbonate and hypokalemia with electrolyte-related clinical manifestations.[64] Polydipsia and polyuria (due to nephrogenic diabetes insipidus) can also be seen. Hypokalemia due to tubular injury by TIN leading to potassium wasting (that enhances aldosterone release) without metabolic acidosis (without distal tubular acidosis) has also been described in Sjögren syndrome.[65] First-line treatment of severe and active TIN-associated Sjögren syndrome is glucocorticoids (prednisone 1 mg/kg/d followed by tapering doses depending on the clinical response). In steroid-dependent cases azathioprine (1–2 mg/kg/d) can be used,[66] and mycophenolate mofetil can also be a therapeutic option.[58] Patients with Sjögren syndrome who have TIN have a better prognosis than those with Sjögren syndrome who develop glomerular diseases, such as membranoproliferative glomerulonephritis or membranous nephropathy; patients with TIN usually do not progress to end-stage renal disease.[67]

TUBULOINTERSTITIAL NEPHRITIS IN IMMUNOGLOBULIN G4–RELATED DISEASE

IgG4-related disease is a systemic disease characterized by cellular infiltrates rich in IgG4-positive plasma cells affecting multiple organs, usually accompanied by fibrosis.[68–70] Clinical manifestations include autoimmune pancreatitis, salivary and lacrimal gland disease, retroperitoneal fibrosis, and chronic periaortitis. Nodular lesions and lymphadenopathies may be seen mimicking malignancies or lymphoma.[71–73] Interstitial lung disease and sclerosing cholangitis can also be present in this multisystem disease. IgG4-related disease commonly affects adjacent structures to the kidney as retroperitoneal fibrosis leading to obstructive nephropathy.[74] Intrinsic renal involvement is found in about 12% of patients[74] whereby the most common intrinsic renal form is TIN. Patients are usually hypocomplementemic.[75,76] Most patients with IgG4-TIN (83%) have another organ affected at the time of diagnosis.[74] Differentiation from other hypocomplementemic TINs, such as SLE-associated interstitial nephritis, can be required.[77] Patients are usually middle-aged and male, with renal manifestations including deterioration of kidney function with a relatively benign urinalysis, low serum complement (C3 and C4), and elevated serum levels of IgG4 (IgG and IgE). Interestingly, 30% to 45% of patients with biopsy-proven IgG4-related disease have normal levels of serum IgG4 (usually in single system disease), hence, the importance of a confirmatory biopsy that includes immunofluorescence staining for IgG subtypes (IgG1–4).[74] Corticosteroids are usually the first line of therapy with a response in most patients. The usual dosage is prednisone 40 mg/d. A response can be seen as early as the first weeks, after which tapering is recommended.[68–70] Relapses are common in this disease. Rituximab may be used to prevent a relapse.[78,79] Other immunosuppressive medications, such as azathioprine or mycophenolate mofetil, have also been used as second-line agents.[8,80]

TUBULOINTERSTITIAL LUPUS NEPHRITIS

SLE is a chronic inflammatory disease that can injure any organ and often affects the kidney. TIN can be present in conjunction with all the glomerular diseases classified by the International Society of Nephrology/Renal Pathology Society,[81] but isolated tubulointerstitial lupus nephritis without glomerular lesions are rare.[82,83] TIN in lupus nephritis is a common finding with or without immune deposits along the tubular basement membrane.[84,85] Histologically, tubular basement membrane immune deposits correlate with serologic activity of SLE but not with prognosis.[85] However, tubular atrophy, interstitial fibrosis, and the grade of severity of TIN in SLE are associated with prognosis, hypertension, and progressive clinical course.[86,87] There can be different grades of severity of tubulointerstitial lesions in different classes of lupus nephritis, most commonly found in class IV lupus nephritis.[87] On the other hand, isolated tubulointerstitial lupus nephritis has predominant TIN clinical features, such as kidney function deterioration with relatively normal urinalysis and signs of tubular dysfunction (metabolic acidosis, hypokalemia, or hyperkalemia).[88,89] Predominant TIN in SLE is usually treated with high-dose steroids.[83]

TUBULOINTERSTITIAL NEPHRITIS IN SYSTEMIC SCLEROSIS

Systemic sclerosis or scleroderma is an immune-mediated disease that is characterized by fibrosis of the skin and of internal organs and vasculopathy. Although uncommon, this disease has high morbidity and mortality.[90] Subclinical renal impairment affects approximately 50% of patients with scleroderma.[91] Scleroderma renal crisis (defined as a thrombotic microangiopathy with accelerated hypertension and progressive kidney injury) is the most prominent renal manifestation, with glomerulonephritis and vasculopathy.[92] TIN may also occur in scleroderma but is much less common. It has been recognized that patients with scleroderma can have increased interstitial extracellular matrix in kidney biopsies and also in autopsy studies. In patients without renal crisis, interstitial fibrosis and tubular atrophy can be present, reflecting chronic changes of scleroderma.[92]

TUBULOINTERSTITIAL NEPHRITIS IN VASCULITIS

TIN may be seen in patients with antineutrophil cytoplasmic antibodies (ANCA) associated vasculitis when the vasculitis affects the renal medulla.[93,94] Drug-induced

Table 4
Differential diagnosis tubulointerstitial nephritis rheumatic cause with drug-induced tubulointerstitial nephritis

	Age	Sex	Clinical Features	Histopathologic Features	Treatment
Sarcoid-related TIN	Young adult	Both	Multisystemic granulomatous affecting any organ, pulmonary infiltrates or adenopathies, hypercalcemia, fever, ACE elevated, TIN	Interstitial nephritis, granulomas 80% cases, no granulomas 20%	Pulses of methylprednisolone and prednisone 1 mg/kg/d Second line: methotrexate, chloroquine, azathioprine, MMF, infliximab
TINU	Young (median 15 y)	Female	Bilateral eye pain or redness, photophobia, dry eyes and decreased acuity, systemic manifestations, TIN	Interstitial nephritis, granulomas can be seen	Prednisone 1 mg/kg/d Usually more prolonged Second line: MMF
TIN in Sjögren	Any	Female	Sicca syndrome, value ocular tests and salival gland biopsy, anti-Ro (SSA), anti-La (SSB), TIN, tubular dysfunction, and electrolyte abnormalities	Interstitial nephritis with more chronic features, granulomas can be present	Prednisone 1 mg/kg/d Second line: azathioprine
IgG4-related disease	Adult	Male	Multiple organs, cholangitis, pancreatitis, salival, lacrimal, retroperitoneal fibrosis, nodular lesions, lung, TIN, hypocomplementemia, IgG4 elevated	Interstitial nephritis, cellular infiltrates rich in IgG4	Prednisone 1 mg/kg/d Second line: rituximab, azathioprine, MMF
Isolated TIN in SLE	Any	Female	SLE clinical features, hypocomplementemia, anti-DNA, TIN	Isolated TIN rare, TIN common with glomerular lupus nephritis in all classes, more frequent in IV	Isolated: prednisone 1 mg/kg/d
TIN in scleroderma	Any	Both	Rare, TIN findings show chronic changes	Chronic TIN, tubular atrophy, and interstitial fibrosis	Treatment of disease or crisis
TIN in vasculitis	Adult and elderly	Both	Predominant TIN seen in drug-induced ANCA vasculitis, very high anti-MPO/PR3 levels	Interstitial nephritis affecting renal medulla	Medication withdrawal
Drug-induced TIN	Elderly and any	Both	Allergic/hypersensitivity manifestations (rash, eosinophilia, fever, arthralgias) more common with antibiotics, rare in NSAIDs and PPI	Interstitial infiltrates with eosinophils, granulomas occasionally seen	To help recovery: rapid removal of the offending drug and early corticosteroids

Abbreviations: ACE, angiotensin-converting-enzyme; anti DNA, anti-double-stranded DNA; MMF, mycophenolate mofetil; PPIs, proton pump inhibitors; PR3, protease 3.

ANCA vasculitis, characterized by very high levels of anti–myeloperoxidase (MPO) ANCA antibodies, is associated with acute interstitial nephritis; drug withdrawal was closely related with recovery of renal function and the disappearance of MPO-ANCAs.[93,95]

SUMMARY

TIN is a relatively common cause of intrinsic kidney injury. Rheumatic diseases are the second most frequent cause of TIN after drug-induced causes. TIN should be suspected in patients with a progressive decline of kidney function, tubular proteinuria (usually less than 1 g/d), and leukocyturia without bacteriuria. Importantly, extrarenal symptoms and hypersensitivity manifestations are keys for diagnosis. Tubular dysfunction and nocturia can be present. This kidney injury is typically nonoliguric but poly-uric even in end stages of renal disease. A first approach when TIN is suspected includes checking medication lists and demonstrating a temporary relationship between initiation of the culprit and symptoms, in which case withdrawal is required. The final diagnosis of TIN is confirmed by a kidney biopsy. The benign urine findings and the subacute kidney failure can often delay the referral to a nephrologist.

In non–drug-related TIN, other causes, such as systemic and rheumatic diseases, have to be considered. Follow-up is mandatory, as renal manifestations may be the initial presentation of a systemic disease. Granulomatous TIN is associated with sarcoidosis, TINU syndrome, and Sjögren syndrome. Although the differential diagnosis can be challenging, certain clinical tips can be helpful (**Table 4**): Hypercalcemia and pulmonary involvement orient to sarcoidosis; uveitis leads to TINU; and sicca syndrome with positive autoantibodies, anti-Ro (SSA) and anti La (SSB), suggests Sjögren syndrome. Hypocomplementemia can be seen in IgG4-related disease and SLE. IgG4 disease may also present with pancreas involvement and high serum levels of IgG4. In SLE, serum autoantibodies and clinical criteria are helpful. Corticosteroids are generally used as a first-line therapy whereby the response is satisfactory in most rheumatologic conditions associated with TIN. Side effects of steroids always have to be considered. Relapses are more frequent with TIN in rheumatic disease compared with drug-induced forms of interstitial nephritis; therefore, not surprisingly, these variants of TIN are more likely to show chronicity and progression to late and end-stage CKD.

ACKNOWLEDGMENTS

The authors would like to thank Teresa Pereda and the division of Renal Pathology of Hospital Costa del Sol for the image in **Fig. 1**.

REFERENCES

1. Joyce E, Glasner P, Ranganathan S, et al. Tubulointerstitial nephritis: diagnosis, treatment, and monitoring. Pediatr Nephrol 2017;32:577–87.
2. Rossert JA, Fischer EA. Acute interstitial nephritis. In: Johnson RJ, Freehally J, editors. Comprehensive clinical nephrology. 2nd edition. Philadelphia: Elsevier Limited; 2003. p. 769.
3. Biermer A. Ein ungervohnlicher Fall von Sharlach. Virchows Arch Pathol Anat 1860;19:537–45.
4. Councilman WT. Acute interstitial nephritis. J Exp Med 1898;3(4–5):189–92.
5. Hodgkins KS, Schnaper HW. Tubulointerstitial injury and the progression of chronic kidney disease. Pediatr Nephrol 2012;27:901–9.

6. Perazella MA, Markowitz GS. Drug-induced acute interstitial nephritis. Nat Rev Nephrol 2010;6:461–70.
7. Muriithi AK, Leung N, Valeri AM, et al. Biopsy-proven acute interstitial nephritis, 1993-2011: a case series. Am J Kidney Dis 2014;64:558–66.
8. Praga M, Sevillano A, Aunon P, et al. Changes in the aetiology, clinical presentation and management of acute interstitial nephritis, an increasingly common cause of acute kidney injury. Nephrol Dial Transplant 2015;30:1472–9.
9. Farrington K, Levison DA, Greenwood RN, et al. Renal biopsy in patients with unexplained renal impairment and normal kidney size. Q J Med 1989;70:221–33.
10. Haas M, Spargo BH, Wit EJ, et al. Etiologies and outcome of acute renal insufficiency in older adults: a renal biopsy study of 259 cases. Am J Kidney Dis 2000; 35:433–47.
11. Praga M, Gonzalez E. Acute interstitial nephritis. Kidney Int 2010;77:956–61.
12. Goicoechea M, Rivera F, Lopez-Gomez JM. Increased prevalence of acute tubulointerstitial nephritis. Nephrol Dial Transplant 2013;28:112–5.
13. Bomback AS, Markowitz GS. Increased prevalence of acute interstitial nephritis: more disease or simply more detection? Nephrol Dial Transplant 2013;28:16–8.
14. Clarkson MR, Giblin L, O'Connell FP, et al. Acute interstitial nephritis: clinical features and response to corticosteroid therapy. Nephrol Dial Transplant 2004;19: 2778–83.
15. Coppo R, Gianoglio B, Porcellini MG, et al. Frequency of renal diseases and clinical indications for renal biopsy in children (report of the Italian National Registry of Renal Biopsies in Children). Group of Renal Immunopathology of the Italian Society of Pediatric Nephrology and Group of Renal Immunopathology of the Italian Society of Nephrology. Nephrol Dial Transplant 1998;13:293–7.
16. Greising J, Trachtman H, Gauthier B, et al. Acute interstitial nephritis in adolescents and young adults. Child Nephrol Urol 1990;10:189–95.
17. Muriithi AK, Leung N, Valeri AM, et al. Clinical characteristics, causes and outcomes of acute interstitial nephritis in the elderly. Kidney Int 2015;87:458–64.
18. Murray T, Goldberg M. Chronic interstitial nephritis: etiologic factors. Ann Intern Med 1975;82:453–9.
19. Gonzalez E, Gutierrez E, Galeano C, et al. Early steroid treatment improves the recovery of renal function in patients with drug-induced acute interstitial nephritis. Kidney Int 2008;73:940–6.
20. Neilson EG. Pathogenesis and therapy of interstitial nephritis. Kidney Int 1989;35: 1257–70.
21. Rossert J. Drug-induced acute interstitial nephritis. Kidney Int 2001;60:804–17.
22. Nolan CR III, Anger MS, Kelleher SP. Eosinophiluria–a new method of detection and definition of the clinical spectrum. N Engl J Med 1986;315:1516–9.
23. Corwin HL, Korbet SM, Schwartz MM. Clinical correlates of eosinophiluria. Arch Intern Med 1985;145:1097–9.
24. Muriithi AK, Nasr SH, Leung N. Utility of urine eosinophils in the diagnosis of acute interstitial nephritis. Clin J Am Soc Nephrol 2013;8:1857–02.
25. Fletcher A. Eosinophiluria and acute interstitial nephritis. N Engl J Med 2008;358: 1760–1.
26. Perazella MA, Bomback AS. Urinary eosinophils in AIN: farewell to an old biomarker? Clin J Am Soc Nephrol 2013;8:1841–3.
27. Michel DM, Kelly CJ. Acute interstitial nephritis. J Am Soc Nephrol 1998;9: 506–15.
28. Kodner CM, Kudrimoti A. Diagnosis and management of acute interstitial nephritis. Am Fam Physician 2003;67:2527–34.

29. Nast CC. Medication-induced interstitial nephritis in the 21st century. Adv Chronic Kidney Dis 2017;24:72–9.
30. Rodriguez-Iturbe B, Garcia GG. The role of tubulointerstitial inflammation in the progression of chronic renal failure. Nephron Clin Pract 2010;116:c81–8.
31. Bhaumik SK, Kher V, Arora P, et al. Evaluation of clinical and histological prognostic markers in drug-induced acute interstitial nephritis. Ren Fail 1996;18: 97–104.
32. Su T, Gu Y, Sun P, et al. Etiology and renal outcomes of acute tubulointerstitial nephritis: a single-center prospective cohort study in China. Nephrol Dial Transplant 2018;33(7):1180–8.
33. Perazella MA. Clinical approach to diagnosing acute and chronic tubulointerstitial disease. Adv Chronic Kidney Dis 2017;24:57–63.
34. Hilderson I, Van LS, Wauters A, et al. Treatment of renal sarcoidosis: is there a guideline? Overview of the different treatment options. Nephrol Dial Transplant 2014;29:1841–7.
35. Berliner AR, Haas M, Choi MJ. Sarcoidosis: the nephrologist's perspective. Am J Kidney Dis 2006;48:856–70.
36. Mahevas M, Lescure FX, Boffa JJ, et al. Renal sarcoidosis: clinical, laboratory, and histologic presentation and outcome in 47 patients. Medicine (Baltimore) 2009;88:98–106.
37. Brause M, Magnusson K, Degenhardt S, et al. Renal involvement in sarcoidosis–a report of 6 cases. Clin Nephrol 2002;57:142–8.
38. Robson MG, Banerjee D, Hopster D, et al. Seven cases of granulomatous interstitial nephritis in the absence of extrarenal sarcoid. Nephrol Dial Transplant 2003;18:280–4.
39. Thumfart J, Muller D, Rudolph B, et al. Isolated sarcoid granulomatous interstitial nephritis responding to infliximab therapy. Am J Kidney Dis 2005;45:411–4.
40. Javaud N, Belenfant X, Stirnemann J, et al. Renal granulomatoses: a retrospective study of 40 cases and review of the literature. Medicine (Baltimore) 2007; 86:170–80.
41. Bijol V, Mendez GP, Nose V, et al. Granulomatous interstitial nephritis: a clinicopathologic study of 46 cases from a single institution. Int J Surg Pathol 2006; 14:57–63.
42. Adams AL, Cook WJ. Granulomatous interstitial nephritis secondary to histoplasmosis. Am J Kidney Dis 2007;50:681–5.
43. Singer DR, Evans DJ. Renal impairment in sarcoidosis: granulomatous nephritis as an isolated cause (two case reports and review of the literature). Clin Nephrol 1986;26:250–6.
44. Joss N, Morris S, Young B, et al. Granulomatous interstitial nephritis. Clin J Am Soc Nephrol 2007;2:222–30.
45. Moudgil A, Przygodzki RM, Kher KK. Successful steroid-sparing treatment of renal limited sarcoidosis with mycophenolate mofetil. Pediatr Nephrol 2006;21: 281–5.
46. Veltkamp M, Drent M, Baughman RP. Infliximab or biosimilars in sarcoidosis; to switch or not to switch? Sarcoidosis Vasc Diffuse Lung Dis 2016;32:280–3.
47. Mackensen F, Smith JR, Rosenbaum JT. Enhanced recognition, treatment, and prognosis of tubulointerstitial nephritis and uveitis syndrome. Ophthalmology 2007;114:995–9.
48. Dobrin RS, Vernier RL, Fish AL. Acute eosinophilic interstitial nephritis and renal failure with bone marrow-lymph node granulomas and anterior uveitis. A new syndrome. Am J Med 1975;59:325–33.

49. Li C, Su T, Chu R, et al. Tubulointerstitial nephritis with uveitis in Chinese adults. Clin J Am Soc Nephrol 2014;9:21–8.

50. Tan Y, Yu F, Qu Z, et al. Modified C-reactive protein might be a target autoantigen of TINU syndrome. Clin J Am Soc Nephrol 2011;6:93–100.

51. Yoshioka K, Takemura T, Kanasaki M, et al. Acute interstitial nephritis and uveitis syndrome: activated immune cell infiltration in the kidney. Pediatr Nephrol 1991;5: 232–4.

52. Gafter U, Kalechman Y, Zevin D, et al. Tubulointerstitial nephritis and uveitis: association with suppressed cellular immunity. Nephrol Dial Transplant 1993;8: 821–6.

53. Sessa A, Meroni M, Battini G, et al. Acute renal failure due to idiopathic tubulo-intestinal nephritis and uveitis: "TINU syndrome". Case report and review of the literature. J Nephrol 2000;13:377–80.

54. Mandeville JT, Levinson RD, Holland GN. The tubulointerstitial nephritis and uveitis syndrome. Surv Ophthalmol 2001;46:195–208.

55. Rosenbaum JT. Bilateral anterior uveitis and interstitial nephritis. Am J Ophthalmol 1988;105:534–7.

56. Takemura T, Okada M, Hino S, et al. Course and outcome of tubulointerstitial nephritis and uveitis syndrome. Am J Kidney Dis 1999;34:1016–21.

57. van LR, Assmann KJ. Acute tubulo-interstitial nephritis with uveitis and favourable outcome after five months of continuous ambulatory peritoneal dialysis (CAPD). Neth J Med 1988;33:133–9.

58. Preddie DC, Markowitz GS, Radhakrishnan J, et al. Mycophenolate mofetil for the treatment of interstitial nephritis. Clin J Am Soc Nephrol 2006;1:718–22.

59. Maripuri S, Grande JP, Osborn TG, et al. Renal involvement in primary Sjogren's syndrome: a clinicopathologic study. Clin J Am Soc Nephrol 2009;4: 1423–31.

60. Kidder D, Rutherford E, Kipgen D, et al. Kidney biopsy findings in primary Sjogren syndrome. Nephrol Dial Transplant 2015;30:1363–9.

61. Bossini N, Savoldi S, Franceschini F, et al. Clinical and morphological features of kidney involvement in primary Sjogren's syndrome. Nephrol Dial Transplant 2001; 16:2328–36.

62. Goules A, Masouridi S, Tzioufas AG, et al. Clinically significant and biopsy-documented renal involvement in primary Sjogren syndrome. Medicine (Baltimore) 2000;79:241–9.

63. Vidal E, Rogues AM, Aldigier JC. The Tinu syndrome or the Sjogren syndrome? Ann Intern Med 1992;116:93.

64. Pun KK, Wong CK, Tsui EY, et al. Hypokalemic periodic paralysis due to the Sjogren syndrome in Chinese patients. Ann Intern Med 1989;110:405–6.

65. Wrong OM, Feest TG, MacIver AG. Immune-related potassium-losing interstitial nephritis: a comparison with distal renal tubular acidosis. Q J Med 1993;86: 513–34.

66. Kaufman I, Schwartz D, Caspi D, et al. Sjogren's syndrome - not just Sicca: renal involvement in Sjogren's syndrome. Scand J Rheumatol 2008;37:213–8.

67. Goules AV, Tatouli IP, Moutsopoulos HM, et al. Clinically significant renal involvement in primary Sjogren's syndrome: clinical presentation and outcome. Arthritis Rheum 2013;65:2945–53.

68. Saeki T, Kawano M. IgG4-related kidney disease. Kidney Int 2014;85:251–7.

69. Raissian Y, Nasr SH, Larsen CP, et al. Diagnosis of IgG4-related tubulointerstitial nephritis. J Am Soc Nephrol 2011;22:1343–52.

70. Stone JH, Zen Y, Deshpande V. IgG4-related disease. N Engl J Med 2012;366: 539–51.
71. Rudmik L, Trpkov K, Nash C, et al. Autoimmune pancreatitis associated with renal lesions mimicking metastatic tumours. CMAJ 2006;175:367–9.
72. Murashima M, Tomaszewski J, Glickman JD. Chronic tubulointerstitial nephritis presenting as multiple renal nodules and pancreatic insufficiency. Am J Kidney Dis 2007;49:e7–10.
73. Cheuk W, Yuen HK, Chu SY, et al. Lymphadenopathy of IgG4-related sclerosing disease. Am J Surg Pathol 2008;32:671–81.
74. Mann S, Seidman MA, Barbour SJ, et al. Recognizing IgG4-related tubulointerstitial nephritis. Can J Kidney Health Dis 2016;3:34.
75. Watson SJ, Jenkins DA, Bellamy CO. Nephropathy in IgG4-related systemic disease. Am J Surg Pathol 2006;30:1472–7.
76. Saeki T, Nishi S, Imai N, et al. Clinicopathological characteristics of patients with IgG4-related tubulointerstitial nephritis. Kidney Int 2010;78:1016–23.
77. Wallace ZS, Deshpande V, Mattoo H, et al. IgG4-related disease: clinical and laboratory features in one hundred twenty-five patients. Arthritis Rheumatol 2015;67: 2466–75.
78. Khosroshahi A, Bloch DB, Deshpande V, et al. Rituximab therapy leads to rapid decline of serum IgG4 levels and prompt clinical improvement in IgG4-related systemic disease. Arthritis Rheum 2010;62:1755–62.
79. Khosroshahi A, Carruthers MN, Deshpande V, et al. Rituximab for the treatment of IgG4-related disease: lessons from 10 consecutive patients. Medicine (Baltimore) 2012;91:57–66.
80. Khosroshahi A, Stone JH. Treatment approaches to IgG4-related systemic disease. Curr Opin Rheumatol 2011;23:67–71.
81. Weening JJ, D'Agati VD, Schwartz MM, et al. Classification of glomerulonephritis in systemic lupus erythematosus revisited. Kidney Int 2004;65:521–30.
82. Singh AK, Ucci A, Madias NE. Predominant tubulointerstitial lupus nephritis. Am J Kidney Dis 1996;27:273–8.
83. Mori Y, Kishimoto N, Yamahara H, et al. Predominant tubulointerstitial nephritis in a patient with systemic lupus nephritis. Clin Exp Nephrol 2005;9:79–84.
84. Brentjens JR, Sepulveda M, Baliah T, et al. Interstitial immune complex nephritis in patients with systemic lupus erythematosus. Kidney Int 1975;7:342–50.
85. Park MH, D'Agati V, Appel GB, et al. Tubulointerstitial disease in lupus nephritis: relationship to immune deposits, interstitial inflammation, glomerular changes, renal function, and prognosis. Nephron 1986;44:309–19.
86. Alexopoulos E, Seron D, Hartley RB, et al. Lupus nephritis: correlation of interstitial cells with glomerular function. Kidney Int 1990;37:100–9.
87. Yu F, Wu LH, Tan Y, et al. Tubulointerstitial lesions of patients with lupus nephritis classified by the 2003 International Society of Nephrology and Renal Pathology Society system. Kidney Int 2010;77:820–9.
88. Kozeny GA, Barr W, Bansal VK, et al. Occurrence of renal tubular dysfunction in lupus nephritis. Arch Intern Med 1987;147:891–5.
89. DeFronzo RA, Cooke CR, Goldberg M, et al. Impaired renal tubular potassium secretion in systemic lupus erythematosus. Ann Intern Med 1977;86:268–71.
90. Denton CP, Khanna D. Systemic sclerosis. Lancet 2017;390:1685–99.
91. Shanmugam VK, Steen VD. Renal disease in scleroderma: an update on evaluation, risk stratification, pathogenesis and management. Curr Opin Rheumatol 2012;24:669–76.

92. Penn H, Denton CP. Diagnosis, management and prevention of scleroderma renal disease. Curr Opin Rheumatol 2008;20:692–6.
93. Feriozzi S, Muda AO, Gomes V, et al. Cephotaxime-associated allergic interstitial nephritis and MPO-ANCA positive vasculitis. Ren Fail 2000;22:245–51.
94. Sakai N, Wada T, Shimizu M, et al. Tubulointerstitial nephritis with anti-neutrophil cytoplasmic antibody following indomethacin treatment. Nephrol Dial Transplant 1999;14:2774.
95. Kitahara T, Hiromura K, Sugawara M, et al. A case of cimetidine-induced acute tubulointerstitial nephritis associated with antineutrophil cytoplasmic antibody. Am J Kidney Dis 1999;33:E7.

Thrombotic Microangiopathies with Rheumatologic Involvement

Faizan Babar, MD, Scott D. Cohen, MD, MPH*

KEYWORDS

- Thrombotic microangiopathies • Systemic lupus erythematosus
- Antiphospholipid antibody syndrome • Scleroderma

KEY POINTS

- Thrombotic microangiopathies are a heterogeneous group of disorders, of which autoimmune diseases are one subtype.
- Thrombotic microangiopathy is characterized by endothelial cell injury leading to vascular thrombosis and organ ischemia.
- Complement system dysregulation and the development of autoantibodies against the von Willebrand factor cleaving protease ADAMTS13 play a key role in the pathogenesis of thrombotic microangiopathy.
- Systemic lupus erythematosus, antiphospholipid antibody syndrome, and scleroderma are commonly associated with thrombotic microangiopathy.
- Treatment involves immunosuppression to treat the underlying autoimmune disease and the use of renin–angiotensin–aldosterone system inhibitors to treat hypertension associated with chronic thrombotic microangiopathy.

Thrombotic microangiopathy (TMA) is a clinicopathologic diagnosis defined as microangiopathic hemolytic anemia (MAHA) with associated features of thrombocytopenia and end-organ ischemia, including the kidneys, central nervous system, and lungs.[1,2] The kidney is particularly susceptible to the endothelial injury of TMA owing to its highly specialized vascular capillary network, the glomerulus.[3] There is a growing appreciation for the vital role of complement system dysregulation and the development of autoantibodies against the von Willebrand factor cleaving protease, ADAMTS13, in the pathogenesis of TMA[4] (**Fig. 1**).

Renal TMA is characterized by endothelial cell injury leading to vascular thrombosis and organ ischemia. Histologically, TMA presents as fibrin thrombi (fragmented red cells) trapped in glomerular endothelium and mesangium[5] (**Figs. 2–4**). Other light microscopic features include mesangiolysis and mesangial cell interposition leading to glomerular basement duplication characteristic of membranoproliferative

Disclosures: None.
Division of Renal Diseases and Hypertension, Department of Medicine, George Washington University, 2150 Pennsylvania Avenue, Washington, DC 20037, USA
* Corresponding author.
E-mail address: scohen@mfa.gwu.edu

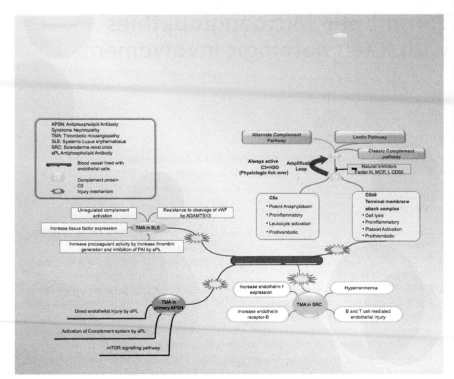

Fig. 1. Pathogenic mechanisms of thrombotic microangiopathy in rheumatic diseases. There is a role for dysregulated complement, resistance to cleavage of von Willebrand's factor by ADAMTS13 and direct endothelial cell injury by antiphospholipid antibody.

glomerulonephritis pattern of injury.[5] In chronic TMA, arteries and arterioles can have intimal proliferation with mucoid changes and entrapped red blood cell fragments or frank necrosis and/or fibrin thrombi.[5] Immunofluorescence studies shows positive staining for fibrin thrombi and occasional nonspecific staining for C3, IgM, or IgG. On electron microscopy, there are features of endothelial cell swelling with loss of

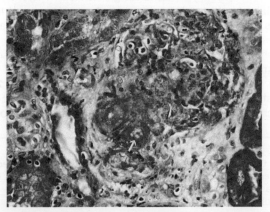

Fig. 2. A 20X Masson trichrome stain. Arteriolar thrombus (*Yellow arrow*) in the glomerulus in a patient with underlying class IV lupus nephritis with thrombotic microangiopathies (TMA). SLE, systemic lupus erythematosus.

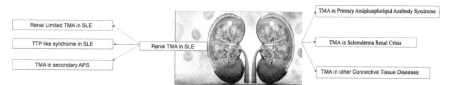

Fig. 3. Classification of thrombotic microangiopathy categorized into infectious, medication related, complement disorders, metabolic disorders, malignancy, thrombotic thrombocytopenic purpura, and autoimmune diseases.

fenestration and trapped fibrin thrombi with fragmented red blood cells.[5] TMA is a heterogeneous entity with a broad differential diagnosis (**Box 1**). This review highlights TMA-related kidney injury associated with rheumatologic diseases.

THROMBOTIC MICROANGIOPATHY IN SYSTEMIC LUPUS ERYTHEMATOUS

Systemic lupus erythematosus (SLE) is an immune complex–mediated autoimmune disease with multiorgan system involvement. Renal involvement is very common in SLE, with almost 50% of patients with SLE developing kidney disease during their lifetime. Kidney injury in the setting of SLE affects all renal compartments, including the glomerulus, tubulointerstitium, and renal vasculature. Glomerular injury is the most common and characterized by immune complex deposits with variable pathologic presentation classified into various categories by the World Health Organization and later by the International Society of Nephrology/Renal Pathology Society classification criteria.[6–8] Interestingly, neither classification system includes TMA. The presentation of TMA in SLE has distinct pathogenesis, risk factors, renal outcomes, and overall prognosis. TMA in SLE may be considered as a separate category across the spectrum of lupus nephritis. The presence of TMA can be further delineated into various categories (see **Box 1**). We discuss each of these subtypes in detail.

RENAL-LIMITED THROMBOTIC MICROANGIOPATHIES IN SYSTEMIC LUPUS ERYTHEMATOSUS

A TMA pattern in lupus nephritis has been described in several observational series.[9–11] In 1 study, TMA lesions were seen in 36 cases of lupus nephritis (24%; n = 148) with or

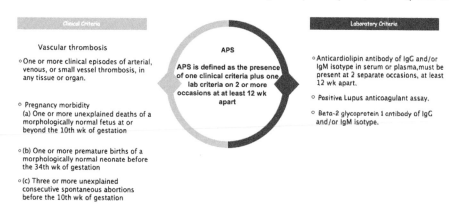

Fig. 4. Revised classification criteria for antiphospholipid antibody syndrome (APS) defined as the presence of one clinical criteria plus 1 laboratory criteria on 2 or more occasions at least 12 weeks apart.

Box 1
Classification of TMA

Infectious Etiology
- Enterohemorrhagic *Escherichia coli*
- *Shigella dysenteriae*
- *Streptococcus pneumoniae*
- Influenza A/H1N1
- Human immunodeficiency virus
- Others: Epstein-Barr virus, cytomegalovirus, parvovirus B19, mycoplasma

TMA with rheumatic diseases
- TMA in systemic lupus erythematosus: renal limited TMA, thrombotic thrombocytopenic purpura-like picture, TMA with positive antiphospholipid antibody syndrome serology
- TMA in primary antiphospholipid antibody syndrome
- TMA in scleroderma renal crisis
- TMA in other autoimmune diseases: rheumatoid arthritis, Still's disease, juvenile dermatomyositis

Drug-induced TMA
- Calcineurin inhibitors
- Ticlopidine
- Clopidogrel
- Quinine
- Tyrosine kinase inhibitors
- Vascular endothelial growth factor inhibitors
- Gemcitabine
- Mitomycin C

Thrombotic thrombocytopenic purpura
- Hereditary
- Autoimmune

Metabolic disorders
- Cobalamin deficiency
- Diacylglycerol kinase epsilon mutation

Disorders of complement regulation
- Atypical hemolytic uremic syndrome
- Hereditary
- Autoimmune
- Pregnancy related
- Transplantation (recurrence in renal allograft)

Malignancy

Abbreviation: TMA, thrombotic microangiopathy.

---

without immune complex renal disease.[9] Positive antiphospholipid antibody syndrome (APS) serology was seen in 2 of the 36 cases.[9] In this series, patients with TMA had a more aggressive renal course with worsening acute kidney injury.

The exact mechanism of TMA associated with SLE is not well-understood. Activation of the different complement pathways by autoantibodies has been described in the pathogenesis of TMA in the setting of SLE.[12,13] Activation of the classic complement pathway is evident with the deposition of C4d and the presence of fibrin microthrombi in glomerular capillaries of patients with SLE.[12,14] Observational studies show an association of infections preceding TMA in the setting of SLE, which supports a role for activation of the classic complement pathway.[13] Recently, activation of the alternate complement pathway is described with TMA in parallel with SLE flares.[15,16] The alternate complement pathway is unique owing to its constant low background activity and autoactivation properties termed the physiologic tick over.[17] Several regulatory proteins, including complement factor H, factor I, and membrane cofactor protein, control alternate complement pathway activity.[18] Genetic mutation or functional deficiency in the presence of autoantibodies against complement regulatory proteins result in uncontrolled activation of the complement pathway.[19] Low complement factor H levels (one of the complement regulatory proteins implicated in the pathogenesis of atypical hemolytic uremic syndrome) are also noted to be decreased in SLE.[9,20] The alternate complement pathway serves as an amplification loop for the classical pathway activation, resulting in the generation of the membrane attack complex C5b-9 causing endothelial cell damage and microthrombi formation.[17] Positive C4d immunostaining and the presence of low complement factor H levels are markers of higher disease activity in TMA related to lupus nephritis.[9]

Patients with TMA injury have distinct clinical presentation. There may be higher degrees of proteinuria compared with other forms of lupus nephritis.[9] The TMA pattern can be found with or without immune complex deposits on pathology. Diffuse proliferative lupus nephritis with subendothelial immune complex deposits (class IV lupus nephritis) is most commonly seen along with TMA lesions.[9,13] Elevated anti-dsDNA titers and hypocomplementemia are not predictive of a TMA pattern of renal injury. Anemia and thrombocytopenia are observed more often with TMA-related lupus nephritis.[13] However, in several reports, TMA injury was only evident on renal biopsies, suggesting isolated renal involvement with no systemic manifestations is possible.[9,10] Long-term renal survival is poor with TMA injury in the setting of lupus nephritis compared with lupus nephritis alone.[9] However, there are mixed results on overall patient survival.[13,21]

THROMBOTIC THROMBOCYTOPENIC PURPURA–LIKE SYNDROME WITH SYSTEMIC LUPUS ERYTHEMATOSUS

Thrombotic thrombocytopenic purpura (TTP) is characterized by the pentad of thrombocytopenia, hemolytic anemia, fever, renal failure, and confusion. Idiopathic TTP carried a high mortality before the introduction of plasma exchange therapy. Classic TTP has been reported in patients with SLE.[10,22,23] Understanding the role of ADAMTS13 is crucial in differentiating idiopathic classic TTP from other TMAs associated with SLE.[24] ADAMTS13 is responsible for the cleavage of large multimers of von Willebrand factor, which prevents platelet aggregation and ultimately thrombosis. Deficiency of ADAMTS13 owing to a genetic mutation in hereditary causes or reduced activity in the presence of an autoantibody inhibitor leads to platelet aggregation and resultant thrombosis. MAHA with SLE is believed to be a distinct entity with poor prognosis.[21] Data from various studies have shown that patients with SLE-associated TTP do not typically have reduced ADAMTS13 activity.[25] Other mechanisms have been proposed for MAHA in the setting of SLE. In 1 in vitro study, the proinflammatory state renders von Willebrand factor resistant to proteolysis mediated by free radical species.[26,27] As a result, oxidized von Willebrand factor might be resistant to cleavage by ADAMTS13 in the proinflammatory state of SLE. Other possible mechanisms of MAHA might be related to antiendothelial antibodies and complement activation with active SLE.[24] Diagnosing MAHA with SLE can be challenging owing to significant overlap in the features, because thrombocytopenia and anemia can be immune mediated with lupus nephritis. Various clinical features may differentiate classic TTP from SLE-associated TTP. Severe acute kidney injury is more likely with secondary TTP associated with SLE compared with classic TTP with renal injury.[28] The prevalence of renal TMAs is likely underestimated owing to lack of biopsy data in patients with severe thrombocytopenia. Other features seen with TTP include a negative direct Coombs test, elevated lactate dehydrogenase, reduced haptoglobin, and the presence of schistocytes on peripheral blood smear. Presence of any one of these systemic features with renal failure should raise the possibility of TTP secondary to SLE.

MANAGEMENT OF THROMBOTIC MICROANGIOPATHIES IN SYSTEMIC LUPUS ERYTHEMATOSUS

The treatment of TMA in the setting of SLE involves immunosuppression to control the disease flare. No specific therapeutic strategy has been described for TMA-related renal injury in SLE. Immunosuppressive medications including corticosteroids, cyclophosphamide, mycophenolate azathioprine, and, rituximab have all been used in TMA-related injury with SLE.[29] Plasma exchange is frequently used to treat TMA-related renal injury.[9,11,21] Response to plasma exchange in combination with immunosuppressive agents has been poor in renal limited TMA in SLE.[9] There are higher treatment failure and relapse rates observed in the TMA-related cohort compared with the non-TMA group of patients with SLE. However, in the TTP-like presentation with SLE, the response to plasma exchange is variable. In 1 observational study plasma exchange combined with corticosteroids showed a positive renal and hematologic response.[11] However, in another observational study treatment failure with plasma exchange was higher in renal TMA with SLE.[28] Cyclophosphamide and mycophenolate mofetil have been used as induction agents in TMA with proliferative lupus nephritis. There is no evidence suggesting the superiority of cyclophosphamide over mycophenolate in TMA with SLE.

Recent insights into the role of the complement system in the pathogenesis of TMA further delineated describing the role of complement inhibitors in TMA-related injury in SLE.[30,31] Eculizumab is a monoclonal antibody that blocks C5a preventing the formation of the terminal MAC complex C5b9.

The role of rituximab in the treatment of TMA secondary to autoimmune diseases is being explored. Rituximab is a monoclonal antibody directed against the CD20 antigen on B cells leading to B-cell apoptosis. Several case reports describe the role of rituximab as an adjunct immunosuppressive agent in TMA-related renal injury secondary to SLE.[32] In refractory cases of TTP-like clinical presentations SLE, rituximab has shown some benefit.[28] One observational study looked at the role of rituximab in TMA with SLE. The study demonstrated an increase in overall patient survival with rituximab use. However, renal survival was unchanged with the addition of rituximab to conventional therapy.[33]

THROMBOTIC MICROANGIOPATHY IN PRIMARY ANTIPHOSPHOLIPID SYNDROME

APS is characterized by vascular thrombosis with positive antiphospholipid antibodies (aPL). APS can be primary or secondary. Secondary APS is defined by positive aPL serology in the setting of other autoimmune disease mainly SLE. Primary APS is defined as the presence of aPLs (lupus anticoagulant, beta 2 glycoprotein, and anticardiolipin antibodies), and vascular thrombosis of arterial or venous type, and spontaneous pregnancy loss. In 1992, standardized criteria were established for definitive APS.[34,35] These criteria were later modified in 2006 and include (1) clinical manifestations of vascular thrombosis or obstetric manifestations and (2) sustained detection of 1 of 3 aPL.[36] However, the clinical spectrum of APS extends beyond the established criteria, with microvascular injury seen in various organs, including the kidneys, nervous system, heart valves, and skin.

Renal histopathologic features of APS include fibrous intimal hyperplasia and severe tubular injury with tubular dilation and pseudothyroidization.[37] There are few data on the prevalence of APS nephropathy (APSN). In a large cohort of patients with APS, the prevalence of renal disease was 2.7%.[38] The exact prevalence of TMA-related injury in APSN is not known. Biopsy series have shown the prevalence of TMA with APSN to be approximately 30%.[37] TMA-related APSN typically presents with acute kidney injury, but may also have subacute presentations. The presence of systemic findings including MAHA and thrombocytopenia are not seen commonly with renal TMA in primary APS.[37] The acute decrease in kidney function with TMA-related renal injury is distinct from the more indolent clinical presentation of renal injury with APS characterized by hypertension, subnephrotic proteinuria, hematuria, and a slow progressive decline in renal function. Extrarenal manifestations of TMA, involving the skin, pulmonary, and central nervous systems, have been seen with catastrophic APS.[39]

Pathogenesis

It is possible that aPL antibodies have direct cytotoxic effect on endothelium, resulting in endothelial injury. The endothelial cell injury leads to platelet aggregation and activation, causing microvascular injury and thrombosis.[40] Complement system involvement in TMA injury is seen in animal models. aPL derived from humans were able to induce complement activation and deposition of the terminal membrane attack complex in glomeruli in mice.[36,41,42] Increased tissue factor expression and complement activation with aPL has been shown to cause increased thrombosis and fetal loss.[41] The role of an activated complement system has also been shown in renal allografts with TMA in the setting of APS.[42] Both C4d staining and the presence of the terminal MAC complex C5b9 have been shown in blood vessels affected by TMA lesions in the renal allograft.[42] A role for the mammalian target of rapamycin pathway in APSN has also been shown to cause a chronic vasculopathy in primary APS.[43] The role of the mammalian target of rapamycin pathway in TMA-related injury needs further research.

THROMBOTIC MICROANGIOPATHY IN SECONDARY ANTIPHOSPHOLIPID SYNDROME

Various observational studies have shown the presence of a TMA pattern as a manifestation of APS with SLE.[8,44] TMA was one of the first vascular injury patterns seen with positive aPL serologies (lupus anticoagulant, anticardiolipin antibodies, beta 2 glycoproteins).[45] Systemic features of MAHA along with a TMA lesion in the kidney have been seen with secondary APS, regardless of underlying lupus glomerulopathy.[46] In 1 observational study regarding biopsy-proven lupus nephritis, 14 of 37 biopsy cases showed features of TMA. Of the cases with TMA findings, 50% had a positive APS serology (n = 14).[46] No association of specific aPL serology with TMA injury has been described. However, observational data suggest a stronger association between lupus anticoagulant and the development of APS in patients with SLE.[10] The exact mechanism of thrombotic microvascular injury with secondary APS is not known. Endothelial dysfunction mediated by aPL and persistent inflammation results in increased thrombin generation, predisposing to increased rates of microvascular thrombosis.[47] The increased procoagulant activity is due to inhibition of the plasminogen activator inhibitor in SLE with positive aPL.[48]

The role of decreased ADAMTS13 activity with antibodies against ADAMTS13 have been described in patients with secondary APS, suggesting a TTP-like picture.[4] These findings may suggest a unique variant of APS with reduced ADAMTS13 activity, presenting with MAHA and renal failure. Clinical presentation in secondary APS is variable. APSN may be seen across various classes of lupus nephritis in the presence of aPL. One study demonstrated an association between APSN with class IV diffuse proliferative lupus nephritis.[44] Accelerated hypertension, nephrotic syndrome, and severe acute kidney injury are seen in acute APSN with SLE. Renal injury owing to TMA is also seen with catastrophic APS involving other organs resulting in noninflammatory vascular thrombosis.[39] The presence of a TMA lesion in APS portends a poor prognosis.[39] Long-term follow-up has shown worsening renal function owing to progression from acute microvascular thrombosis to progressive glomerulosclerosis and fibrocellular intimal proliferation.[49]

MANAGEMENT OF THROMBOTIC MICROANGIOPATHIES WITH ANTIPHOSPHOLIPID ANTIBODY SYNDROME

There is limited evidence for the management of APS vasculopathy. The optimal treatment of primary APSN is unclear. Angiotensin-converting enzyme inhibitors are used as first-line therapy for blood pressure control.[10,47] Chronic anticoagulation to prevent microvascular thrombosis and immunosuppression with steroids to deplete pathogenic aPLs are cornerstones in the management.[50] However, the role of anticoagulation in APSN is unclear, because some patients experience a continued decline in renal function despite optimal anticoagulation.[51]

The growing appreciation for the role of dysregulated complement system activation in TMA related to APSN has led to clinical studies exploring a potential role for eculizumab. Several case reports demonstrated the effectiveness of eculizumab in primary and secondary APSN.[30] The combination of complement blockade therapy with plasma exchange and high-dose corticosteroids is a potentially effective strategy, specifically in catastrophic APS.[42,52] Eculizumab has also been proven to be effective in TMA with catastrophic APS that does not respond to plasmapheresis.[53] Likewise, B-cell depletion with rituximab is another effective therapeutic option in treating patients with catastrophic APS with good hematologic and renal recovery, although data are limited.[54]

THROMBOTIC MICROANGIOPATHY IN SCLERODERMA

Scleroderma can also present with TMA and is termed scleroderma renal crisis (SRC). SRC is considered a rheumatologic emergency requiring prompt diagnosis and treatment. SRC is characterized by acute kidney injury and systemic MAHA with or without accelerated hypertension.[55,56] The renal histopathology of SRC is characterized by intimal proliferation, thickening, and vascular thrombosis resulting in luminal narrowing and glomerular ischemic injury.[57] Renal biopsy findings in SRC overlap with pathologic features of malignant hypertension and other rheumatologic diseases with TMA. However, thrombotic lesions in SRC are mostly confined to small vessels, including arteries and arterioles compared with glomeruli. The exact pathogenesis of TMA in SRC is unknown. The role of both B-cell–mediated and T-cell–mediated immunity in endothelial injury has been described in animal models of SRC.[58–60] The role of autoantibodies against RNA polymerase I, II, and III causing endothelial injury has also been shown.[61,62] In addition to antibody-mediated endothelial injury, overexpression of endothelin-1 and its receptor endothelin-B have been seen in cases of SRC.[63] Risk factors for SRC include diffuse cutaneous manifestations, prior use of corticosteroids, and the presence of antitopoisomerase antibodies.[64] Patients with SRC present with severe acute kidney injury with or without accelerated hypertension as a result of hyperreninemia.[55,56] Systemic features of MAHA (anemia, thrombocytopenia, and evidence of hemolysis) are seen in 50% to 60% of patients with SRC.[65] In 1 observational study, a higher association of MAHA was noted with normotensive SRC.[56] Other clinical features seen in SRC include headaches, blurred vision, and cardiac involvement.[66] Observational studies have shown improved renal outcomes in patients with dialysis-dependent SRC who are hypertensive compared with those who are normotensive. The exact reason for the poor renal outcomes in normotensive patients is unknown; however, this outcome may reflect increased cardiac involvement.[56] N-Terminal pro-brain natriuretic peptide may be a potential biomarker in determining outcomes in SRC.[67,68] Elevated N-terminal pro-brain natriuretic peptide has been associated with poor renal outcomes.[67,68] However, pro-brain natriuretic peptide is cleared renally and elevated levels are associated with decreases in the glomerular filtration rate.

No clear association exists between the systemic manifestations of MAHA and renal outcomes. In 1 observational study, the presence of MAHA was associated with poor renal outcomes.[68] However, another study did not show any association of MAHA with renal recovery.[56]

The diagnosis of SRC can be challenging owing to the significant overlap in clinical features with other causes of TMA. The diagnosis of SRC relies on strong clinical suspicion in cases of accelerated hypertension and acute kidney injury, progressive cutaneous involvement with systemic sclerosis, positive autoantibodies against topoisomerase I and II, and a prior history of steroid use in the previous 15 days.[64]

TREATMENT OF SCLERODERMA RENAL CRISIS

The introduction of angiotensin-converting enzyme inhibitors for the treatment of SRC led to a significant decrease in mortality. At a single medical center, the 1-year mortality rate decreased from 85% to 24%.[69] Angiotensin-converting enzyme inhibitors significantly improve blood pressure for many patients and, in some cases, may also lead to regression of cutaneous manifestations of scleroderma.[70] Despite the known clinical effectiveness of angiotensin-converting enzyme inhibitors in SRC, there has been no randomized trial to validate the effectiveness of angiotensin-converting enzyme inhibitors.

The role of angiotensin receptor blockers as monotherapy for SRC is unclear. Higher rates of renal failure and suboptimal blood pressure control have been reported with angiotensin receptor blocker monotherapy for SRC.[71,72] Increased expression of endothelin-mediated endothelial injury has led to an exploration of the therapeutic effectiveness of endothelin receptor antagonists in SRC. The efficacy of bosentin (an endothelin receptor blocker) in SRC has been described.[70,73,74] Endothelin receptor antagonists have shown promising results in controlling blood pressure and improving renal function in SRC. Other novel agents like aliskiren, a direct renin antagonist, have also shown promise in controlling blood pressure.[74] However, combination of renin–angiotensin–aldosterone system inhibitors is not recommended given clinical trial data showing higher rates of acute kidney injury and hyperkalemia in other patient populations.[75,76]

Immunosuppression has not been shown to be effective in SRC. Prednisone at doses of greater than 15 mg/d is a risk factor to precipitate SRC.[77] Similarly, cyclosporine can increase nephrotoxicity in this setting and can trigger renal crisis. Plasmapheresis might be effective in cases of severe TMA with SRC. Further investigation is needed to evaluate the role of the complement inhibitor eculizumab in SRC. Currently no data exist for the use of eculizumab in SRC.

THROMBOTIC MICROANGIOPATHY IN OTHER RHEUMATIC DISEASES

Renal TMA has also been reported in rheumatoid arthritis, adult Still's disease, and dermatomyositis.[78] Renal involvement is rarely noted in patients with these connective tissue diseases; however, case reports have described renal TMA with systemic features of MAHA. Positive antiphospholipid serology and ADAMTS13 deficiency have been reported in several cases.[79,80] The presence of APS antibodies or ADAMTS13 deficiency might explain the development of TMA in rheumatoid arthritis and dermatomyositis. No distinct pathogenesis of TMA has been described in the literature for rheumatoid arthritis or dermatomyositis. Treatment consisted of plasmapheresis and immunosuppression including steroids and cyclophosphamide.[78,81] Eculizumab was used in 1 patient with TMA with juvenile dermatomyositis who experienced a subsequent improvement in renal function.[82]

SUMMARY

There are a variety of autoimmune diseases associated with the development of TMA, including SLE, scleroderma, and APS. The pathogenesis is distinct from classic TTP-associated with deficiency of ADAMTS13. TMA is more common in the setting of SLE and APS. Treatment options focus on control of the underlying connective tissue disease and may include plasmapheresis as well as biologic therapies including rituximab and eculizumab. Control of blood pressure with renin–angiotensin–aldosterone system inhibition is a cornerstone in the management of chronic TMA. Additional studies are needed to determine the optimal treatment approach in patients with autoimmune diseases and TMA (**Fig. 5**).

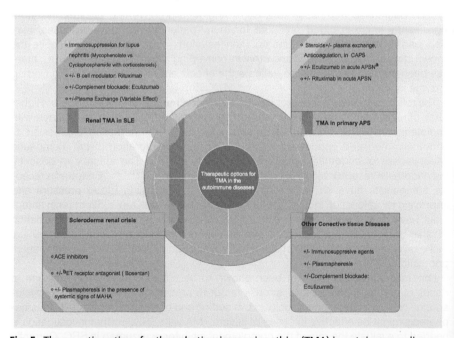

Fig. 5. Therapeutic options for thrombotic microangiopathies (TMA) in autoimmune diseases. Treatment options consist of immunosuppression for the underlying rheumatic disease including cyclophosphamide, mycophenolate mofetil, corticosteroids, rituximab, eculizumab, and plasma exchange. Anticoagulation is essential in the setting of primary antiphospholipid antibody syndrome. Angiotensin-converting enzyme (ACE) inhibitors are first-line therapy for scleroderma renal crisis. APSN, antiphospholipid antibody syndrome nephropathy; CAPS, Catastrophic Antiphospholipid Syndrome; ET, Endothelin Antagonist; MAHA, microangiopathic hemolytic anemia; SLE, systemic lupus erythematosus. [a] Acute antiphospholipid antibody syndrome ephropathy. [b] ET Endothelin receptor.

ACKNOWLEDGMENTS

The authors wish to thank Mary Fidler, MD, Mayo Clinic, Department of Pathology for provision of clinical photomicrographs.

REFERENCES

1. Go RS, Winters JL, Leung N, et al. Thrombotic microangiopathy care pathway: a consensus statement for the mayo clinic complement alternative pathway-thrombotic microangiopathy (CAP-TMA) disease-oriented group. Mayo Clin Proc 2016;91(9):1189–211.
2. George JN, Nester CM. Syndromes of thrombotic micro-angiopathy. N Engl J Med 2014;371:654–66.
3. Kerr H, Richards A. Complement-mediated injury and protection of endothelium: lessons from atypical haemolytic uraemic syndrome. Immunobiology 2012; 217(2):195–203.
4. Austin SK, Starke RD, Lawrie AS, et al. The VWF/ADAMTS-13 axis antibodies and ADAMTS-13 dysfunction. Br J Haematol 2008;141:536–44.
5. Lusco MA, Fogo AB, Najafian B, et al. AJKD atlas of renal pathology: thrombotic microangiopathy. Am J Kidney Dis 2016;68(6):e33–4.
6. Weening JJ, D'Agati VD, Schwartz MM, et al. The classification of glomerulonephritis in systemic lupus erythematosus revisited. J Am Soc Nephrol 2004;15:241–50.
7. Churg J, Sobin LH. Renal disease: classification and atlas of glomerular disease. Tokyo: Igaku-Shoin; 1982.
8. Churg J, Bernstein J, Glassock RJ. Renal disease: classification and atlas of glomerular diseases. 2nd edition. New York: Igaky- Shoin; 1995.
9. Song D, Wu LH, Wang FM, et al. The spectrum of renal thrombotic microangiop-athy in lupus nephritis. Arthritis Res Ther 2013;1(15):R12.
10. Daugas E, Nochy D, Huong DL, et al. Antiphospholipid syndrome nephropathy in systemic lupus erythematosus. J Am Soc Nephrol 2002;13(1):42–52.
11. Nesher G, Vaughn VE, Terry TL, et al. Thrombotic microangiografthic hemolytic anemia in systemic lupus erythematosus. Review article. Semin Arthritis Rheum 1994;24(3):165–72.
12. Cohen D, Koopmans M, Kremer Hovinga IC, et al. Potential for glomerular C4d as an indicator of thrombotic microangiopathy in lupus nephritis. Arthritis Rheum 2008;58(8):2460–9.
13. Chen MH, Chen MH, Chen WS, et al. Thrombotic microangiopathy in systemic lupus erythematosus: a cohort study in North Taiwan. Rheumatology 2011; 50(4):768–75.
14. Shen Y, Chen X, Sun C, et al. Association between anti-β2 glycoprotein antibodies and renal glomerular C4d deposition in lupus nephritis patients with glomerular mi-crothrombosis: a prospective study of 155 cases. Lupus 2010;19:1195–203.
15. Li S, Liu Z, Zen C, et al. Peritubular capillary C4d deposition in lupus nephritis different from antibody-mediated renal rejection. Lupus 2007;16:875–80.
16. Sato N, Ohsawa I, Nagamachi S, et al. Significance of glomerular activation of the alternative pathway and lectin pathway in lupus nephritis. Lupus 2011;20:1378–86.
17. Lachmann PJ. The amplification loop of the contents complement pathways. Adv Immunol 2009;104:115–49.
18. Estaller C, Weiss EH, Schwaeble W, et al. Human complement factor H: two factor H proteins are derived from alternatively spliced transcripts. Eur J Immunol 1991; 21:799–802.

19. Bao L, Haas M, Quigg RJ, et al. Complement factor H deficiency accelerates development of lupus nephritis. J Am Soc Nephrol 2010;22:285–95.

20. Lee BH, Kwak SH, Shin JI, et al. Atypical hemolytic uremic syndrome associated with complement factor H autoantibodies and CFHR1/CFHR3 deficiency. Pediatr Res 2009;66:336–40.

21. Musio F, Bohen EM, Yuan CM, et al. Review of thrombotic thrombocytopenic purpura in the settings of systemic lupus erythematosus. Semin Arthritis Rheum 1998;28(1):1–19.

22. Lim GT, Kim SS, Park SH, et al. Thrombotic thrombocytopenic purpura-like syndrome associated with systemic lupus erythematosus–combined treatment with plasmapheresis and fresh frozen plasma infusion. J Korean Med Sci 1992;7(1): 66–70.

23. Roca-Tey R, Anglés R, Palomar M. Systemic lupus erythematosus and thrombotic thrombocytopenic purpura. Med Clin (Barc) 1994;102(2):75–6.

24. Lansigan F, Isufi I, Tagoe E. Microangiopathic hemolytic anemia resembling thrombotic thrombocytopenia purpura, in systemic lupus erythematosus: the role of ADAMTS-13. Rehumatology (Oxford) 2011;50:824–9.

25. Mannucci PM, Vanoli M, Forza I, et al. Von Willebrand factor cleaving protease (ADAMTS-13) in 123 patients with connective tissue diseases (systemic lupus erythematosus and systemic sclerosis). Haematologica 2003;88(8):914–8.

26. Lancellotti S, De Filippis V, Pozzi N, et al. Formation of methionine sulfoxide by peroxynitrite at position 1606 of vWF inhibits cleavage by ADAMTS-13. a new prothrombotic mechanism in a disease associated with oxidative stress. Free Radic Biol Med 2010;48(3):446–56.

27. Chen J, Fu X, Wang Y, et al. Oxidative modification of von Willebrand factor by neutrophil oxidants inhibits its cleavage by ADAMTS13. Blood 2010;115(3): 706–12.

28. Letchumanan P, Ng HJ, Lee LH, et al. A comparison of thrombotic thrombocytopenia purpura in an inception cohort of patients with and without systemic lupus erythematosus. Rheumatology (Oxford) 2009;48(4):399–403.

29. Hamasaki K, Miura T, Kanda H, et al. Systemic lupus erythematosus and thrombotic thrombocytopenia purpura: a case report and literature review. Clin Rheumatol 2003;22:355–8.

30. De Holanda MI, Porto LC, Wagner T, et al. Use of eculizumab in a systemic lupus erythematosus patient presenting thrombotic microangiopathy and heterozygous deletion in CFHR1-CFHR3. A case report and systematic review. Clin Rheumatol 2017;36(12):2859–67.

31. El-Husseini A, Hannan S, Awad A, et al. Thrombotic microangiopathy in systemic lupus erythematosus: efficacy of eculizumab. Am J Kidney Dis 2015;65(1):127–30.

32. Gharbi CH, Philippe B, Sabria R, et al. Rapidly progressive lupus nephritis and concomitant thrombotic microangiopathy. Clin Exp Nephrol 2010;14(5):487–91.

33. Sun F, Wang X, Wu W, et al. TMA secondary to SLE: rituximab improves overall but not renal survival. Clin Rheumatol 2018;37(1):213–8.

34. Levine JS, Branch DW, Rauch J. The antiphospholipid syndrome. N Engl Med 2002;346:752–63.

35. Hughson MD, Nadasdy T, McCarty GA, et al. Renal thrombotic microangiopathy in patients with systemic lupus erythematosus and the antiphospholipid syndrome. Am J Kidney Dis 1992;20:150–8.

36. Miyakis S, Lockshin MD, Atsumi T, et al. International consensus statement on an update of the classification criteria for definite antiphospholipid syndrome (APS). J Thromb Haemost 2006;4:295–306.

37. Nochy D, Daugas E, Droz D, et al. The intrarenal vascular lesions associated with primary antiphospholipid syndrome. Arthritis Rheum 2002;46(4):1019–27.

38. Cervera R, Piette JC, Font J, et al. Antiphospholipid syndrome: clinical and immunologic manifestations and patterns of disease expression in a cohort of 1,000 patients Euro-Phospholipid Project Group. Arthritis Rheum 2002;46(4):1019–27.

39. Stratta P, Canavese C, Ferrero S, et al. Catastrophic antiphospholipid syndromes in systemic lupus erythematosus. Ren Fail 1999;21(1):49–61.

40. Lanir N, Zilberman M, Yron I, et al. Reactivity patterns of antiphospholipid antibodies and endothelial cells: effect of antiendothelial antibodies on cell migration. J Lab Clin Med 1998;131:548–56.

41. Seshan SV, Franzke CW, Redecha P, et al. Role of tissue factor in a mouse model of thrombotic microangiopathy induced by antiphospholipid antibodies. Blood 2009;114:1675–83.

42. Hadaya K, Ferrari-Lacraz S, Fumeaux D, et al. Eculizumab in acute recurrence of thrombotic microangiopathy after renal transplantation. Am J Transplant 2011; 11(11):2523–7.

43. Canaud G, Bienaime F, Tabarin F, et al. Inhibition of the mTORC pathway in the antiphospholipid syndrome. N Engl J Med 2014;371:303–12.

44. Miranda JM, Jara LJ, Calleja C, et al. Clinical significance of antiphospholipid syndrome nephropathy (APSN) in patients with systemic lupus erythematosus SLE. Reumatol Clin 2009;5(5):209–13.

45. Kant KS, Pollack VE, Weiss MA, et al. Glomerular thrombosis in systemic lupus erythematosus: prevalence and significance. Medicine 1981;60:71–80.

46. Frampton G, Hicks J, Cameron JS. Significance of anti-phospholipid antibodies in patients with lupus nephritis. Kidney Int 1991;39:1225–31.

47. Musial J, Swadzba J, Szceklik A. Adaptive mechanism of counterbalancing enhanced thrombogenesis in antiphospholipid syndrome. Thromb Haemost 1994;71:424–7.

48. Yamazaki M, Asakura H, Jokaji H, et al. Plasma levels of lipoprotein are elevated in patients with antiphospholipid antibody syndrome. Thromb Haemost 1994;71:424–7.

49. Banfi G, Bertani T, Boeri V, et al. Renal vascular lesions as a marker of poor prognosis in patients with lupus nephritis Gruppo Italiano per lo Studio della Nefrite Lupica (GISNEL). Am J Kidney Dis 1991;18(2):240–8.

50. Sinico RA, Cavazzana I, Nuzzo M, et al. Renal involvement in primary antiphospholipid syndrome: retrospective analysis of 160 patients. Clin J Am Soc Nephrol 2010;5(7):1211–7.

51. Bienaime F, Legendre C, Terzi F, et al. Antiphospholipid syndrome and kidney disease. Kidney Int 2017;91(1):34–44.

52. Lonze BE, Singer AL, Montgomery RA. Eculizumab and renal transplantation in a patient with CAPS. N Engl J Med 2010;362:1744–5.

53. Shapira I, Andrade D, Allen SL, et al. A brief report: induction of sustained remission in recurrent catastrophic antiphospholipid syndrome via inhibition of terminal complement with eculizumab. Arthritis Rheum 2012;64:2719–23.

54. Vieregge GB, Harrington TJ, Andrews D, et al. Catastrophic antiphospholipid syndrome with severe acute thrombotic microangiopathy and hemorrhagic complications. Case Rep Med 2013;2013:915309.

55. Asamoah-Odei E. Scleroderma renal crisis in a normotensive patient internal medicine–nephrology, Christiana Care Health Services, Christiana Care Health System, Newark, Delaware, USA. Kidney Int Rep 2016;1(4):311–5.

56. Helfrich D, Banner B, Virginia D, et al. Renal failure in systemic sclerosis. Arthritis Rheumatol 1989;32(9):1128–34.
57. Batal I, Domsic RT, Medsger TA Jr, et al. Scleroderma renal crisis: a pathology perspective. Int J Rheumatol 2010;2010:543704.
58. Sakkas LI. New developments in the pathogenesis of systemic sclerosis. Autoimmunity 2005;38(2):113–6.
59. Chizzolini C. Update on pathophysiology of scleroderma with special reference to immunoinflammatory events. Ann Med 2007;39(1):42–53.
60. Sato S, Fujimoto M, Hasegawa MK, et al. Altered B lymphocyte function] induces systemic a to immunity in systemic sclerosis. Mol Immunol 2004; 41(12):1123–33.
61. Chang M, Wang RJ, Yangco DT, et al. Analysis of autoantibodies against RNA polymerases using immunoaffinity-purified RNA polymerase I, II, and III antigen in an enzyme-linked immunosorbent assay. Clin Immunol Immunopathol 1998; 89(1):71–8.
62. Santiago M, Baron M, Hudson M, et al. Antibodies to RNA polymerase III in systemic sclerosis detected by ELISA. J Rheumatol 2007;34(7):1528–34.
63. Kobayashi H, Nishimaki T, Kaise S, et al. Immunohistological study of endothelin-1 and endothelin-A and B receptors in two patients with scleroderma renal crisis. Clin Rheumatol 1999;18(5):425–7.
64. Denton CP, Lapadula G, Mouthon L, et al. UK Scleroderma Study Group (UKSSG) guidelines on the diagnosis and management of scleroderma renal crisis. Rheumatology (Oxford) 2009;48(Suppl 3):iii32–5. Renal complications and scleroderma renal crisis.
65. Penn H, Howie AJ, Kingdon EJ, et al. Scleroderma renal crisis: patient characteristics and long-term outcomes. QJM 2007;100(8):485–94.
66. Steen VD, Medsger TA. Long-term outcomes of scleroderma renal crisis. Ann Intern Med 2000;133:600–3.
67. Chighizola CB, Pregnolato F, Meroni PL, et al. N-terminal pro Brain Natriuretic Peptide as predictor of outcome in scleroderma renal crisis. Clin Exp Rheumatol 2016;34(Suppl 100(5)):122–8.
68. Medsger TA Jr, Masi AT, Rodnan GP, et al. Survival with systemic sclerosis (scleroderma). A life-table analysis of clinical and demographic factors in 309 patients. Ann Intern Med 1971;75:369–76.
69. Steen VD, Costantino JP, Shapiro AP, et al. Outcome of renal crisis in systemic sclerosis: relation to availability of angiotensin converting enzyme (ACE) inhibitors. Ann Intern Med 1990;113:352–7.
70. Steen VD. Scleroderma renal crisis. Rheum Dis Clin North Am 2003;29:315–33.
71. Caskey FJ, Thacker EJ, Johnston PA, et al. Failure of losartan to control blood pressure in scleroderma renal crisis. Lancet 1997;349(9052):620.
72. Steen V, DeMarco P. Complications in the use of angiotensin receptor blockers in the treatment of scleroderma renal crisis. Arthritis Rheum 2001;44:397.
73. Penn H, Quillinan N, Khan K, et al. Targeting the endothelin axis in scleroderma renal crisis: rationale and feasibility. QJM An Int J Med 2013;106(9):839–48.
74. Dhaun N, MacIntyre IM, Bellamy CO, et al. Endothelin receptor antagonism and renin inhibition as treatment options for scleroderma kidney. Am J Kidney Dis 2009;54(4):726–31.
75. Fried LF, Emanuele N, Zhang JH, et al. Combined angiotensin inhibition for the treatment of diabetic nephropathy. N Engl J Med 2013;369:1892–903.
76. Mann JF, Schmieder RE, McQueen M, et al. ONTARGET investigators. Lancet 2008;372(9638):547–53.

77. Steen VD, Medsger TA Jr. Case-control study of corticosteroids and other drugs that either precipitate or protect from the development of scleroderma renal crisis. Arthritis Rheum 1998;41:1613–9.
78. Sakthirajan R, Dhanapriya J, Dineshkumar T, et al. Thrombotic microangiopathy: an unusual cause of renal failure in rheumatoid arthritis. Indian J Nephrol 2017; 27(1):81–3.
79. Matsuyama T, Kuwana M, Matsumoto M, et al. Heterogeneous pathogenic processes of thrombotic microangiopathies in patients with connective tissue diseases. Thromb Haemost 2009;102:371–8.
80. Nomura M, Okada J, Tateno S, et al. Renal thrombotic microangiopathy in a patient with rheumatoid arthritis and antiphospholipid syndrome: successful treatment with cyclophosphamide pulse therapy and anticoagulant. Intern Med 1994;33:484–7.
81. Kfoury Baz EM, Mahfouz RA, Masri AF. Thrombotic thrombocytopenic purpura in a patient with rheumatoid arthritis treated by plasmapheresis. Ther Apher 1999; 3(4):314–6.
82. Vanoni F, Jorgensen C, Parve P. A difficult case of juvenile dermatomyositis complicated by thrombotic microangiopathy and Purtscher-like retinopathy. From 18th Pediatric Rheumatology European Society (PReS) Congress Bruges, Belgium, 14–8 Sep. 2011. Abstract

Anti–Glomerular Basement Membrane Disease

Kavita Gulati, MB BCh, BAO, BSc[a,b], Stephen P. McAdoo, MBBS, PhD[a,b,*]

KEYWORDS

- Goodpasture syndrome • Vasculitis • Rapidly progressive glomerulonephritis
- Pulmonary hemorrhage • Plasma exchange

KEY POINTS

- Anti–glomerular basement membrane (GBM) disease often presents with rapidly progressive glomerulonephritis with or without lung hemorrhage. It is rare to present with lung hemorrhage alone.
- Antibodies are generally directed at E_A or E_B epitopes found within the noncollagenous (NC1) domain of the $\alpha3$ chain of type IV collagen.
- Renal and patient survival in untreated anti-GBM is poor, although intensive therapy provides improved outcomes in patients with alveolar hemorrhage or rapidly progressive glomerulonephritis not requiring dialysis at outset.
- Relapses are uncommon in patients with anti-GBM disease.
- Patients who are double positive for antineutrophil cytoplasm antibody and anti-GBM have more relapsing disease and often need maintenance immunosuppressive therapy.

Anti–glomerular basement membrane (anti-GBM) disease is a rare, life-threatening, small vessel vasculitis that can affect both the glomerular and pulmonary capillaries.[1] It usually presents as a rapidly progressive glomerulonephritis (RPGN), with or without pulmonary hemorrhage. Rare cases have been reported to present with pulmonary hemorrhage alone or with a more indolent course.

It is an immune complex–mediated disease, facilitated by antibodies directed against intrinsic antigens in the basement membranes of both pulmonary and renal vasculature. These autoantibodies are detectable by serum immunoassay or are

Disclosure Statement: None.
[a] Renal and Vascular Inflammation Section, Department of Medicine, Imperial College London, Commonwealth Building, Hammersmith Hospital Campus, Du Cane Road, London W12 0NN, UK; [b] Vasculitis Clinic, Imperial College Healthcare NHS Trust, Hammersmith Hospital, Du Cane Road, London W12 0HS, UK
* Corresponding authors. Renal and Vascular Inflammation Section, Imperial College London, Commonwealth Building, Hammersmith Hospital Campus, Du Cane Road, London W12 0NN, UK.
E-mail address: s.mcadoo@imperial.ac.uk

Rheum Dis Clin N Am 44 (2018) 651–673
https://doi.org/10.1016/j.rdc.2018.06.011
0889-857X/18/© 2018 Elsevier Inc. All rights reserved.

seen as classic linear polyclonal immunoglobulin (Ig) G deposits on immunofluorescence staining of the GBM on analysis of kidney biopsy samples.

NOMENCLATURE

The term Goodpasture syndrome was the eponymous name given by Stanton and
Tange[2] to a case series of 9 patients presenting with pulmonary hemorrhage associated with glomerulonephritis. This name was in acknowledgment of an earlier case
report by Goodpasture[3] describing a fatal case of renopulmonary syndrome after influenza in 1919. However, the latter may not have referred to anti-GBM disease because
there was also a description of a splenic vasculitic granuloma. Furthermore, at that
time the culprit autoantibody had yet to be identified.

However, the term Goodpasture syndrome is still used widely in literature to describe
the clinical constellation of both pulmonary hemorrhage and glomerulonephritis,
regardless of the underlying cause. The term Goodpasture disease is used to describe
renopulmonary syndrome in patients with detectable anti-GBM antibodies.

For the purpose of this article, the nomenclature is restricted to using anti-GBM disease as per the Chapel Hill Consensus.[1] Anti-GBM antibody is the term used to
describe the circulating factor; however, it is clear that these antibodies target both
glomerular and alveolar basement membranes (and potentially others in the retina,
choroid plexus, and cochlea). These antibodies tend to be IgG autoantibodies against
the noncollagenous (NC1) domain of the alpha 3 chain of type IV collagen in the basement membrane.

EPIDEMIOLOGY

Anti-GBM disease is a rare disorder, with an estimated frequency of 1 to 2 cases per
million population per year in European populations. A recent study from Ireland was
the first to report a national disease incidence (of 1.64 per million population per year).[4]
It is rare to find cases of anti-GBM disease in African populations, but it has been well
described in other white and Asian populations.

However, anti-GBM disease is a fairly common cause of RPGN.[5] Detectable antibodies or classic histologic findings are found in 10% to 15% of cases of RPGN,
although this varies across different populations, with one Japanese study showing
that only 6.6% of RPGN cases were attributable to anti-GBM disease.[6]

Anti-GBM disease seems to have a bimodal distribution, with younger patients (20–
30 years old) being more frequently male and presenting with renopulmonary syndrome, whereas older patients (60–70 years old) have a female predominance with
renal involvement only.[7]

PREDISPOSING FACTORS

Like many autoimmune diseases, there are strong positive and protective associations
with human leukocyte antigen (HLA) polymorphisms in anti-GBM disease, and in
particular with major histocompatibility complex class II genes. There is a hierarchy
of associations with particular DRB1 alleles: for example, DRB1*1501 is a strong susceptibility allele, whereas the presence of DRB1*01 confers a dominant-negative protective effect.[8] However, the susceptibility alleles are common in healthy populations,
whereas disease is exceedingly rare, thus suggesting that additional factors, whether
genetic or environmental, contribute to disease pathogenesis in humans.

Seasonal distribution and outbreaks of disease have been previously
described,[7,9,10] as well as clusters linked anecdotally to influenza outbreaks.[11,12] In

addition, the recent Irish study described both temporal and spatial clustering of cases,[4] which together suggest environmental factors such as infection may be important in provoking disease.

Other putative environmental triggers include inhalation of pulmonary irritants such as cigarette smoke or hydrocarbons.[13,14] It is suggested that these irritants may increase pulmonary capillary permeability, thus predisposing to alveolar hemorrhage in individuals who develop anti-GBM antibodies. They may also have a role in the initiation of the autoimmune response by releasing or modifying pathogenic autoantigens within the alveolar basement membrane.

Anti-GBM disease has been reported concurrently with several other renal diseases, including antineutrophil cytoplasm antibody (ANCA)--associated vasculitis (AAV), IgA nephropathy, and membranous glomerulonephritis.[15,16] There are also case reports of disease occurring after lithotripsy for renal stones.[17,18] It has been suggested that these conditions may likewise initiate a local inflammatory response within the kidney that then results in the generation of an immune-mediated reaction to GBM antigens and development of anti-GMB disease.

PATHOGENESIS
The Autoantigen

The glomerular and alveolar basement membranes, like all basement membranes, are lamellar extracellular matrices composed of 4 major macromolecules: laminin, nidogen, heparin sulfate proteoglycan, and type IV collagen. The collagen IV family consists of 6 genetically distinct α-chains ($\alpha1$–6) that trimerize with each other to make specific triple-helical protomers: $\alpha1\alpha1\alpha2$, $\alpha3\alpha4\alpha5$, and $\alpha5\alpha5\alpha6$. The expression of the $\alpha3\alpha4\alpha5$ protomer is almost exclusively restricted to the glomerular and alveolar basement membranes (with the $\alpha1\alpha1\alpha2$ protomer being most abundantly expressed elsewhere). In the GBM, these $\alpha3\alpha4\alpha5$ protomers polymerize end to end via their C-terminal NC1 domains to form hexameric NC1 structures (**Fig. 1**). The quaternary structure of this hexamer is stabilized by hydrophobic and hydrophilic interactions across the planar surfaces of opposing trimers and reinforced by sulfilimine bonds cross-linking opposing domains. The $\alpha3\alpha4\alpha5$ protomers likewise associate via their N-terminal 7S domains to complete a latticelike network that is essential for glomerular structure and function. The target of the autoimmune response in anti-GBM disease was first identified as a 27-kDa protein in collagenase-solubilized GBM preparations and subsequently shown to be the non-collagenase domain of the $\alpha3$ chain: $\alpha3(IV)NC1$.[19,20] Immunization with either collagenase-solubilized or recombinant forms of this protein from various species induces disease in several animal models, confirming the universal antigenicity of this protein.

Humoral immunity

Anti-GBM disease is considered a prototypic antibody-mediated condition, following the seminal observation of disease induction following passive transfer of autoantibody from humans to squirrel monkeys.[21] All patients with typical anti-GBM disease have antibodies reactive to $\alpha3(IV)NC1$, and a proportion also show reactivity of $\alpha4$ or $\alpha5$ chains, purported to arise secondarily because of a process of epitope spreading.[22] Two key B-cell epitopes within $\alpha3(IV)NC1$ are recognized, designated E_A (incorporating residues 17–31 toward the amino terminus) and E_B (residues 127–141 toward the carboxy terminus).[23] In disease, antibodies tend to be of the IgG1 and IgG3 subclasses, and their titer and avidity have been associated with disease

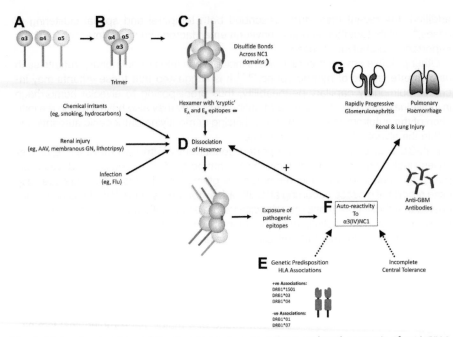

Fig. 1. Molecular structure of the Goodpasture autoantigen and pathogenesis of anti-GBM disease. Individual α3, α4, and α5 collagen IV chains, with globular C-terminal noncollagenous domains (A); these trimerize to form trimeric protomers (B), and then organize end to end to form hexameric NC1 structures cross-linked by disulfide bonds, and within which the pathogenic E_A and E_B epitopes on the α3 chain are sequestered (C). Disruption of disulfide bonds and dissociation of the hexamer (caused by proposed inflammatory or chemical insults) results in exposure of these epitopes (D), which, in genetically susceptible individuals (E), permits a fulminant anti-GBM response to develop (F), with both humoral and cellular effectors contributing to renal and pulmonary injury (G). GN, glomerulonephritis.

severity.[24–27] Once bound in the kidney, these antibodies can initiate a local inflammatory response via both complement-dependent and Fc receptor-dependent mechanisms. Consistent with an antibody-mediated disease process, copy number variation and polymorphisms in genes encoding FcRγ receptors have been associated with disease susceptibility in Asian populations.[28,29] However, it is notable that low-level natural autoantibodies that recognize the same epitopes can be identified in healthy individuals, although they tend to be of different subclasses (Ig2 and IgG4 dominant).[30] In addition, the presence of circulating anti-GBM antibodies can predate the onset of clinical disease by several months.[31] These observations suggest that additional factors contribute to disease pathogenesis.

Cellular immunity

The strong HLA association, and the detection of high-affinity, class-switched autoantibody, indicates a requirement for T-cell help in the generation of anti-GBM antibodies. Peripheral CD4+ cells from patients have been shown to proliferate in response to α3(IV)NC1 (as do cells from healthy individuals, but at much lower frequency), and the frequency of autoreactive CD4+ T cells has been shown to correlate with disease activity.[32,33]

Studies in experimental models of anti-GBM disease also suggest that directly nephritogenic T-cell responses may contribute to disease pathogenesis. In early avian models, mononuclear cells could transfer disease to bursectomized birds,[34] and B-cell deficient mice develop glomerular injury following immunization with α3(IV)NC1.[35] Disease has also been transferred by CD4+ T cells from nephritic rats, expanded in vitro by stimulation with α3(IV)NC1, without detectable antibody responses, suggesting directly injurious responses by cellular effectors.[36] In a series of elegant experiments using HLA-transgenic mice, Ooi and colleagues[37] identified an immunodominant T-cell epitope within α3(IV)NC1 that can induce both autoantibody production and glomerulonephritis in mice expressing the human *DRB1*1501* susceptibility allele (but not in mice expressing the protective *DRB1*01* allele). In addition, CD4+ T-cell clones generated from *DRB1*1501* transgenic mice and specific for the immunodominant T-cell epitope transferred disease to naive animals. In a rat model, immunization with an immunodominant T-cell epitope resulted in glomerular injury, followed by the expansion of B-cell responses to distinct α3(IV)NC1 epitopes in renal draining lymph nodes.[38] It has thus been suggested that T cell–mediated glomerular injury may be the inciting event in anti-GBM disease, which then triggers de novo internal immunization to B-cell epitopes released from damaged GBM and subsequent autoantibody production required for full expression of disease. Direct evidence of this phenomenon in humans is lacking, although historical case reports of patients who developed glomerulonephritis before the deposition of anti-GBM antibodies, and the detection of an early T-cell infiltrate in pathology studies,[39,40] suggests that cell-mediated injury may occur in at least a subset of patients.

Tolerance and autoimmunity

α3(IV)NC1 is expressed in human thymus,[33,41] although the finding of natural autoantibodies and autoreactive T cells in healthy individuals suggests central tolerance to the antigen is incomplete. However, additional immune checkpoints must be broken for disease to develop. Of note, the B-cell epitopes within native α3(IV)NC1 are cryptic, being sequestered within the quaternary structure of the hexameric NC1 arrangement, such that they remain protected from immune surveillance in normal circumstances. It has been shown that patient-derived anti-GBM antibodies do not bind cross-linked α3α4α5 hexamers until they are dissociated, and this process of conformational transformation is thought to be critical to disease pathogenesis by exposing hidden epitopes to immune detection, and allowing the binding of pathogenic autoantibodies[22] (see **Fig. 1**). This process may explain the association of anti-GBM disease with other disorders that disrupt or modify the structure of the glomerular (eg, ANCA vasculitis, lithotripsy) or alveolar (eg, smoking) basement membrane, and of the induction of humoral responses following T cell–mediated glomerular injury.

Alternative mechanisms that induce reactivity to self-antigens in anti-GBM disease have been proposed, based on observations in experimental models, including processes of so-called molecular mimicry and autoantigen complementarity following immunization with foreign peptides.[42,43] Reactivity to microbial peptides in a proportion of patients with anti-GBM disease was recently described,[44] although causality is not established in humans.

Relapses are rare in anti-GBM disease, suggesting that immune tolerance can be reinstated as disease resolves. This suggestion is supported by the finding of an expanding population of CD25+ antigen-specific T cells in patients after their acute presentation that may suppress responses to α3(IV)NC1.[45] In addition, further work by Ooi and colleagues[46] using their HLA-transgenic mouse model showed that immunization with the immunodominant T-cell epitope of α3(IV)NC1 differentially induced conventional or tolerogenic/suppressor T-cell responses when presented on the *DRB1*1501* susceptibility and *DRB1*01* resistance alleles, respectively, suggesting a novel mechanism for the dominant-negative protective effect of some HLA associations in human disease.[46]

CLINICAL PRESENTATION

Patients typically present with RPGN, which is usually defined as greater than 50% loss of glomerular filtration rate occurring over 3 months, although in anti-GBM disease the deterioration may be much more rapid, occurring within days to weeks, and a brief prodrome of less than 2 weeks' duration is typical. In the early stages, symptoms may be nonspecific, although, as the disease progresses, features of overt renal failure with oligoanuria and fluid overload may develop. Approximately 50% of patients have an indication for renal replacement therapy at the point of diagnosis. Symptoms of frank hematuria and loin pain are recognized.

Bedside urinalysis may identify hematuria, proteinuria, and leukocyturia in cases of RPGN. Proteinuria is often in the subnephrotic range, presumably because of the severe reduction in glomerular blood flow that occurs in crescentic glomerulonephritis. Urine microscopy, ideally performed on a fresh urine specimen, is required to confirm erythrocyturia, and the presence of red blood cell casts is pathognomonic for glomerulonephritis (whereas leukocyte or epithelial cell casts are nonspecific).

Diffuse alveolar hemorrhage, presenting with dyspnea, cough, hemoptysis, or overt respiratory failure, is present in 40% to 60% of patients at presentation. There is an increased frequency of lung involvement in current smokers.[13]

A differential diagnosis for renopulmonary syndromes is given in **Table 1**. Extrarenal/pulmonary manifestations in anti-GBM disease are unusual, and their presence should alert to the possibility of double positivity with detectable ANCAs. Anti-GBM disease is generally not a relapsing-remitting condition, although infrequent cases have been described.[47,48]

Table 1 Differential diagnosis for renopulmonary syndrome	
ANCA-associated vasculitis	Granulomatosis with polyangiitis Microscopic polyangiitis Eosinophilic granulomatosis with polyangiitis
Immune-complex small vessel vasculitis	Systemic lupus erythematosus Cryoglobulinemic vasculitis Henoch Schönlein purpura/IgA vasculitis
Mixed connective tissue disease	Systemic sclerosis Dermatomyositis/polymyositis
Antiphospholipid syndromes	With vasculitis or with pulmonary embolism
Infectious disease	Specific infections with renal and lung involvement; eg, legionella, mycoplasma, leptospirosis, Hantavirus, cytomegalovirus, tuberculosis Respiratory tract infection with associated acute kidney injury
Primary renal disease leading to lung disease mimicking renopulmonary syndrome	Acute kidney injury with pulmonary edema ± uremic hemoptysis Nephrotic syndrome with pulmonary venous thromboembolism Opportunistic pneumonia in patients receiving immunosuppression for renal disease

DIAGNOSIS

Diagnosis is made from a typical clinical history, positive serologic testing, and/or the demonstration of linear IgG deposits along the GBM on renal biopsy.

SEROLOGY TESTING

Circulating anti-GBM antibodies were first described using indirect immunofluorescence techniques on normal human or primate kidney.[49] The development of solid-phase assays (eg, radioimmunoassay or enzyme-linked immunosorbent assay [ELISA]) quickly followed, and in current practice a variety of such assays are available, which may use native human or animal GBM isolates, or more commonly recombinant α3(IV)NC1 preparations. These assays are generally accepted to have a high sensitivity and specificity,[50] although it is recognized that between 5% and 10% of patients with demonstrable anti-GBM antibody on renal biopsy are negative by conventional serum assays. As summarized in a recent commentary by Glassock,[51] this may be caused by:

- Intrinsic sensitivity of the chosen assay
- Isotype or subclass of antibody not being detectable (eg, IgA, IgG4)
- Antibody disappearance before clinical resolution
- The so-called immunologic sink: high-affinity antibodies rapidly bind tissue and are removed from circulation, with only low-affinity antibodies remaining
- Absence of relevant epitopes in antigens used in the detection assay
- T lymphocytes, complement, or other mediators causing tissue damage rather than a predominantly antibody-mediated process

These cases show that serologic tests, although useful for rapid diagnoses, should not be the sole means of excluding a diagnosis of anti-GBM disease and reinforce the importance of performing a renal biopsy when possible.

RENAL BIOPSY FINDINGS

Severe glomerular injury is evident on light microscopy with disruption of the GBMs caused by fibrinoid necrosis and consequent crescent formation (**Fig. 2**). Crescents

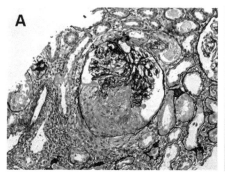
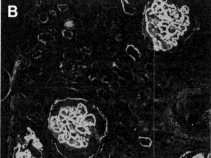

Fig. 2. Renal pathology in anti-GBM disease. (*A*) Light microscopy showing acute, cellular crescent formation and resultant compression of the underlying glomerular tuft (Jones methenamie silver stain, original magnification x 200). (*B*) Immunofluorescence microscopy, showing strong linear staining for IgG along glomerular basement membranes (anti human IgG-FITC, original magnification X 200).

are usually widespread and of similar age and activity, reflecting the acuity of disease onset. Diagnostic lesions are seen on immunofluorescence microscopy, where there is strong linear GBM staining for polyclonal IgG. Rarer cases of linear staining for either IgA or IgM have been described. Complement components, indicating activation of the classic pathway by deposited antibody, may also been seen in GBM. Electron-dense deposits are not typically seen on electron microscopy. Asynchronous crescent formation, or the presence of necrotizing vasculitis in larger blood vessels on renal biopsy, is not typical of anti-GBM disease and should alert to the possibility of a concomitant ANCA-mediated process.

TREATMENT AND OUTCOMES

Given the pathogenic capability of anti-GBM antibodies, their rapid removal with plasma exchange has become a central component of disease therapy. Successful treatment of anti-GBM disease using the combination of plasma exchange along with cytotoxics and corticosteroids was first described in 1976. In Lockwood's[52] seminal study, plasma exchange was associated with rapid removal of circulating autoantibodies, resolution of lung hemorrhage, and salvage of kidney function in patients who were not requiring dialysis at presentation. A subsequent small randomized controlled trial likewise showed a more rapid decrease in anti-GBM titers when plasma exchange was added to immunosuppressive therapy, with a trend toward improved renal outcome (although groups were poorly matched by histopathologic severity).[53] Several observational studies support the use of plasma exchange, with improved outcomes compared with cohorts treated with immunosuppression alone, including a large contemporaneous Chinese study of almost 200 patients.[54]

The largest published series to systematically use plasma exchange comes from our center[55]: we recommend daily large-volume (4 L) exchanges for 5% human albumin to ensure rapid antibody removal. Plasma exchange treatments should be continued for at least 14 days or until autoantibodies become undetectable. Patients should be monitored for rebound antibody production, and plasma exchange reinstated should this occur. Exchange against fresh frozen plasma is recommended if there is bleeding risk (alveolar hemorrhage, recent biopsy) and patients should be monitored carefully for development of coagulopathy, hypofibrinogenemia, and thrombocytopenia. Using this approach, most lung hemorrhage (>90%) responds to treatment, and most patients not requiring immediate dialysis have good renal prognosis. Based on these findings, both the American Society for Apheresis (ASFA) and the Kidney Disease Improving Global Outcomes (KDIGO) guidelines recommend inclusion of plasma exchange in therapeutic regimens for anti-GBM disease in this setting.[56,57]

In addition to plasma exchange, medical therapy with immunosuppression and corticosteroids is required to prevent ongoing autoantibody production and to ameliorate end-organ damage. Daily oral cyclophosphamide (eg, 2 mg/kg/d) is most commonly used, although pulsed intravenous regimens are used at some centers, based on published experience in ANCA-associated vasculitis that suggest equivalent efficacy for initial treatment of disease.[58] However, a recent multicenter study from France suggested that use of intravenous cyclophosphamide was associated with poorer patient survival in anti-GBM disease,[59] such that daily oral dosing may remain the preferred option in these cases. The duration of immunosuppressive therapy is not clearly defined, although it is usually continued for 2 to 3 months, along with a tapering course of oral corticosteroids for 6 to 9 months (eg, initial dose 1 mg/kg/d). Because anti-GBM disease rarely relapses, maintenance therapy beyond this time point is not usually required, unless there is a concomitant disorder, such as ANCA-associated vasculitis.

Table 2
Rituximab use in native anti-glomerular basement membrane disease

Reference	Case Details	Indications for Rituximab	Treatments	Outcome
Arzoo et al,[85] 2002	73 F Alveolar hemorrhage Lung biopsy: anti-GBM disease Hematuria, no renal biopsy	Relapsing disease	CS, AZA, PEX, CYC RTX: 6 × weekly 375 mg/m²	23 mo: Resolution of DAH Independent renal function Undetectable Ab
Wechsler et al,[86] 2008	55 M Biopsy-proven RPGN; no RRT at outset (biopsy also showed acute TIN and IgA deposition)	Standard regimen contraindicated (type 1 diabetes, HIV positive, recurrent septic arthritis)	CS, MMF, IVIG RTX: 4 × weekly 375 mg/m²	16 mo: Independent renal function Undetectable Ab
Schless et al,[87] 2009 2 cases	18 F Biopsy-proven RPGN, RRT at outset Alveolar hemorrhage	Nonresponse to standard regimen	CS, PEX, CYC RTX: 1 × 1 g	10 wk: RRT dependent Undetectable Ab (leukoencephalopathy)
	20 M Biopsy-proven RPGN, RRT at outset	Nonresponse to standard regimen	CS, PEX, CYC RTX: 1 × 1 g	3 mo: Independent renal function Undetectable Ab
Mutsaers et al,[88] 2010	20 F Oliguric RPGN	Nonresponse to standard regimen	CS, CYC, PEX RTX: 2 × 2 weekly 375 mg/m²	2 mo: Independent renal function Undetectable Ab

(continued on next page)

Table 2
(continued)

Reference	Case Details	Indications for Rituximab	Treatments	Outcome
Shah et al, 2012[89] 3 cases	54 M RPGN, RRT at outset Alveolar hemorrhage	Bone marrow suppression (CYC)	CS, CYC, PEX RTX: 4 × weekly 375 mg/m²	49 mo: RRT dependent Undetectable Ab
	64 M Biopsy-proven RPGN, RRT at outset (also MPO-ANCA positive)	Thrombocytopenia (CYC)	CS, CYC RTX: 4 × weekly 375 mg/m²	37 mo: Independent renal function Undetectable Abs
	17 M Hemoptysis Biopsy-proven RPGN, no RRT at outset	Patient choice (concerns about fertility)	CS, PEX RTX: 2 × weekly 375 mg/m²	33 mo: Independent renal function Undetectable Ab
Syeda et al,[90] 2013	68 F Biopsy-proven RPGN, RRT at outset (also MPO-ANCA positive)	TTP (CYC)	CS, CYC, PEX RTX: 4 × weekly 375 mg/m²	24 mo: RRT dependent Undetectable Abs
Bandak et al,[91] 2014	24 M Biopsy-proven RPGN, RRT at outset	Nonresponse to standard regimen	CS, CYC, PEX RTX: 1 × 1 g	9 mo: Independent renal function Undetectable Ab
Narayanan et al,[92] 2014	21 M Biopsy-proven RPGN, RRT at outset Alveolar hemorrhage	100% cellular crescents To reduce IS burden	CS, PEX RTX: 2 × doses	4 mo: RRT dependent Low-level Ab

Touzot et al,[93] 2015 8 cases	21 F Biopsy-proven RPGN, RRT at outset Alveolar hemorrhage	Severity of initial presentation	CS, CYC, PEX RTX: 4 × weekly 375 mg/m²	3 mo: Independent renal function Undetectable Ab
	46 F Biopsy-proven RPGN, RRT at outset	Nonresponse to standard regimen	CS, CYC, PEX RTX: 4 × weekly 375 mg/m²	12 mo: RRT dependent Undetectable Ab
	16 F Biopsy-proven RPGN, RRT at outset Pulmonary hemorrhage, on ECMO	Severity of initial presentation	CS, MMF, CYC, PEX RTX: 4 × weekly 375 mg/m²	10 mo: Independent renal function Undetectable Ab
	65 M Biopsy-proven RPGN, no RRT at outset	Nonresponse to standard regimen	CS, MMF, CYC, PEX RTX: 4 × weekly 375 mg/m²	56 mo: Independent renal function Undetectable Ab
	19 F Biopsy-proven RPGN, no RRT at outset	Nonresponse to standard regimen	CS, CYC, PEX RTX: 4 × weekly 375 mg/m²	39 mo: Independent renal function Undetectable Ab
	22 M Biopsy-proven RPGN, no RRT at outset Alveolar hemorrhage	Relapsing disease	CS, CYC, PEX RTX: 4 × weekly 375 mg/m²	12 mo: Independent renal function Undetectable Ab
	21 ? Biopsy-proven RPGN, no RRT at outset	Severity of disease	CS, CYC, PEX RTX: 4 × weekly 375 mg/m²	93 mo: Independent renal function Undetectable Ab
	17 F Biopsy-proven RPGN, no RRT at outset Alveolar hemorrhage	Relapsing disease	CS, CYC, PEX RTX: 4 × weekly 375 mg/m²	6 mo: RRT dependent Undetectable Ab
Huang et al,[94] 2016	84 M Biopsy-proven RPGN, no RRT at outset Pulmonary fibrosis/lung vasculitis (nonhemorrhagic) Also MPO-ANCA positive	Heparin-induced thrombocytopenia (PEX) Nonresponse to standard regimen	CS, CYC, PEX, MMF RTX: 4 × weekly 700 mg	4.5 mo: Independent renal function Undetectable Abs

Abbreviations: Ab, antibodies; AZA, azathioprine; CS, corticosteroids; CYC, cyclophosphamide; DAH, diffuse alveolar hemorrhage; ECMO, extracorporeal membrane oxygenation; F, female; HIV, human immunodeficiency virus; IS, immunosuppression; IVIG, intravenous Ig; M, male; MMF, mycophenolate mofetil; MPO, myeloperoxidase; PEX, plasma exchange; RRT, renal replacement therapy; RTX, rituximab; TIN, tubular interstitial nephritis; TTP, thrombotic thrombocytopenic purpura.

Rituximab is an effective treatment of several other autoantibody-associated glomerular diseases, although published experience in anti-GBM disease is limited (**Table 2**), and it has most commonly been used as adjunctive or second-line therapy in resistant cases. It seems to be associated with immunologic response, although clinical outcomes are variable. At present, there is insufficient evidence to recommend its first-line use in the treatment of anti-GBM disease; however, it may be considered if there are compelling contraindications to cyclophosphamide therapy or as adjunctive treatment in severe disease.

With intensive combination therapy, most patients with lung hemorrhage respond to treatment (>90%).[55] Similarly, in patients presenting with RPGN but not requiring immediate dialysis, renal recovery is sustained at 1 year in most cases (95% if presenting creatinine level <500 μmol/L; 82% if presenting creatinine level >500 μmol/L). However, in patients presenting with an immediate need for renal replacement therapy, several studies have shown that fewer than 10% of patients recover independent function (**Table 3**), and so the decision to treat these patients, in the absence of lung hemorrhage, remains contentious. These studies have attempted to identify predictors of patient and renal outcome, although direct comparisons are challenging because of differences in treatment schedules, definitions, and methods of analysis.

In the Hammersmith series, no patient with 100% glomerular crescents and dialysis dependence at presentation recovered therapy, and so current guidelines do not recommend treatment in these cases.[60] A more recent study by van Daalen and colleagues[61] examined outcomes of a worldwide, multicenter cohort treated with comparable intensive regimens. One-hundred and twenty-three patients were followed up for a median of 3.9 years, making it the largest histopathologic study in anti-GBM disease to date. It confirmed previous observations of most favorable outcomes in patients presenting with creatinine levels of less than 500 μmol/L. Independent predictors of end-stage renal disease (ESRD) were dialysis requirement at presentation, reduced proportion of normal glomeruli, and increased interstitial infiltrate on kidney biopsy. Of note, no patient with 100% crescents or greater than 50% sclerotic glomeruli recovered renal function.

Another notable, although small, study from 2 centers in the United Kingdom, showed oligoanuria at presentation as the strongest predictor of poor renal survival and nonrecovery from dialysis[62] (and in keeping with the original observations of Lockwood[52]).

The decision to treat patients with indicators of adverse renal prognosis, in the absence of lung hemorrhage, therefore requires careful consideration on an individualized basis. Taking these studies into account, the authors currently suggest that intensive treatment be considered in anti-GBM disease in which there is:

- Clinically evident alveolar hemorrhage (regardless of renal status)
- RPGN and dialysis is not required
- If RPGN and dialysis is required, consider treatment if:
  ○ Less than 100% glomerular crescents on biopsy
  ○ Less than 50% glomerulosclerosis on biopsy
  ○ There are other features on renal biopsy to account for renal dysfunction (eg, severe acute tubular injury)
  ○ Nonoliguric
  ○ Recent onset of dialysis requirement
  ○ Double-positive ANCA disease present (discussed later)

LONG-TERM OUTCOMES

When patients survive their initial illness with preserved renal function, their prognosis is generally favorable, and the progression toward ESRD seems to be slow in series with

Table 3

Outcomes studies in anti–glomerular basement membrane disease (including studies describing >40 patients and reported after 2000)

Centers	Period	Cases (n)	ANCA Double Positive (%)	RRT at Diagnosis (%)	Treatment Modality (%)	Recovery from RRT (%)	Patient Survival (%)	Renal Survival (%)	Associations/Comments
6 centers worldwide[61]	1986–2015	123	32	56	PEX 33 CYC 80 CS 96	9	83 at 5 y	34 at 5 y	Improved renal outcomes post-2007. No patients with 100% crescents or >50% glomerulosclerosis recovered renal function if dialysis dependent at diagnosis. Predictors of ESRD during follow-up: • RRT at presentation • Percentage normal glomeruli • Extend of interstitial infiltrate on kidney biopsy
80 centers France[59]	1983–2006	122	15	68	PEX 100 CYC 84 CS 97	2	86 at 1 y	38 at 1 y	Predictors of overall mortality: • Age>60 y • Fewer plasma exchanges • Use of alternative immunosuppression Independent renal function at 1 y (in surviving patients) predicted by presenting creatinine <500 µmol/L only
4 centers Europe[81]	2000–2013	78	47	60	PEX 85 CYC 95 CS 99	17 (29 if ANCA+)	86 at 1 y	49 at 1 y	Predictors of renal and patient survival • Age • RRT at presentation Double-positive patients had trend toward higher rates of recovery from RRT and overall intermediate renal outcome

(continued on next page)

Table 3 (continued)

Centers	Period	Cases (n)	ANCA Double Positive (%)	RRT at Diagnosis (%)	Treatment Modality (%)	Recovery from RRT (%)	Patient Survival (%)	Renal Survival (%)	Associations/Comments
365 centers Japan[6]	1989–2000	47	13	60	PEX 55 CYC 36 CS 85	NA	77 at 6 mo	21 at 6 mo	Most patients presented with advanced disease and not all treated; no clear predictors of patient or renal survival identified
1 center China[54]	1998–2008	176	22	NA	PEX + CYC + CS 43 CYC + CS 34 CS 23	NA	73 at 1 y	25 at 1 y	Combination treatment with PEX + CYC + CS improved both renal and patient survival compared with CYC + CS or CS alone. Double-positive patients had poorer overall survival, although comparable renal survival
2 centers United Kingdom[62]	1999–2011	43	21	81	PEX + CYC + CS 74 Low-dose CS or no treatment 26	5.7	88 at 1 y	16 at 1 y	Predictors of renal survival at 3 mo: • Nonoliguric at presentation • Percentage glomerular crescents
1 center United Kingdom[55]	1975–2000	71	Excluded	55	PEX + CYC + CS 100 (those not treated were excluded)	5	77 at 1 1y	53 at 1 y	All patients who required immediate RRT and had 100% glomerular crescents remained RRT dependent. Age was not associated with patient or renal outcome

Abbreviations: ESRD, end-stage renal disease; NA, not available.

long-term follow-up. Relapses are very uncommon and usually associated with continued exposure to environmental triggers, such as pulmonary irritants. In patients who have progressed to ESRD because of anti-GBM disease, their overall survival seems to be comparable with patients with other causes of ESRD.[63] Renal transplant after anti-GBM disease is usually successful, provided it is delayed for at least 6 months after achieving seronegativity for circulating autoantibodies, and recurrent disease in renal allografts is very uncommon under modern immunosuppressive regimens.[63,64] Timing of transplants in patients who are seronegative at presentation remains unclear, because these patients have no circulating biomarkers to confirm disease remission.

ANTI–GLOMERULAR BASEMENT MEMBRANE DISEASE AFTER ALEMTUZUMAB THERAPY

Secondary autoimmune phenomena after alemtuzumab, an anti-CD52 lymphocyte-depleting treatment for relapsing-remitting multiple sclerosis (MS), are common.[65] Autoimmune thyroid disease occurred in up to 30% of patients in controlled trials, and there are case reports of both membranous nephropathy and anti-GBM disease following treatment.[66,67] It has been proposed that T-cell reconstitution after alemtuzumab is driven largely by homeostatic expansion of cells that have escaped deletion (rather than by thymopoiesis), resulting in a T-cell pool that is enriched for autoreactive cells.[68] Anti-GBM disease has not been reported when alemtuzumab is used for other indications other than MS (eg, renal transplant), perhaps because of the use of maintenance immunosuppression, or because of the shared HLA susceptibilities in MS and anti-GBM disease. Careful monitoring of patients for renal disorder after treatment with alemtuzumab is needed in order to facilitate early detection and treatment.[69] The authors recommend conventional treatment of anti-GBM disease occurring in this setting.

ANTI–GLOMERULAR BASEMENT MEMBRANE DISEASE IN PREGNANCY

Anti-GBM disease related to pregnancy is exceptionally rare; a systematic review in 2014 identified 8 cases in the literature,[70] and there are a small number of subsequent case reports.[71,72] Disease was most commonly diagnosed in the second trimester, and although 6 of 8 cases in the review resulted in live births, the rate of adverse fetal and maternal outcomes was high. Steroids and plasma exchange may be used safely in pregnancy, and judicious use of cyclophosphamide may be considered from the second trimester, when the risk of fetal abnormalities is reduced after organogenesis.[72] Azathioprine may be considered as an alternative immunosuppressant, although it is unlikely to be sufficiently potent for early disease control. Transplacental transfer of ANCAs has been implicated in neonatal renopulmonary syndrome,[73] and it is notable that anti-GBM antibodies were shown in 2 of 5 neonates tested, although none had evidence of kidney or lung disease.

DOUBLE-SEROPOSITIVE PATIENTS

The concurrence of both ANCA and anti-GBM antibodies is well recognized and occurs at a much higher frequency than would be expected by chance alone given the rarity of the individual diseases. This phenomenon was first reported within a few years of the first description of ANCA,[74,75] and it is clear that the autoantibodies are antigenically distinct and that double positivity is not caused by a cross-reactive anomaly.[76] In larger series, between 20% and 40% of patients with anti-GBM disease have concurrent ANCA (see **Table 3**), directed against myeloperoxidase in most.

Several studies have characterized the clinical features and outcomes of these cases, with conflicting results, although many are limited by small sample size and heterogeneity of disease severity at presentation and treatments used.[15,27,62,77–80] The authors recently analyzed the outcomes of 37 double-positive patients who received intensive treatment at 4 centers in Europe, and compared their clinical features with parallel cohorts of single-positive anti-GBM disease and ANCA-associated vasculitis cases.[81] Double-positive patients had similar age distribution to AAV patients, and presented with longer prodromes and more extrarenal disease manifestations than single-positive anti-GBM patients, suggesting that AAV may have occurred first and acted as a trigger for the development anti-GBM autoreactivity. The severity of renal and lung disease at presentation was comparable between anti-GBM and double-positive cases, although there was a tendency for greater recovery from dialysis

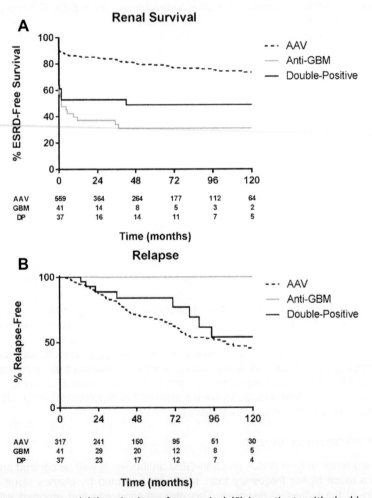

Fig. 3. Long-term renal (A) and relapse-free survival (B) in patients with double-positive ANCA and anti-GBM disease, compared with parallel single-positive anti-GBM and AAV cases. (*From* McAdoo SP, Tanna A, Hruskova Z, et al. Patients double-seropositive for ANCA and anti-GBM antibodies have varied renal survival, frequency of relapse, and outcomes compared to single-seropositive patients. Kidney Int 2017;92(3):698; with permission.)

and better long-term renal survival in the latter. This observation should be interpreted with care, although it may suggest that a subset of double-positive patients may be more responsive to initial disease treatment, even when presenting with adverse indicators. During long-term follow-up, patients with AAV and double-positive patients had a similar risk of relapse, although no patient with single-positive anti-GBM disease had recurrence of disease (**Fig. 3**). Relapses in double-positive patients tended to occur in PR3-ANCA cases and were associated with anticipatory increases in ANCA titer, highlighting the need to consider maintenance immunosuppressive therapy and careful follow-up in these cases.

ATYPICAL ANTI–GLOMERULAR BASEMENT MEMBRANE DISEASE

Atypical anti-GBM disease is a term that has been used variably to describe cases with classic linear IgG staining on renal biopsy but uncharacteristic clinicopathologic features. Nasr and colleagues[82] recently described 20 such cases; all had bright linear GBM staining for immunoglobulin on kidney biopsy, although none had detectable α3(IV)NC1 antibodies by commercial ELISA, and none had lung hemorrhage. Most had had only mild renal insufficiency, although all had proliferative glomerular changes on renal biopsy but without diffuse crescent formation. Treatment was with heterogeneous immunosuppression (and generally did not include plasma exchange), and both patient and renal survival at 1 year were favorable, at 93% and 85%, respectively. Of note, GBM staining was IgM dominant in 2 cases, and IgA dominant in another. In addition, half of patients had restriction for either kappa or lambda lights on immunofluorescence testing, although none had glomerular capillary wall deposits on electron microscopy (that would be expected in proliferative glomerulonephritis with monoclonal immunoglobulin deposits), nor did they have identified features of an underlying plasma cell dyscrasia. Several other case reports and small series have similarly described atypical cases, with similarly indolent renal disease and seronegativity by conventional assay. One recent report describes a case of florid anti-GBM with kappa-light chain restriction on GBM staining in association with a circulating paraprotein,[83] thus suggesting that anti-GBM disease may occur within the spectrum of monoclonal gammopathy of renal significance. Several mechanisms for the unusual pattern of renal injury in these cases have been proposed, including differences in antibody isotype or subclasses, varied antigenic targets, and differential pathogenicity in antibodies related to their ability to fix complement or recruit inflammatory cells.[84] The term atypical, therefore, is likely to include a variety of different disease processes, and further work is clearly needed to fully understand the multiple facets and full spectrum of anti-GBM disease.

SUMMARY

1. Anti-GBM disease often presents with rapidly progressive glomerulonephritis with or without lung hemorrhage. It is rare to present with lung hemorrhage alone.
2. Antibodies are generally directed at E_A or E_B epitopes found within the NC1 domain of the α3 chain of type IV collagen.
3. Renal and patient survival in untreated anti-GBM is poor, although intensive therapy provides improved outcomes in patients with alveolar hemorrhage or rapidly progressive glomerulonephritis not requiring dialysis at outset.
4. Relapses are uncommon in patients with anti-GBM disease.
5. Patients who are double positive for ANCA and anti-GBM have more relapsing disease and often need maintenance immunosuppressive therapy.

REFERENCES

1. Jennette JC, Falk RJ, Bacon PA, et al. 2012 revised international Chapel Hill Consensus Conference nomenclature of vasculitides. Arthritis Rheum 2013; 65(1):1–11.
2. Stanton MC, Tange JD. Goodpasture's syndrome (pulmonary haemorrhage associated with glomerulonephritis). Australas Ann Med 1958;7(2):132–44.
3. Goodpasture E. The significance of certain pulmonary lesions in relation to the etiology of influenza. Am J Med Sci 1919;158:863–70.
4. Canney M, O'Hara PV, McEvoy CM, et al. Spatial and temporal clustering of anti-glomerular basement membrane disease. Clin J Am Soc Nephrol 2016;11(8):1392–9.
5. Jennette JC. Rapidly progressive crescentic glomerulonephritis. Kidney Int 2003; 63(3):1164–77.
6. Hirayama K, Yamagata K, Kobayashi M, et al. Anti-glomerular basement membrane antibody disease in Japan: part of the nationwide rapidly progressive glomerulonephritis survey in Japan. Clin Exp Nephrol 2008;12(5):339–47.
7. Savage CO, Pusey CD, Bowman C, et al. Antiglomerular basement membrane antibody mediated disease in the British Isles 1980-4. Br Med J 1986; 292(6516):301–4.
8. Fisher M, Pusey CD, Vaughan RW, et al. Susceptibility to anti-glomerular basement membrane disease is strongly associated with HLA-DRB1 genes. Kidney Int 1997;51(1):222–9.
9. Fischer EG, Lager DJ. Anti-glomerular basement membrane glomerulonephritis: a morphologic study of 80 cases. Am J Clin Pathol 2006;125(3):445–50.
10. Williams PS, Davenport A, McDicken I, et al. Increased incidence of anti-glomerular basement membrane antibody (anti-GBM) nephritis in the Mersey Region, September 1984-October 1985. Q J Med 1988;68(257):727–33.
11. Perez GO, Bjornsson S, Ross AH, et al. A mini-epidemic of Goodpasture's syndrome clinical and immunological studies. Nephron 1974;13(2):161–73.
12. Wilson CB, Smith RC. Goodpasture's syndrome associated with influenza A2 virus infection. Ann Intern Med 1972;76(1):91–4.
13. Donaghy M, Rees AJ. Cigarette smoking and lung haemorrhage in glomerulonephritis caused by autoantibodies to glomerular basement membrane. Lancet 1983;2(8364):1390–3.
14. Bombassei GJ, Kaplan AA. The association between hydrocarbon exposure and anti-glomerular basement membrane antibody-mediated disease (Goodpasture's syndrome). Am J Ind Med 1992;21(2):141–53.
15. Rutgers A, Slot M, van Paassen P, et al. Coexistence of anti-glomerular basement membrane antibodies and myeloperoxidase-ANCAs in crescentic glomerulonephritis. Am J kidney Dis 2005;46(2):253–62.
16. Jia XY, Hu SY, Chen JL, et al. The clinical and immunological features of patients with combined anti-glomerular basement membrane disease and membranous nephropathy. Kidney Int 2014;85(4):945–52.
17. Xenocostas A, Jothy S, Collins B, et al. Anti-glomerular basement membrane glomerulonephritis after extracorporeal shock wave lithotripsy. Am J kidney Dis 1999;33(1):128–32.
18. Guerin V, Rabian C, Noel LH, et al. Anti-glomerular-basement-membrane disease after lithotripsy. Lancet 1990;335(8693):856–7.
19. Saus J, Wieslander J, Langeveld JP, et al. Identification of the Goodpasture antigen as the alpha 3(IV) chain of collagen IV. J Biol Chem 1988;263(26):13374–80.

20. Turner N, Mason PJ, Brown R, et al. Molecular cloning of the human Goodpasture antigen demonstrates it to be the alpha 3 chain of type IV collagen. J Clin Invest 1992;89(2):592–601.

21. Lerner RA, Glassock RJ, Dixon FJ. The role of anti-glomerular basement membrane antibody in the pathogenesis of human glomerulonephritis. J Exp Med 1967;126(6):989–1004.

22. Pedchenko V, Bondar O, Fogo AB, et al. Molecular architecture of the Goodpasture autoantigen in anti-GBM nephritis. N Engl J Med 2010;363(4):343–54.

23. Netzer KO, Leinonen A, Boutaud A, et al. The Goodpasture autoantigen. Mapping the major conformational epitope(s) of alpha3(IV) collagen to residues 17-31 and 127-141 of the NC1 domain. J Biol Chem 1999;274(16):11267–74.

24. Zhao J, Yan Y, Cui Z, et al. The immunoglobulin G subclass distribution of anti-GBM autoantibodies against rHalpha3(IV)NC1 is associated with disease severity. Hum Immunol 2009;70(6):425–9.

25. Segelmark M, Butkowski R, Wieslander J. Antigen restriction and IgG subclasses among anti-GBM autoantibodies. Nephrol Dial Transplant 1990;5(12):991–6.

26. Cui Z, Zhao MH. Avidity of anti-glomerular basement membrane autoantibodies was associated with disease severity. Clin Immunol 2005;116(1):77–82.

27. Segelmark M, Hellmark T, Wieslander J. The prognostic significance in Goodpasture's disease of specificity, titre and affinity of anti-glomerular-basement-membrane antibodies. Nephron Clin Pract 2003;94(3):c59–68.

28. Zhou XJ, Lv JC, Bu DF, et al. Copy number variation of FCGR3A rather than FCGR3B and FCGR2B is associated with susceptibility to anti-GBM disease. Int Immunol 2010;22(1):45–51.

29. Zhou XJ, Lv JC, Yu L, et al. FCGR2B gene polymorphism rather than FCGR2A, FCGR3A and FCGR3B is associated with anti-GBM disease in Chinese. Nephrol Dial Transplant 2010;25(1):97–101.

30. Cui Z, Zhao MH, Segelmark M, et al. Natural autoantibodies to myeloperoxidase, proteinase 3, and the glomerular basement membrane are present in normal individuals. Kidney Int 2010;78(6):590–7.

31. Olson SW, Arbogast CB, Baker TP, et al. Asymptomatic autoantibodies associate with future anti-glomerular basement membrane disease. J Am Soc Nephrol 2011;22(10):1946–52.

32. Zou J, Hannier S, Cairns LS, et al. Healthy individuals have Goodpasture autoantigen-reactive T cells. J Am Soc Nephrol 2008;19(2):396–404.

33. Salama AD, Chaudhry AN, Ryan JJ, et al. Goodpasture's disease, CD4(+) T cells escape thymic deletion and are reactive with the autoantigen alpha3(IV)NC1. J Am Soc Nephrol 2001;12(9):1908–15.

34. Bolton WK, Tucker FL, Sturgill BC. New avian model of experimental glomerulonephritis consistent with mediation by cellular immunity. Nonhumorally mediated glomerulonephritis in chickens. J Clin Invest 1984;73(5):1263–76.

35. Dean EG, Wilson GR, Li M, et al. Experimental autoimmune Goodpasture's disease: a pathogenetic role for both effector cells and antibody in injury. Kidney Int 2005;67(2):566–75.

36. Wu J, Hicks J, Borillo J, et al. CD4(+) T cells specific to a glomerular basement membrane antigen mediate glomerulonephritis. J Clin Invest 2002;109(4):517–24.

37. Ooi JD, Chang J, O'Sullivan KM, et al. The HLA-DRB1*15:01-restricted Goodpasture's T cell epitope induces GN. J Am Soc Nephrol 2013;24(3):419–31.

38. Robertson J, Wu J, Arends J, et al. Activation of glomerular basement membrane-specific B cells in the renal draining lymph node after T cell-mediated glomerular injury. J Am Soc Nephrol 2005;16(11):3256–63.

39. Bolton WK, Innes DJ Jr, Sturgill BC, et al. T-cells and macrophages in rapidly progressive glomerulonephritis: clinicopathologic correlations. Kidney Int 1987; 32(6):869–76.

40. Nolasco FE, Cameron JS, Hartley B, et al. Intraglomerular T cells and monocytes in nephritis: study with monoclonal antibodies. Kidney Int 1987;31(5):1160–6.

41. Wong D, Phelps RG, Turner AN. The Goodpasture antigen is expressed in the human thymus. Kidney Int 2001;60(5):1777–83.

42. Arends J, Wu J, Borillo J, et al. T cell epitope mimicry in antiglomerular basement membrane disease. J Immunol 2006;176(2):1252–8.

43. Reynolds J, Preston GA, Pressler BM, et al. Autoimmunity to the alpha 3 chain of type IV collagen in glomerulonephritis is triggered by 'autoantigen complementarity'. J Autoimmun 2015;59:8–18.

44. Li JN, Jia X, Wang Y, et al. Plasma from patients with anti-glomerular basement membrane disease could recognize microbial peptides. PLoS One 2017;12(4): e0174553.

45. Salama AD, Chaudhry AN, Holthaus KA, et al. Regulation by CD25+ lymphocytes of autoantigen-specific T-cell responses in Goodpasture's (anti-GBM) disease. Kidney Int 2003;64(5):1685–94.

46. Ooi JD, Petersen J, Tan YH, et al. Dominant protection from HLA-linked autoimmunity by antigen-specific regulatory T cells. Nature 2017;545(7653):243–7.

47. Liu P, Waheed S, Boujelbane L, et al. Multiple recurrences of anti-glomerular basement membrane disease with variable antibody detection: can the laboratory be trusted? Clin Kidney J 2016;9(5):657–60.

48. Gu B, Magil AB, Barbour SJ. Frequently relapsing anti-glomerular basement membrane antibody disease with changing clinical phenotype and antibody characteristics over time. Clin Kidney J 2016;9(5):661–4.

49. McPhaul JJ Jr, Dixon FJ. The presence of anti-glomerular basement membrane antibodies in peripheral blood. J Immunol 1969;103(6):1168–75.

50. Sinico RA, Radice A, Corace C, et al. Anti-glomerular basement membrane antibodies in the diagnosis of Goodpasture syndrome: a comparison of different assays. Nephrol Dial Transplant 2006;21(2):397–401.

51. Glassock RJ. Atypical anti-glomerular basement membrane disease: lessons learned. Clin Kidney J 2016;9(5):653–6.

52. Lockwood CM, Rees AJ, Pearson TA, et al. Immunosuppression and plasma-exchange in the treatment of Goodpasture's syndrome. Lancet 1976;1(7962): 711–5.

53. Johnson JP, Moore J Jr, Austin HA 3rd, et al. Therapy of anti-glomerular basement membrane antibody disease: analysis of prognostic significance of clinical, pathologic and treatment factors. Medicine (Baltimore) 1985; 64(4):219–27.

54. Cui Z, Zhao J, Jia XY, et al. Anti-glomerular basement membrane disease: outcomes of different therapeutic regimens in a large single-center Chinese cohort study. Medicine (Baltimore) 2011;90(5):303–11.

55. Levy JB, Turner AN, Rees AJ, et al. Long-term outcome of anti-glomerular basement membrane antibody disease treated with plasma exchange and immunosuppression. Ann Intern Med 2001;134(11):1033–42.

56. Schwartz J, Padmanabhan A, Aqui N, et al. Guidelines on the use of therapeutic apheresis in clinical practice-evidence-based approach from the writing

committee of the American Society for Apheresis: the seventh special issue. J Clin Apher 2016;31(3):149–62.

57. Kidney Disease: Improving Global Outcomes (KDIGO) Glomerulonephritis Work Group. KDIGO clinical practice guideline for glomerulonephritis. Kidney Int Suppl 2012;2:139–274.

58. de Groot K, Harper L, Jayne DR, et al. Pulse versus daily oral cyclophosphamide for induction of remission in antineutrophil cytoplasmic antibody-associated vasculitis: a randomized trial. Ann Intern Med 2009;150(10):670–80.

59. Huart A, Josse AG, Chauveau D, et al. Outcomes of patients with Goodpasture syndrome: a nationwide cohort-based study from the French Society of Hemapheresis. J Autoimmun 2016;73:24–9.

60. Booth A, Harper L, Hammad T, et al. Prospective study of TNFalpha blockade with infliximab in anti-neutrophil cytoplasmic antibody-associated systemic vasculitis. J Am Soc Nephrol 2004;15(3):717–21.

61. van Daalen EE, Jennette JC, McAdoo SP, et al. Predicting outcome in patients with Anti-GBM glomerulonephritis. Clin J Am Soc Nephrol 2018;13(1):63–72.

62. Alchi B, Griffiths M, Sivalingam M, et al. Predictors of renal and patient outcomes in anti-GBM disease: clinicopathologic analysis of a two-centre cohort. Nephrol Dial Transplant 2015;30(5):814–21.

63. Tang W, McDonald SP, Hawley CM, et al. Anti-glomerular basement membrane antibody disease is an uncommon cause of end-stage renal disease. Kidney Int 2013;83(3):503–10.

64. Briggs JD, Jones E. Renal transplantation for uncommon diseases. Scientific Advisory Board of the ERA-EDTA Registry. European Renal Association-European Dialysis and Transplant Association. Nephrol Dial Transplant 1999; 14(3):570–5.

65. Costelloe L, Jones J, Coles A. Secondary autoimmune diseases following alemtuzumab therapy for multiple sclerosis. Expert Rev Neurother 2012;12(3):335–41.

66. Clatworthy MR, Wallin EF, Jayne DR. Anti-glomerular basement membrane disease after alemtuzumab. N Engl J Med 2008;359(7):768–9.

67. Meyer D, Coles A, Oyuela P, et al. Case report of anti-glomerular basement membrane disease following alemtuzumab treatment of relapsing-remitting multiple sclerosis. Mult Scler Relat Disord 2013;2(1):60–3.

68. Jones JL, Thompson SA, Loh P, et al. Human autoimmunity after lymphocyte depletion is caused by homeostatic T-cell proliferation. Proc Natl Acad Sci U S A 2013;110(50):20200–5.

69. Sprangers B, Decoo D, Dive D, et al. Management of adverse renal events related to alemtuzumab treatment in multiple sclerosis: a Belgian consensus. Acta Neurol Belg 2018;118(2):143–51.

70. Thomson B, Joseph G, Clark WF, et al. Maternal, pregnancy and fetal outcomes in de novo anti-glomerular basement membrane antibody disease in pregnancy: a systematic review. Clin Kidney J 2014;7(5):450–6.

71. Qin J, Song G, Liu Q. Goodpasture's syndrome in early pregnancy: a case report. Exp Ther Med 2018;15(1):407–11.

72. Nelson-Piercy C, Agarwal S, Lams B. Lesson of the month: selective use of cyclophosphamide in pregnancy for severe autoimmune respiratory disease. Thorax 2016;71(7):667–8.

73. Schlieben DJ, Korbet SM, Kimura RE, et al. Pulmonary-renal syndrome in a newborn with placental transmission of ANCAs. Am J kidney Dis 2005;45(4):758–61.

74. O'Donoghue DJ, Short CD, Brenchley PE, et al. Sequential development of systemic vasculitis with anti-neutrophil cytoplasmic antibodies complicating anti-glomerular basement membrane disease. Clin Nephrol 1989;32(6):251–5.

75. Jayne DR, Marshall PD, Jones SJ, et al. Autoantibodies to GBM and neutrophil cytoplasm in rapidly progressive glomerulonephritis. Kidney Int 1990;37(3):965–70.

76. Short AK, Esnault VL, Lockwood CM. Anti-neutrophil cytoplasm antibodies and anti-glomerular basement membrane antibodies: two coexisting distinct autoreactivities detectable in patients with rapidly progressive glomerulonephritis. Am J kidney Dis 1995;26(3):439–45.

77. Bosch X, Mirapeix E, Font J, et al. Prognostic implication of anti-neutrophil cytoplasmic autoantibodies with myeloperoxidase specificity in anti-glomerular basement membrane disease. Clin Nephrol 1991;36(3):107–13.

78. Levy JB, Hammad T, Coulthart A, et al. Clinical features and outcome of patients with both ANCA and anti-GBM antibodies. Kidney Int 2004;66(4):1535–40.

79. Lindic J, Vizjak A, Ferluga D, et al. Clinical outcome of patients with coexistent antineutrophil cytoplasmic antibodies and antibodies against glomerular basement membrane. Ther Apher Dial 2009;13(4):278–81.

80. Srivastava A, Rao GK, Segal PE, et al. Characteristics and outcome of crescentic glomerulonephritis in patients with both antineutrophil cytoplasmic antibody and anti-glomerular basement membrane antibody. Clin Rheumatol 2013;32(9):1317–22.

81. McAdoo SP, Tanna A, Hruskova Z, et al. Patients double-seropositive for ANCA and anti-GBM antibodies have varied renal survival, frequency of relapse, and outcomes compared to single-seropositive patients. Kidney Int 2017;92(3):693–702.

82. Nasr SH, Collins AB, Alexander MP, et al. The clinicopathologic characteristics and outcome of atypical anti-glomerular basement membrane nephritis. Kidney Int 2016;89(4):897–908.

83. Vankalakunti M, Nada R, Kumar A, et al. Circulating monoclonal IgG1-kappa antibodies causing anti-glomerular basement membrane nephritis. Indian J Nephrol 2017;27(4):327–9.

84. Rosales IA, Colvin RB. Glomerular disease with idiopathic linear immunoglobulin deposition: a rose by any other name would be atypical. Kidney Int 2016;89(4):750–2.

85. Arzoo K, Sadeghi S, Liebman HA. Treatment of refractory antibody mediated autoimmune disorders with an anti-CD20 monoclonal antibody (rituximab). Ann Rheum Dis 2002;61(10):922–4.

86. Wechsler E, Yang T, Jordan SC, et al. Anti-glomerular basement membrane disease in an HIV-infected patient. Nat Clin Pract Nephrol 2008;4(3):167–71.

87. Schless B, Yildirim S, Beha D, et al. Rituximab in two cases of Goodpasture's syndrome. NDT Plus 2009;2(3):225–7.

88. Mutsaers P, Selten H, van Dam B. Additional antibody suppression from rituximab added to conventional therapy in severe, refractory anti-GBM nephritis. NDT Plus 2010;3(4):421–2.

89. Shah Y, Mohiuddin A, Sluman C, et al. Rituximab in anti-glomerular basement membrane disease. QJM 2012;105(2):195–7.

90. Syeda UA, Singer NG, Magrey M. Anti-glomerular basement membrane antibody disease treated with rituximab: a case-based review. Semin Arthritis Rheum 2013;42(6):567–72.

91. Bandak G, Jones BA, Li J, et al. Rituximab for the treatment of refractory simultaneous anti-glomerular basement membrane (anti-GBM) and membranous nephropathy. Clin Kidney J 2014;7(1):53–6.
92. Narayanan M, Casimiro I, Pichler R. A unique way to treat Goodpasture's disease. BMJ Case Rep 2014;2014 [pii:bcr2014206220].
93. Touzot M, Poisson J, Faguer S, et al. Rituximab in anti-GBM disease: a retrospective study of 8 patients. J Autoimmun 2015;60:74–9.
94. Huang J, Wu L, Huang X, et al. Successful treatment of dual-positive anti-myeloperoxidase and anti-glomerular basement membrane antibody vasculitis with pulmonary-renal syndrome. Case Rep Nephrol Dial 2016;6(1):1–7.

Autoimmune Kidney Diseases Associated with Chronic Viral Infections

Joshua D. Long, BA, Stephanie M. Rutledge, MBBS,
Meghan E. Sise, MD, MS*

KEYWORDS

- Hepatitis C virus • Hepatitis B virus • Human immunodeficiency virus
- Mixed cryoglobulinemia syndrome • Glomerulonephritis • Direct-acting antivirals
- Interferon

KEY POINTS

- Hepatitis B virus infection can cause both membranous nephropathy and polyarteritis nodosa.
- Hepatitis C virus infection can cause cryoglobulinemic glomerulonephritis and is associated with other autoimmune kidney diseases, including membranous nephropathy, fibrillary glomerulopathy, immunotactoid glomerulopathy, and immunoglobulin A nephropathy.
- Patients with human immunodeficiency virus (HIV) infection may be affected by HIV-associated nephropathy and HIV-associated immune complex diseases.
- Treatment of kidney diseases that occur in the setting of chronic viral infection relies first on controlling viral replication with antiviral medications.
- Immunosuppression is typically needed only in severe presentations of virally associated autoimmune kidney diseases.

INTRODUCTION

Although hepatitis B virus (HBV), hepatitis C virus (HCV), and human immunodeficiency virus (HIV) are ubiquitous in medicine today and in the general public's consciousness, the renal consequences of these diseases receive far less attention. A variety of different mechanisms lead to the development of immune-mediated

Disclosures: S.M. Rutledge and J.D. Long have no conflicts of interest to declare and no grants or other funding to disclose. M.E. Sise has received grant support from Gilead Sciences (GS-US-337-4063), Abbvie, and Merck & Co. She has participated in scientific advisory board meetings for Abbvie and Merck & Co and is a Scientific Consultant to Abbvie.
Department of Medicine, Division of Nephrology, Massachusetts General Hospital, 55 Fruit Street, GRB 7, Boston, MA 02114, USA
* Corresponding author. 165 Cambridge Street, Suite 302, Boston, MA 02114.
E-mail address: msise@partners.org

kidney damage in each of these viral infections. Although most treatment trials and observational studies in these populations are small, important information can be gleaned from them, giving clinicians the tools they need to best treat the different presentations of each of these diseases in patients.

HEPATITIS B VIRUS INFECTION

HBV, a member of the Hepadnaviridae family, is a small, enveloped, hepatotropic, noncytopathic DNA virus that is a leading cause of chronic liver disease and hepatocellular carcinoma worldwide.[1,2] Despite the advent of successful vaccination strategies in the early 1980s, it is estimated that more than 300 million people worldwide are infected with HBV.[1,2] The virus remains a severe public health issue, especially in Asia, Africa, and South America, where the virus is endemic.[3] HBV infection may lead to an asymptomatic carrier state, or may have clinical manifestations ranging from acute hepatitis, fulminant hepatitic failure, or chronic hepatitis that leads to cirrhosis.[3] Antiviral therapies (**Table 1**) are necessary to prevent the progression of chronic HBV infection to hepatocellular carcinoma or cirrhosis.[1]

Hepatitis B Virus–Associated Kidney Diseases: Membranous Nephropathy

Mechanism/pathogenesis of hepatitis B virus–membranous nephropathy

Membranous nephropathy (MN) is among the most common causes of nephrotic syndromes in adults across the world. MN occurs in an idiopathic form and secondary forms; HBV-related MN (HBV-MN) is an important cause of secondary MN in HBV-endemic areas, particularly in children, but it also affects adults.[4] HBV-MN was first described by Combes and colleagues[5] in 1971, who demonstrated HBsAg antibody complexes in the glomerular basement membrane of an adult who developed MN after a posttransfusion HBV infection. Renal biopsies from all 21 patients with HBV-MN in one study exhibited diffuse granular deposition of hepatitis B e-antigen (HBeAg), immunoglobulin (Ig)G, and C3 along the glomerular capillary walls.[6] Mesangial abnormalities and deposits are more likely to be observed in cases of secondary MN, like HBV-MN, than in idiopathic MN.[7] Characteristic kidney biopsy findings are demonstrated in **Fig. 1**.

The exact pathogenic mechanism by which some individuals develop MN from HBV infection remains unknown, but the leading hypothesis suggests that, like other forms of secondary MN, circulating immune complexes may be passively trapped in the subepithelial space (**Fig. 2**).[6,8] All 3 major HBV antigens (HBsAg, HBcAg, and HBeAg) have been identified by immunofluorescence in the glomerular capillary wall and mesangium in HBV-MN.[9–18] These complexes, in the subepithelial and mesangial space, then may locally activate the complement cascade and recruit inflammatory cells.[11,16,17,19,20] Alternatively, it has been suggested that HBV viral replication itself may occur and damage endothelial tissues, leading to immune complex formation.[21] Finally, some have suggested that HBV infection causes the induction of autoantibodies to intrinsic glomerular antigens,[16] as some patients with HBV-MN do have Phospholipase A2 Receptor (PLA2R) staining of immune deposits.[22] It is important to stain biopsies and perform PLA2R antibody testing to exclude the possibility of concomitant HBV and primary MN. A genetic predisposition to HBV-MN may result from impaired cell-mediated immunity and inadequate interferon (IFN)-α production may lead to inadequate clearance of antigen-antibody complexes.[23–26] These theories suggest that a chronic HBV infection itself is not sufficient for the development of HBV-MN. Instead, it is likely that

Table 1
Antiviral agents used to treat hepatitis B virus infection

Agent	Mechanism of Action	Benefits	Downsides
IFN (PEG-IFN preferred over IFN-α)	• Augments innate immunity • Induces genes that interfere with HBV lifecycle	• Finite duration of treatment (typically ~1 y) • Does not promote viral resistance • Virologic response is usually lasting after stopping therapy	• Need for subcutaneous injections • Significant side-effect profile[a]
Lamivudine	Suppression of replication by inhibiting HBV polymerase	• Low cost • Administered orally • Good safety profile • Also treats HIV infection	• Resistance is common, no longer used as monotherapy[187] • Dose adjustment needed for renal failure • Long-term therapy needed
Entecavir	Suppression of HBV replication by inhibiting HBV polymerase	• Potent antiviral activity • Administered orally • Low rate of drug resistance • No dose adjustment needed for renal failure	• Possible effect on sex organs[188] • Cannot be used in patients with resistance to lamivudine • Long-term therapy needed
Tenofovir (TDF or TAF)	Suppression of HBV replication by inhibiting HBV polymerase	• Can be used as initial therapy or also in patients with resistance to other oral nucleos(t)ide analogs • Also has activity against HIV infection • Does not promote viral resistance • TAF can be used in patients with renal impairment	• TDF is not safe in patients with chronic kidney disease • TDF may lead to bone demineralization • TAF has less renal and bone toxicity than TDF • Long-term therapy needed

Abbreviations: HBV, hepatitis B virus; HIV, human immunodeficiency virus; IFN, interferon; PEG, pegylated; TAF, tenofovir alafenamide (newer formulation); TDF, tenofovir disoproxil fumarate (older formulation).

[a] Common interferon side effects include fatigue, anemia, seizure, psychiatric symptoms, flulike symptoms, headache, myalgia, abdominal pain, insomnia, weakness, thrombocytopenia, neutropenia.

immunologic, genetic, and environmental factors must align in specifically vulnerable individuals.[24]

Management/treatment of hepatitis B virus–membranous nephropathy
Vaccination to prevent HBV infection is an extremely important strategy to prevent HBV-MN, and for this reason, the disease is extremely rare in parts of the world

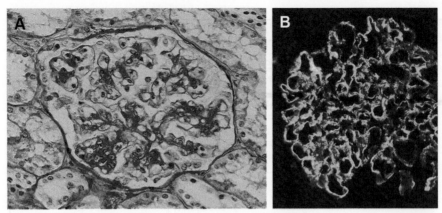

Fig. 1. (*A*, original magnification x 400) Periodic acid-Schiff staining in a case of HBV-associated MN. Periodic acid-Schiff staining shows both mild glomerular basement membrane thickening as well as increase of mesangial matrix and mesangial hypercellularity. (*B*) Immunofluorescence staining in a case of HBV-associated MN IgG. Immunofluorescent staining with anti-human IgG demonstrates granular staining along the capillary walls and mesangial staining. Electron microscopy demonstrates mesangial and subepithelial location of deposits as well as diffuse podocyte foot process effacement (not shown).

with effective vaccination strategies. For those with established HBV-MN, treatment recommendations are based on small case series and uncontrolled observations. The optimal antiviral strategies are largely extrapolated from randomized trials in patients with HBV infection without HBV-MN. Antiviral therapies approved for chronic

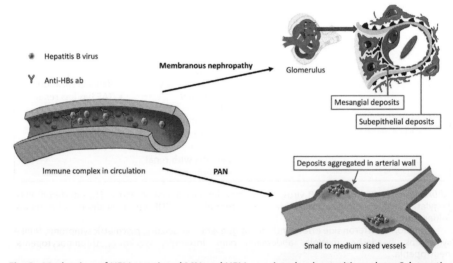

Fig. 2. Mechanism of HBV-associated MN and HBV-associated polyarteritis nodosa. Schematic representation of the hypothesized pathogenesis of HBV-MN and HBV-PAN. HBs ab, Hepatitis B surface antibody. In HBV-MN circulating immune complexes deposit in the subepithelial and mesangial space. Subepithelial deposits lead to glomerular basement membrane thickening and podocyte foot process effacement leading to nephrotic syndrome. In HBV-PAN, it is hypothesized that circulating immune complexes are deposited in the small-medium vessel walls, preferentially at branch points leading to inflammation and aneurysm formation (although it is possible that immune complexes form in situ in the vessel walls).

HBV include pegylated interferon (PEG-IFN) and the nucleotide/nucleoside analogs shown in **Table 1**.[27] The goal of antiviral therapy is the suppression of HBV DNA and clearance of both HBe and HBs antigen.[28]

Although the natural course of HBV-MN in children often involves remission and preservation of renal function, adults with HBV-MN typically develop disease progression with a low probability of spontaneous remission; therefore, immediate antiviral treatment is recommended.[28]

Interferon-based therapies for hepatitis B virus–membranous nephropathy Antiviral therapy for HBV-MN has historically relied on PEG-IFN, which has an immunomodulatory effect in addition to its suppression of HBV replication. IFN is still used as first-line therapy in some patients with favorable virologic characteristics; however, side effects are common and include flulike symptoms, fatigue, anemia, leukopenia, neuropsychiatric effects, and the potential of triggering other autoimmune diseases. Although IFN is less well tolerated than nucleot(s)ide antiviral agents, it is more likely to result in sustained remission. If IFN is not effective or not tolerated, it is recommended that patients switch to nucleotide/nucleoside analogs.

A retrospective report examined 15 patients with HBV-related glomerulonephritis treated with IFN-α subcutaneously for 16 weeks, including 10 with HBV-MN, 4 with HBV-associated membranoproliferative glomerulonephritis (MPGN), and 1 with a nondiagnostic biopsy. Seroconversion of HBeAg to anti-HBe antibodies was observed in 8 of 15 patients, as was long-term resolution of proteinuria in most patients who had a virologic response (7 of 8 virologic responders).[29] Patients with HBV-MN were more likely to respond than those with HBV-MPGN. A separate randomized trial on the effect of IFN-α in children with HBV-MN who had been unresponsive to prior corticosteroid treatment demonstrated resolution of proteinuria in 20 of 20 of the patients, who were treated 3 times a week for 12 months. By the end of the third month, all patients were free of proteinuria. HBeAg seroconversion occurred in most by 1 year.[30] Other studies using IFN exist, but with smaller sample sizes and varying results.[6,15,25]

Oral nucleotide/nucleoside analog therapies for hepatitis B virus–membranous nephropathy infection Nucelot(s)ide analogs directly suppress HBV replication and have far fewer side effects than IFN-based therapies; however, the downside is that long-term therapy is needed. Lamivudine has been studied in HBV-MN, is usually well tolerated, and typically results in reduction of HBV DNA levels and a reduction of proteinuria.[31–33] In by far the largest single study on treatment of patients with HBV-MN with lamivudine, Tang and colleagues[4] noted disappearance of circulating HBV DNA along with reduction of proteinuria (4.9 ± 2.4 g/d to median 0.19 g/d within 3 years); 6 of 10 patients with HBV-MN who were treated went into complete remission (proteinuria level <0.3 g/24 hours) within 12 months. Renal outcomes were improved, with cumulative 3-year renal survival (end-stage renal disease [ESRD] as primary endpoint) 100% in the treated group and only 58% in untreated patients, who also experienced significant proteinuria within a year.[4] However, prolonged lamivudine monotherapy commonly leads to viral resistance in up to 20% of patients per year of treatment due to its low mutational barrier to resistance; thus, newer nucleot(s)ide analogs are now standard of care for antiviral management of HBV.[28,31,34,35]

Entecavir, a newer guanosine nucleoside analog with a higher barrier to resistance, is considered first line for HBV infection (see **Table 1**).[36,37] A retrospective study of 42 adults with HBV-MN compared entecavir monotherapy (19 patients) with entecavir therapy with tacrolimus (23 patients). The probability of proteinuria remission in the tacrolimus + entecavir group was 69% after 12 weeks and 87% after 24 weeks. In the entecavir monotherapy group, remission was reached in only 42% by 24 weeks. The mean time to partial or complete remission in the entecavir plus tacrolimus group was 18.6 weeks compared with 34.3 weeks in the entecavir-alone group. HBV DNA titer was observed to be reduced in all patients with active HBV replication and none of the HBV carriers in the tacrolimus + entecavir group showed evidence of HBV reactivation. Tacrolimus combined with entecavir may be an effective strategy to induce remission of HBV-MN.[38]

Other immunosuppressive agents, such as corticosteroids or plasmapheresis, have little utility in HBV-MN given the effectiveness of antiviral therapies to decrease HBV replication. Although tacrolimus was used in one study discussed previously, there is an important concern that immunosuppression may be harmful through induction of HBV replication and may cause liver damage and deterioration of renal lesions, thus antiviral therapy alone is considered first line in managing HBV-MN.[39–41]

Polyarteritis Nodosa Caused by Hepatitis B Virus Infection

Mechanism/pathogenesis of hepatitis B virus–polyarteritis nodosa

Polyarteritis nodosa (PAN) is a rare necrotizing vasculitis that predominately targets medium and small-sized arteries, causing inflammation and necrosis of the artery walls, often at their branch points, leading to microaneurysm formation and organ infarction.[13,42–44] HBV was first associated with the development of PAN in 1970 by Trepo and Thivolet.[45] Effective vaccination protocols and improved safety of blood products achieved via thorough screening have substantially decreased the prevalence of HBV-PAN worldwide today; however, it is estimated that 1% of patients with chronic HBV infection may develop PAN (HBV-PAN).[46]

The renal vasculature is affected in approximately 70% to 80% of cases of PAN, and clinical manifestations may range from malignant hypertension and proteinuria to renal insufficiency and hemorrhage/infarct due to microaneurysms.[47,48] Renal infarcts may produce microhematuria or macrohematuria, mild to moderate proteinuria, or, alternatively, may be clinically silent.[49] HBV-PAN is not a cause of acute glomerulonephritis[49]; however, multiple renal infarcts or uncontrolled hypertension can lead to impaired renal function,[47,50] yet ESRD from HBV-PAN is uncommon.[49]

The exact mechanism of HBV-PAN is not well understood, but it is believed to be immunopathogenic (see **Fig. 2**).[51] HBV replicates efficiently only in hepatocytes and it is generally presumed that the extrahepatic manifestations of HBV, including PAN, are secondary immunologic disorders that arise from either circulating or in situ formation of immune complexes of HBV antigens and their corresponding antibodies.[52–54] It is clear that almost all cases of HBV-PAN are associated with HBe antigenemia and high HBV replication.[55] What is unclear is why antigen-antibody complexes deposit in the arterial wall, but one theory is that a cross-reaction occurs between arterial wall antigens and the antigen that initiated the disease process.[51] HBs antigen and antibody immune complexes have been detected in the vascular lesions of patients with HBV-PAN.[13] The immune complexes activate the complement cascade, attracting and recruiting polymorphonuclear neutrophils, resulting in blood vessel damage and vasculitis.[51,56] Active disease is marked by low serum complement levels.[57] Serum antineutrophilic cytoplasmic antibodies are rarely present in HBV-PAN.[56,58–60]

Management/treatment of hepatitis B virus–polyarteritis nodosa

Treatment should be initiated as soon as possible after a diagnosis of HBV-PAN is made because of the severe consequences of this disease, which can be life-threatening.[61] Early attempts to use corticosteroids and other immunosuppressive agents in patients with HBV-PAN promoted viral persistence and replication, thus increasing the risk of chronic hepatitis and cirrhosis.[62,63] Currently recommended strategies rely primarily on antiviral therapies to promote HBV seroconversion and lead to lower probability of relapse than immunosuppressant therapy alone.[55,61] Controlling viral replication with antiviral agents has proven to be an effective strategy in curing the disease's vasculitic effects.[57] The European League Against Rheumatism has recommended that a combination of antiviral therapy, plasma exchange, and glucocorticoids should be used for severe cases of HBV-PAN.[64–67] The rationale behind this strategy is twofold. First, initial corticosteroid therapy and plasma exchange are implemented to rapidly control the most severe life-threatening manifestations of PAN common during the first weeks of the disease. Second, abruptly stopping corticosteroid treatment may enhance immunologic clearance of HBV-infected hepatocytes and favors the seroconversion of HBe antigen to anti-HBe antibody with antiviral therapy.[55] This strategy has resulted in a strong correlation between inhibition of viral replication and resolution of all clinical symptoms.[55] However, it should be noted that plasma exchange comes with the risk of catheter-associated infections.[67]

For milder cases of HBV-PAN, that is, cases without severe ulcerative or gangrenous lesions of the extremities, acute kidney injury, polyneuropathy, central nervous system involvement, mesenteric arteritis, or myocardial ischemia, it is unclear whether corticosteroid treatment and plasma exchange are necessary additions to antiviral therapy, or whether antiviral therapy alone is sufficient. For these patients, the risks of immunosuppression and plasma exchange may outweigh the benefits.

An early study evaluating the effectiveness of lamivudine in patients with HBV-PAN showed that 90% of patients achieved clinical recovery within 6 months and two-thirds of these patients showed HBe seroconversion within 9 months.[67] Although there are many compelling reasons why lamivudine may be superior to alpha-IFN in treating patients with HBV-PAN, resistance mutations against lamivudine are common and can reduce its effectiveness in up to 20% of treated patients per year.[28] Newer antivirals (see **Table 1**) have also been suggested as possible treatment options for this disease,[49,68–71] but minimal data are available on treatment with these agents in patients with HBV-PAN.

Even once the symptoms of HBV-PAN resolve, it is important to ensure a virologic response to HBV treatment, otherwise the symptoms of PAN can relapse. However, those who achieve both a vasculitic and virologic response to treatment can be considered cured, and clinical relapses are uncommon.

HEPATITIS C VIRUS INFECTION

HCV is the most common chronic viral infection in the world; in 2015 it affected approximately 71 million people worldwide and 3.5 million people in the United States.[72] HCV is a blood-borne, single-stranded RNA virus belonging to the flavivirus family, and its genome encodes a single polyprotein containing 10 proteins. HCV is categorized into 6 major genotypes, each with multiple subtypes. After initial infection with HCV, roughly 20% of patients will mount an immune response that successfully eradicates the virus, while the remaining 80% develop a chronic infection with persistently elevated HCV RNA. During the chronic phase, HCV infects hepatocytes causing immune dysfunction, chronic hepatitis, and after 20 to 30 years of HCV infection, individuals may develop cirrhosis, which can lead to the need for liver transplantation or result in hepatocellular carcinoma or death.[73,74] Beyond causing liver disease, HCV infection is associated with numerous extrahepatic manifestations, including kidney disease.

Hepatitis C Virus–Associated Kidney Diseases: Cryoglobulinemic Glomerulonephritis

Mechanism/pathogenesis of hepatitis C virus–related cryoglobulinemic glomerulonephritis

One common extrahepatic manifestation of chronic HCV infection is cryoglobuline-mia.[75–77] Cryoglobulins are proteins that circulate in the serum, precipitate below core body temperature, and dissolve on rewarming.[78,79] Circulating cryoglobulins are commonly detected in HCV-infected patients; up to 50% of patients with chronic HCV will have detectable serum cryoglobulins at some point during their infection; however, only 2% to 3% develop the vasculitic symptoms that characterize hepatitis C–related mixed cryoglobulinemic syndrome (HCV-MCS). Common presentations of HCV-MCS include skin rash (palpable purpura), weakness, neuropathy, and arthralgia, as well as hematuria and proteinuria due to cryoglobulinemic glomerulonephritis (GN). Serologic abnormalities commonly include a positive rheumatoid factor (RF) and hypocomplementemia in most cases.[80–82]

Typical renal manifestations of cryoglobulinemic GN include hypertension, protein-uria, microscopic hematuria, renal insufficiency, and even nephrotic syndrome.[83] Light microscopy shows a membranoproliferative pattern of GN (MPGN) due to deposition of mesangial and subendothelial immune complexes, which leads to glomerular hypercel-lularity, thickening of the glomerular basement membrane, and a "double-contoured" appearance.[84,85] The presence of "pseudothrombi," large eosinophilic, intraglomerular periodic acid-Schiff stain–positive deposits, is pathognomonic for cryoglobulinemic GN. Electron microscopy typically reveals subendothelial deposits.[86] Immunofluores-cence confirms mesangial and capillary wall deposition of IgM, IgG, and C3.[87] Vasculitis of the small and medium-sized renal arteries may be seen in approximately 33% with cryoglobulinemic GN.[86,88] Significant podocyte injury can be seen in approximately 20% of these patients, who typically present with nephrotic-range proteinuria.[86,88,89] Milder forms of cryoglobulinemic GN, referred to as mesangioproliferative GN, are char-acterized by an increase in the mesangial matrix without significant subendothelial infil-tration of leukocytes.[88] These patients typically have a mild clinical course.

Several other glomerular diseases have been associated with chronic HCV infec-tion. MN is a much less common renal manifestation of HCV and whether HCV is truly causal is not well understood, as most studies showing a possible association were done before routine testing of PLA2R. Unlike patients with MPGN, patients with MN commonly present with nephrotic syndrome, typically have normal complement levels, and no elevation of RF or serum cryoglobulin levels.[90,91] Fibrillary glomerulone-phritis and immunotactoid glomerulopathy have been associated with HCV infection; these diseases are characterized by organized immune deposits within the mesan-gium and capillary walls.[92–95] The clinical presentation of fibrillary and immunotactoid GN is typically nephrotic-range proteinuria, hematuria, hypertension, and acute or chronic renal insufficiency; the cases presented in the literature typically had a very poor prognosis.[96–98] Finally, IgA nephropathy can occur in patients with HCV-related cirrhosis due to impaired clearance of IgA and IgA-containing immune com-plexes by the injured Kupffer cells in the liver. This secondary form of IgA nephropathy is typically clinically silent or causes only hematuria, but in a minority of causes it may cause significant hematuria, proteinuria, and renal insufficiency.[99]

Management/treatment of hepatitis C virus–related cryoglobulinemic glomerulonephritis

The goals of treatment of HCV-MCS are to eradicate HCV infection and cure the symptoms of MCS; as such, antiviral therapy is the cornerstone of management of cryoglobulinemic GN. The association between IFN and resolution of cryoglobuline-mic GN was established by Johnson and colleagues[100] when they treated 4 patients with cryoglobulinemic GN with IFN-α monotherapy, and all patients experienced a reduction in proteinuria. Most studies of IFN-based therapies demonstrated that sustained clinical benefit was limited to patients who successfully cleared HCV RNA.[101,102] However, IFN-based therapies rarely led to a sustained virologic response (SVR), or cure, in patients with HCV-MCS and cryoglobulinemic GN; IFN-α monotherapy achieved SVR in 4% to 27% of patients with HCV-MCS and a moderate complete clinical response rate of 27% to 62%.[101–106] The combination of pegylated IFN-α with ribavirin (RBV) was more efficacious, resulting in SVR rates of 18% to 54% and complete clinical response rates of 44% to 77%, although relapse rates were still as high as 60%. As a result, improvement in kidney manifestations were seen in only 50% of patients treated with IFN-based therapies, and most had recurrent cryoglobulinemic GN symptoms if HCV viremia relapsed.[101,105,107–113]

Because of the poor efficacy of IFN-based therapies, immunosuppression that targets the downstream B-cell arm of autoimmunity was historically necessary to prevent progression of cryoglobulinemic GN. Rituximab, an anti-CD20 monoclonal antibody, used with or without corticosteroids, is highly effective at decreasing the production of cryoglobulins and treating the inflammatory renal lesions seen in cryoglobulinemic GN.[114–117] Rituximab-based immunosuppression is generally considered safe in HCV infection and it does not reduce the efficacy of IFN-based antiviral therapy in clearing HCV infection.[108,118] Complete clinical response with the addition of rituximab may be seen in 54% to 73% of treated patients, although relapse rates may be as high as 39%.[108,119,120] Multiple prospective studies have shown that when rituximab was added to IFN and RBV-based antiviral therapy, it shortened the time to clinical remission and led to better renal response rates and higher rates of cryoglobulin clearance.[108,120,121] Even when used in the absence of concurrent antiviral therapy in patients intolerant to IFN, rituximab-based immunosuppressive therapy improved clinical symptoms of HCV-MCS.[122,123] Multiple studies have shown stable transaminases and no increase in HCV viremia during rituximab therapy, suggesting it is safe in patients with cryoglobulinemic GN and liver disease.[121–123] Thus, in the era of IFN-based therapy for HCV, 2008 guidelines recommended initiation of antiviral therapy and rituximab-based immunosuppression at the time of diagnosis of HCV-MCS, particularly in cases of cryoglobulinemic GN.[124]

Direct-acting antiviral therapies (DAAs) have revolutionized the management of HCV infection, rapidly transforming it into a curable disease. DAAs target the nonstructural proteins that make up the replicative machinery of HCV. There are 3 approved classes of DAAs: NS3/4A protease inhibitors, NS5A protein inhibitors, and NS5B polymerase inhibitors. The general approach for curative treatment is to target multiple components of the viral replicative machinery with agents from 2 or more classes and inhibit them for 8 to 24 weeks; this is sufficient to achieve cure in the vast majority of patients (>95%). Regimen selection and treatment duration is determined by the potency of the regimen, HCV genotype, and whether the patient has cirrhosis or prior HCV treatment experience. Up-to-date HCV treatment guidelines can be found at HCVguidelines.org.[125] All of the DAA regimens currently approved by the Food and Drug Administration (FDA) can be used in patients with estimated glomerular filtration rate (eGFR) >30 mL/min per 1.73 m^2, but there are only 3 regimens that have been approved for patients with eGFR less than 30 mL/min per 1.73 m^2 or those on dialysis (**Table 2**). These include (1) paritaprevir/ritonavir/ombitasvir and dasabuvir, (2) elbasvir and grazoprevir, or (3) glecaprevir and pibrentasvir.[124,126–128] Sofosbuvir-based DAA combination therapies are generally not recommended in patients with eGFR less

Table 2 Direct-acting antiviral combinations approved by the Food and Drug Administration		
DAA Combination	**Genotype**	**Safety if eGFR <30**
Sofosbuvir/Simeprevir (SOF/SIM)	1	Sofosbuvir not approved if GFR <30 Simeprevir largely hepatically metabolized
Sofosbuvir/Daclatasvir (SOF/DAC)	1–3	Sofosbuvir not approved if GFR <30 Simeprevir largely hepatically metabolized
Sofosbuvir/Ledipasvir (SOF/LDV)	1, 4	Sofosbuvir not approved if GFR <30 Ledipasvir largely hepatically metabolized
Ombitasvir/Paritaprevir/ Ritonavir + Dasabuvir (PrOD) Ombitasvir/Paritaprevir/Ritonavir (PrO)	1 4	Safe and effective in advanced/ ESRD on hemodialysis
Grazoprevir/Elbasvir (GRZ/ELB)	1, 4	Safe and effective in advanced/ ESRD on hemodialysis
Sofosbuvir/Velpatasvir (SOF/VEL)	Pan-Genotypic	Sofosbuvir not approved if GFR <30 Velpatasvir largely hepatically metabolized
Glecaprevir/Pibrentasvir (GLE/PIB)	Pan-Genotypic	Safe and effective in advanced/ ESRD on hemodialysis Glecaprevir and pibrentasvir largely hepatically metabolized

Abbreviations: DAA, direct-acting antiviral; eGFR, estimated glomerular filtration rate; ESRD, end-stage renal disease; GFR, glomerular filtration rate.

than 30 mL/min per 1.73 m^2, because the parent drug and its active metabolite GS-331007 accumulate in renal disease.[129–132] In the past 2 years, "pan-genotypic" therapies that effectively function against the major viral genotypes 1 to 6 have been approved by the FDA (see **Table 2**).[127,133]

DAAs have also had an important impact on recommendations for management of HCV-MCS and cryoglobulinemic GN. Several centers have published their experience with novel DAA therapies in HCV-MCS, including agents such as sofosbuvir, simeprevir, telaprevir, boceprevir, daclatasvir, ledipasvir, asunaprevir, dasabuvir, paritaprevir, and ombitasvir. Studies demonstrate that DAA regimens achieve SVR in 95% (297 of 313) of patients with HCV-MCS, which is similar to cure rates in the general population with HCV.[134–145] There are currently no reports of HCV-MCS treated with more recently approved DAAs, such as sofosbuvir/velpatasvir/voxilaprevir, elbasvir/grazoprevir, glecaprevir/pibrentasvir, or sofosbuvir/velpatasvir, but there is no reason to believe that these agents would be less effective in HCV-MCS. The complete clinical remission rate of HCV-MCS symptoms after IFN-free DAA therapy has ranged widely between studies, but across all studies, 85% of patients were reported to have either a partial (20%) or complete clinical response (65%).[134–140,146] Achieving clinical remission was tied to SVR status, but there were several cases of complete clinical response in patients who relapsed virologically.[118,134–137,142,145,147,148]

Because cryoglobulinemic GN affects fewer than half of patients with HCV-MCS, each published series of DAAs in HCV-MCS included only a handful of patients with cryoglobulinemic GN, summarized in **Table 3**. In summary, of 9 studies that evaluated response of cryoglobulinemic GN to treatment with DAA, 17 (33%) of 52 patients showed complete resolution of GN and 15 (29%) of 52 showed improvement in renal parameters. These studies have led to a change in the Kidney Disease: Improving Global Outcomes 2017 guidelines for management of cryoglobulinemic GN in the context of HCV infection.[149] It is now recommended that DAAs be used as first-line therapy and that immunosuppression be reserved only for those patients with severe manifestations or those who do not enter remission after achieving SVR with DAA therapy. Initiation of immunosuppression (rituximab and steroids ± plasmapheresis) in the

Table 3
Virologic and clinical outcomes in patients with cryoglobulinemic glomerulonephritis treated with direct-acting antivirals

Reference	DAA Regimens Used	Partial Remission (PR)/Complete Remission (CR), %	% Receiving Concurrent Immunosuppression
Cornella et al,[147] 2015	TVR + IFN + RBV SOF + IFN + RBV 100% SVR rate	2/3 (67%) CR	3/3 (100%)
Saadoun et al,[118] 2015	BOC/TVR + IFN + RBV SVR not reported	5/7 (71%) PR 0/7 (0%) CR	4/7 (57%)
Sise et al,[143] 2016	SOF + SIM, SOF + RBV 86% SVR rate	4/7 (57%) PR 0/7 (0%) CR	2/7 (29%)
Gragnani et al,[142] 2016	SOF-based DAA therapy 100% SVR rate	1/4 (25%) PR 3/4 (75%) CR	1/4 (25%)
Saadoun et al,[139] 2016	SOF + RBV 80% SVR rate	4/5 (80%) PR 0/5 (0%) CR	2/5 (40%)
Saadoun et al,[134] 2017	SOF + DAC 100% SVR rate	1/5 (20%) PR 4/5 (80%) CR	ND
Gragnani et al,[138] 2017	SOF + DAC SOF + RBV PROD 100% SVR rate	0/3 (0%) CR	ND
Emery et al,[135] 2017	SOF + RBV SOF + SIM PROD + -RBV SOF + LDV + -RBV SVR not reported	3/10 (30%) CR	4/10 (40%)
Bonacci et al,[136] 2017	SOF + LDV, SOF + SIM, SIM + DAC, SOF + DAC, ASV + DAC + IFN + RBV 100% SVR rate	5/7 (71%) CR	2/7 (29%)

Clinical response to DAA therapy in patients with cryoglobulinemic glomerulonephritis. Clinical and virologic outcomes in the 52 patients with MCS and renal involvement who were treated with DAA therapy. The SVR rate was 94%; 17 (33%) of 52 showed complete resolution (CR) of GN and 15 (29%) of 52 demonstrated PR. Forty-two percent (18/43) required concurrent immunosuppression.

Abbreviations: ASV, asunaprevir; BOC, boceprevir; DAA, direct-acting antiviral; DAC, daclatasvir; GN, glomerulonephritis; IFN, interferon; LDV, ledipasvir; ND, not done; PROD, ombitasvir-paritaprevir-ritonavir and dasabuvir; RBV, ribavirin; SIM, simeprevir; SOF, sofosbuvir; SVR, sustained virologic response; TVR, telaprevir.

small minority of patients who present with rapidly progressive glomerulonephritis, severe systemic vasculitis, or symptomatic nephrosis is still recommended. Again, DAA therapy should be selected based on the eGFR; there is no specific preferred DAA regimen in cases of rapidly progressive glomerulonephritis or nephrotic syndrome.

Little is known about the effect of IFN or DAA-based treatment on the other HCV-associated glomerular diseases. There are 2 case reports of patients with HCV-related IgA nephropathy who had resolution of proteinuria after treatment with IFN with or without RBV.[150,151] There is also a case report of a patient with HCV and fibrillary glomerulonephritis who had an improvement in renal function following treatment with IFN.[92]

HUMAN IMMUNODEFICIENCY VIRUS INFECTION

Today, approximately 38.8 million people live with HIV worldwide, with approximately 833,000 of them residing in the United States.[152] Uncontrolled HIV infection is an important cause of morbidity, including systemic organ damage, direct damage of many tissues via mononuclear cell infection and activation, and the development of cancers and opportunistic infections due to reduced cell-mediated immunity.[153] Approximately 1 million people died from HIV in 2016.[154] Potent, combination antiretroviral (ARV) therapy has significantly decreased the morbidity and mortality of HIV infection.[155] However, HIV has adverse effects metabolically and on multiple organ systems, and cardiovascular disease and chronic kidney disease are more common, even in patients who are undergoing ARV therapy.[156–159]

Human Immunodeficiency Virus–Associated Kidney Diseases: Human Immunodeficiency Virus–Associated Nephropathy

Mechanism/pathogenesis of human immunodeficiency virus–associated nephropathy
HIV infection has been associated with multiple forms of kidney failure related to the direct effect of the virus on the kidney cells, dysfunction resulting from opportunistic infections and sepsis, and ARV medication nephrotoxicity.[160–162] HIV-associated nephropathy (HIVAN) was first described in 1984,[163] and is a podocytopathy that results either in patients with advanced disease or with high viremia associated with the acute phase of infection.[164] Patients affected by HIVAN are typically of West African descent.[165] The histopathologic findings in HIVAN are a collapsing form of focal segmental glomerulosclerosis (FSGS), characterized by collapse of the glomerular tuft and pseudocrescent formation; microcystic tubular dilatation and interstitial inflammation are also commonly observed (**Fig. 3**). Most individuals present with nephrotic-range proteinuria and many experience a rapid decline in kidney function due to the collapsing FSGS lesion. Peripheral edema is less common in patients with HIVAN than in primary FSGS or other causes of nephrotic syndrome not related to HIV infection.[166]

Much of the pathogenesis of HIVAN has been defined via a validated HIV transgenic mouse model (Tg26 or TgFVB), which, on the permissive FVBN/J genetic background, recapitulates the phenotypic and molecular features of human disease. Studies in this model suggest that expression of HIV genes, specifically Nef and VPr, within kidney cells leads to podocyte dedifferentiation and proliferation.[167] There is an extremely strong association between HIVAN and West African descent, and HIVAN is considered on the spectrum of *APOL1*-related diseases.[168,169] *APOL1*-related kidney diseases include primary focal segmental glomerulosclerosis, HIVAN, and nondiabetic chronic kidney disease (CKD) occurring in patients of West African descent who have 2 high-risk alleles for *APOL1* on chromosome 22. Papeta and colleagues[169]

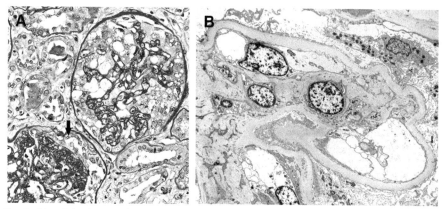

Fig. 3. (*A*, original magnification x 400) Periodic acid-Schiff stain of a kidney biopsy of a patient with HIVAN. Collapse of the glomerular capillary tuft with reactive podocytes and "pseudocrescent" formation (*arrow*) are shown. (*B*, original magnification × 20, 000) Electron microscopy of a kidney biopsy of a patient with HIVAN. Electron microscopy demonstrates widespread podocyte foot process effacement.

confirmed the association of *APOL1* haplotypes with risk of HIVAN and idiopathic FSGS in African American individuals (odds ratio 10.9, $P = 10^{-9}$).

Management/treatment of human immunodeficiency virus–associated nephropathy
Effective ARV therapy has decreased the incidence of HIVAN dramatically.[170–172] Patients with biopsy-proven HIVAN who have not begun ARV therapy should begin immediately.[173] Observational studies suggest that renal survival is improved in patients with HIVAN on ARV therapy compared with those not treated with ARV therapies.[174] Angiotensin-converting enzyme (ACE)-inhibitor therapy should begin in any patient with hypertension or proteinuria.[175] Glucocorticoid therapy is generally not recommended as first-line therapy for HIVAN, but some have used it in patients who have progressive disease despite treatment with ARV therapy and ACE inhibitors, or in patients whose biopsies show a very significant interstitial inflammatory infiltrate; however, adverse event rates in patients with HIVAN treated with glucocorticoids are high. Outcomes in HIVAN are poor, with 2 recent series showing that most progress to ESRD despite ARV therapy.[166,176] Fortunately, in the era of ARV therapy, survival for HIV-infected patients on dialysis and post–kidney transplant outcomes are similar to HIV-negative patients.[177]

Human Immunodeficiency Virus–Associated Immune Complex Diseases (Human Immunodeficiency Virus Immune Complex Kidney Disease and Others)

A myriad of other forms of immune-mediated glomerular diseases can be seen in patients with HIV infection, highlighting the importance of renal biopsy in the diagnosis of unexplained worsening renal function or proteinuria/hematuria in patients with HIV infection. An association with MN, IgA nephropathy, and MPGN has been reported in small series, although whether HIV is causative or merely coexisting is unknown.

A lupuslike glomerulonephritis with characteristic "full-house" immunofluorescence also haas been described in patients with HIV infection. The "ball-in-cup" basement membrane reaction around the large deposits seen in this disease may be pathognomonic. This specific form of glomerulonephritis is often referred to as HIV immune complex kidney disease (HIVICK). It appears that the racial make-up of patients with HIVICK mirrors the local demographics of the overall patient cohorts, thus suggesting no strong racial/genetic predisposition to this disease, unlike what is seen in HIVAN.[178,179] Treatment of HIVICK and other immune-mediated glomerulopathies in patients with HIV includes ensuring the patient's viral load is suppressed with ARV therapy, and then using a similar immunosuppressant strategy as recommended for uninfected patients with the same underlying pathologic lesion found on biopsy.

Antiretroviral Therapy Nephrotoxicity

Although ARV therapy is highly effective at controlling HIV replication, multiple common ARVs may be nephrotoxic. Early-generation nucleoside or nucleotide analog reverse-transcriptase inhibitors, such as didanosine, caused severe mitochondrial toxicity leading to lactic acidosis, renal failure, and rhabdomyolysis. Newer formulations, such as tenofovir disoproxil fumarate (TDF), a nucleotide analog reverse-transcriptase inhibitor widely used as first-line ARV therapy and prophylaxis for HIV infection, can cause proximal renal tubular epithelial cell dysfunction, leading to acute kidney injury and Fanconi syndrome.[161,180] The mechanism of TDF nephrotoxicity is via adverse effects on mitochondrial function by inhibition of mitochondrial DNA polymerase.[181] Kidney biopsies from patients with TDF nephrotoxicity show varying degrees of renal tubular injury and ultrastructural changes that include dysplastic, enlarged, or reduced numbers of mitochondria.[182] Guidelines from the Infectious Disease Society of American/HIV Medicine Association now recommend that TDF should be avoided in patients with predialysis CKD if eGFR <60 mL/min per 1.73 m^2.[173] Tenofovir alafenamide is a newer prodrug of tenofovir that leads to much lower plasma levels of tenofovir, and is associated with significantly less nephrotoxicity and bone demineralization than TDF.[183]

Protease inhibitors, including indinavir and atazanavir, may precipitate causing kidney stones or intratubular crystal deposition and can lead to obstructive renal failure.[184–186] Because these stones are often predominantly composed of the medication itself and not calcium, they may be radiolucent and are easily missed on ultrasound or computed tomography scans.

SUMMARY

Chronic viral infections can lead to immune-mediated kidney disease. Control of the kidney disease relies primarily on treatment of viremia with antiviral agents; however, immunosuppression also may be needed in severe cases. Fortunately, in the current era, HBV, HCV, and HIV infection can be controlled with potent antiviral agents in most cases. More clinical trials are needed to determine first-line therapies for patients who develop autoimmune kidney diseases in the context of chronic viral infections and to define when adjunctive immunosuppressive therapy is warranted.

ACKNOWLEDGMENTS

The authors would like to acknowledge Ivy Rosales and A. Bernard Collins for supplying original photographs of patient kidney biopsies for **Figs. 1** and **3**, and Xavier Fernando Vela Parada for original illustration of **Fig. 2**.

REFERENCES

1. You CR, Lee SW, Jang JW, et al. Update on hepatitis B virus infection. World J Gastroenterol 2014;20(37):13293–305.

2. Liang TJ. Hepatitis B: the virus and disease. Hepatology 2009;49(5 Suppl): S13–21.

3. Sunbul M. Hepatitis B virus genotypes: global distribution and clinical importance. World J Gastroenterol 2014;20(18):5427–34.

4. Tang S, Lai FM, Lui YH, et al. Lamivudine in hepatitis B-associated membranous nephropathy. Kidney Int 2005;68(4):1750–8.

5. Combes B, Shorey J, Barrera A, et al. Glomerulonephritis with deposition of Australia antigen-antibody complexes in glomerular basement membrane. Lancet 1971;2(7718):234–7.

6. Lai KN, Li PK, Lui SF, et al. Membranous nephropathy related to hepatitis B virus in adults. N Engl J Med 1991;324(21):1457–63.

7. Chan TM. Hepatitis B and renal disease. Curr Hepat Rep 2010;9(2):99–105.

8. Li P, Wei RB, Tang L, et al. Clinical and pathological analysis of hepatitis B virus-related membranous nephropathy and idiopathic membranous nephropathy. Clin Nephrol 2012;78(6):456–64.

9. Takekoshi Y, Tanaka M. Hepatitis B virus-associated glomerulonephritis in children. In: Murakami K, Kitagawa T, Yabuta K, et al, editors. Recent advances in pediatric nephrology. New York: Excerpta Medica; 1987.

10. Takekoshi Y, Tanaka M, Miyakawa Y, et al. Free "small" and IgG-associated "large" hepatitis B e antigen in the serum and glomerular capillary walls of two patients with membranous glomerulonephritis. N Engl J Med 1979;300(15): 814–9.

11. Hirose H, Udo K, Kojima M, et al. Deposition of hepatitis B e antigen in membranous glomerulonephritis: identification by F(ab')2 fragments of monoclonal antibody. Kidney Int 1984;26(3):338–41.

12. Nagy J, Bajtai G, Brasch H, et al. The role of hepatitis B surface antigen in the pathogenesis of glomerulopathies. Clin Nephrol 1979;12(3):109–16.

13. Michalak T. Immune complexes of hepatitis B surface antigen in the pathogenesis of periarteritis nodosa. A study of seven necropsy cases. Am J Pathol 1978; 90(3):619–32.

14. Lai KN, Lai FM, Lo S, et al. IgA nephropathy associated with hepatitis B virus antigenemia. Nephron 1987;47(2):141–3.

15. Chung DR, Yang WS, Kim SB, et al. Treatment of hepatitis B virus associated glomerulonephritis with recombinant human alpha interferon. Am J Nephrol 1997;17(2):112–7.

16. Johnson RJ, Couser WG. Hepatitis B infection and renal disease: clinical, immunopathogenetic and therapeutic considerations. Kidney Int 1990;37(2):663–76.

17. Couser WG, Salant DJ. In situ immune complex formation and glomerular injury. Kidney Int 1980;17(1):1–13.

18. Couser WG, Abrass CK. Pathogenesis of membranous nephropathy. Annu Rev Med 1988;39:517–30.

19. Milner LS, Dusheiko GM, Jacobs D, et al. Biochemical and serological characteristics of children with membranous nephropathy due to hepatitis B virus infection: correlation with hepatitis B e antigen, hepatitis B DNA and hepatitis D. Nephron 1988;49(3):184–9.

20. Ito H, Hattori S, Matusda I, et al. Hepatitis B e antigen-mediated membranous glomerulonephritis. Correlation of ultrastructural changes with HBeAg in the serum and glomeruli. Lab Invest 1981;44(3):214–20.

21. Mason A, Theal J, Bain V, et al. Hepatitis B virus replication in damaged endothelial tissues of patients with extrahepatic disease. Am J Gastroenterol 2005; 100(4):972–6.

22. Xie Q, Li Y, Xue J, et al. Renal phospholipase A2 receptor in hepatitis B virus-associated membranous nephropathy. Am J Nephrol 2015;41(4–5):345–53.

23. Ikeda T, Lever AM, Thomas HC. Evidence for a deficiency of interferon production in patients with chronic hepatitis B virus infection acquired in adult life. Hepatology 1986;6(5):962–5.

24. Bhimma R, Coovadia HM. Hepatitis B virus-associated nephropathy. Am J Nephrol 2004;24(2):198–211.

25. Bhimma R, Coovadia HM, Kramvis A, et al. Treatment of hepatitis B virus-associated nephropathy in black children. Pediatr Nephrol 2002;17(6):393–9.

26. Vaughan RW, Zurowska A, Moszkowska G, et al. HLA-DRB and -DQB1 alleles in Polish patients with hepatitis B associated membranous nephropathy. Tissue Antigens 1998;52(2):130–4.

27. Mesquita M, Lasser L, Langlet P. Long-term (7-year-) treatment with lamivudine monotherapy in HBV-associated glomerulonephritis. Clin Nephrol 2008;70(1): 69–71.

28. Moon JY, Lee SH. Treatment of hepatitis B virus-associated membranous nephropathy: lamivudine era versus post-lamivudine era. Korean J Intern Med 2012;27(4):394–6.

29. Conjeevaram HS, Hoofnagle JH, Austin HA, et al. Long-term outcome of hepatitis B virus-related glomerulonephritis after therapy with interferon alfa. Gastroenterology 1995;109(2):540–6.

30. Lin CY. Treatment of hepatitis B virus-associated membranous nephropathy with recombinant alpha-interferon. Kidney Int 1995;47(1):225–30.

31. Gan SI, Devlin SM, Scott-Douglas NW, et al. Lamivudine for the treatment of membranous glomerulopathy secondary to chronic Hepatitis B infection. Can J Gastroenterol 2005;19(10):625–9.

32. Khedmat H, Taheri S. Hepatitis B virus-associated nephropathy: an International Data Analysis. Iran J Kidney Dis 2010;4(2):101–5.

33. Fabrizi F, Dixit V, Martin P. Meta-analysis: anti-viral therapy of hepatitis B virus-associated glomerulonephritis. Aliment Pharmacol Ther 2006;24(5):781–8.

34. Buster EH, Janssen HL. Antiviral treatment for chronic hepatitis B virus infection–immune modulation or viral suppression? Neth J Med 2006;64(6):175–85.

35. Lok AS, Heathcote EJ, Hoofnagle JH. Management of hepatitis B: 2000–summary of a workshop. Gastroenterology 2001;120(7):1828–53.

36. Chang TT, Gish RG, de Man R, et al. A comparison of entecavir and lamivudine for HBeAg-positive chronic hepatitis B. N Engl J Med 2006;354(10):1001–10.

37. Yokosuka O, Kurosaki M, Imazeki F, et al. Management of hepatitis B: consensus of the Japan Society of Hepatology 2009. Hepatol Res 2011;41(1): 1–21.

38. Wang L, Ye Z, Liang H, et al. The combination of tacrolimus and entecavir improves the remission of HBV-associated glomerulonephritis without enhancing viral replication. Am J Transl Res 2016;8(3):1593–600.

39. Lai KN, Tam JS, Lin HJ, et al. The therapeutic dilemma of the usage of corticosteroid in patients with membranous nephropathy and persistent hepatitis B virus surface antigenaemia. Nephron 1990;54(1):12–7.

40. Taskapan H, Oymak O, Dogukan A, et al. Transformation of hepatitis B virus-related membranous glomerulonephritis to crescentic form. Clin Nephrol 2000;54(2):161–3.

41. Lai FM, Tam JS, Li PK, et al. Replication of hepatitis B virus with corticosteroid therapy in hepatitis B virus related membranous nephropathy. Virchows Arch A Pathol Anat Histopathol 1989;414(3):279–84.

42. Jennette JC, Falk RJ, Bacon PA, et al. 2012 revised International Chapel Hill consensus conference nomenclature of vasculitides. Arthritis Rheum 2013; 65(1):1–11.

43. Guillevin L. Infections in vasculitis. Best Pract Res Clin Rheumatol 2013;27(1): 19–31.

44. Lai KN, Lai FM. Clinical features and the natural course of hepatitis B virus-related glomerulopathy in adults. Kidney Int Suppl 1991;35:S40–5.

45. Trepo C, Thivolet J. Hepatitis associated antigen and periarteritis nodosa (PAN). Vox Sang 1970;19(3):410–1.

46. Drueke T, Barbanel C, Jungers P, et al. Hepatitis B antigen-associated periarteritis nodosa in patients undergoing long-term hemodialysis. Am J Med 1980; 68(1):86–90.

47. Lhote F, Cohen P, Guillevin L. Polyarteritis nodosa, microscopic polyangiitis and Churg-Strauss syndrome. Lupus 1998;7(4):238–58.

48. Howard T, Ahmad K, Swanson JA, et al. Polyarteritis nodosa. Tech Vasc Interv Radiol 2014;17(4):247–51.

49. Hernandez-Rodriguez J, Alba MA, Prieto-Gonzalez S, et al. Diagnosis and classification of polyarteritis nodosa. J Autoimmun 2014;48-49:84–9.

50. Pagnoux C, Seror R, Henegar C, et al. Clinical features and outcomes in 348 patients with polyarteritis nodosa: a systematic retrospective study of patients diagnosed between 1963 and 2005 and entered into the French Vasculitis Study Group Database. Arthritis Rheum 2010;62(2):616–26.

51. Levin S, Graber J, Ehrenwald E, et al. Polyarteritis nodosa-induced pancreatico-duodenal artery aneurysmal rupture. Int J Angiol 2015;24(1):63–6.

52. Heermann KH, Gerlich WH. Immunology of hepatitis B virus infections. Rheumatol Int 1989;9(3–5):167–73.

53. Calabrese LH. The rheumatic manifestations of infection with the human immunodeficiency virus. Semin Arthritis Rheum 1989;18(4):225–39.

54. Lidar M, Lipschitz N, Langevitz P, et al. The infectious etiology of vasculitis. Autoimmunity 2009;42(5):432–8.

55. Trepo C, Guillevin L. Polyarteritis nodosa and extrahepatic manifestations of HBV infection: the case against autoimmune intervention in pathogenesis. J Autoimmun 2001;16(3):269–74.

56. Guillevin L, Lhote F, Cohen P, et al. Polyarteritis nodosa related to hepatitis B virus. A prospective study with long-term observation of 41 patients. Medicine 1995;74(5):238–53.

57. De Virgilio A, Greco A, Magliulo G, et al. Polyarteritis nodosa: a contemporary overview. Autoimmun Rev 2016;15(6):564–70.

58. Guillevin L, Visser H, Noel LH, et al. Antineutrophil cytoplasm antibodies in systemic polyarteritis nodosa with and without hepatitis B virus infection and Churg-Strauss syndrome–62 patients. J Rheumatol 1993;20(8):1345–9.

59. Shusterman N, London WT. Hepatitis B and immune-complex disease. N Engl J Med 1984;310(1):43–6.

60. Segelmark M, Selga D. The challenge of managing patients with polyarteritis nodosa. Curr Opin Rheumatol 2007;19(1):33–8.

61. Guillevin L, Mahr A, Callard P, et al. Hepatitis B virus-associated polyarteritis nodosa: clinical characteristics, outcome, and impact of treatment in 115 patients. Medicine 2005;84(5):313–22.

62. Guillevin L, Pagnoux C. Therapeutic strategies for systemic necrotizing vasculitides. Allergol Int 2007;56(2):105–11.

63. Puechal X, Guillevin L. Therapeutic immunomodulation in systemic vasculitis: taking stock. Joint Bone Spine 2013;80(4):374–9.

64. Mukhtyar C, Guillevin L, Cid MC, et al. EULAR recommendations for the management of primary small and medium vessel vasculitis. Ann Rheum Dis 2009;68(3):310–7.

65. Guillevin L, Lhote F, Jarrousse B, et al. Polyarteritis nodosa related to hepatitis B virus. A retrospective study of 66 patients. Ann Med Interne (Paris) 1992; 143(Suppl 1):63–74.

66. Guillevin L, Lhote F, Leon A, et al. Treatment of polyarteritis nodosa related to hepatitis B virus with short term steroid therapy associated with antiviral agents and plasma exchanges. A prospective trial in 33 patients. J Rheumatol 1993; 20(2):289–98.

67. Guillevin L, Mahr A, Cohen P, et al. Short-term corticosteroids then lamivudine and plasma exchanges to treat hepatitis B virus-related polyarteritis nodosa. Arthritis Rheum 2004;51(3):482–7.

68. Vigano M, Martin P, Cappelletti M, et al. HBV-associated cryoglobulinemic vasculitis: remission after antiviral therapy with entecavir. Kidney Blood Press Res 2014;39(1):65–73.

69. Enomoto M, Nakanishi T, Ishii M, et al. Entecavir to treat hepatitis B-associated cryoglobulinemic vasculitis. Ann Intern Med 2008;149(12):912–3.

70. Pagnoux C, Cohen P, Guillevin L. Vasculitides secondary to infections. Clin Exp Rheumatol 2006;24(2 Suppl 41):S71–81.

71. Teng GG, Chatham WW. Vasculitis related to viral and other microbial agents. Best Pract Res Clin Rheumatol 2015;29(2):226–43.

72. Division of Viral Hepatitis and National Center for HIV/AIDS VH S, and TB Prevention., Surveillance for Viral Hepatitis - United States, 2015. 2015. Available at: https://www.cdc.gov/hepatitis/statistics/2015surveillance/commentary. htm. Accessed June 19, 2017.

73. Wedemeyer H, He XS, Nascimbeni M, et al. Impaired effector function of hepatitis C virus-specific CD8+ T cells in chronic hepatitis C virus infection. J Immunol 2002;169(6):3447–58.

74. Poynard T, Bedossa P, Opolon P. Natural history of liver fibrosis progression in patients with chronic hepatitis C. The OBSVIRC, METAVIR, CLINIVIR, and DOS-VIRC groups. Lancet 1997;349(9055):825–32.

75. Ferri C, Zignego A, Pileri S. Cryoglobulins. J Clin Pathol 2002;55(1):4–13.

76. Gorevic PD, Frangione B. Mixed cryoglobulinemia cross-reactive idiotypes: implications for the relationship of MC to rheumatic and lymphoproliferative diseases. Seminars in hematology 1991;28(2):79–94.

77. Dammacco F, Sansonno D, Piccoli C, et al. The cryoglobulins: an overview. Eur J Clin Invest 2001;31(7):628–38.

78. Wintrobe MM. Hyperproteinemia associated with multiple myeloma: with report of case in which an extraordinary hyperproteinemia was associated with thrombosis of the retinal veins and symptoms suggesting Raynaud's disease. Bull Johns Hopkins Hosp 1933;52:156–65.

79. Lospalluto J, Dorward B, Miller W Jr, et al. Cryoglobulinemia based on interaction between a gamma macroglobulin and 7S gamma globulin. Am J Med 1962; 32:142–7.

80. Pascual M, Schifferli J. Hepatitis C virus infection and glomerulonephritis, vol. 20. New York: Oxford University Press Inc; 1996.

81. Cicardi M, Cesana B, Del Ninno E, et al. Prevalence and risk factors for the presence of serum cryoglobulins in patients with chronic hepatitis C. J Viral Hepat 2000;7(2):138–43.

82. Trejo O, Ramos-casals M, García-carrasco M, et al. Cryoglobulinemia: study of etiologic factors and clinical and immunologic features in 443 patients from a single center. Medicine 2001;80(4):252–62.

83. Ozkok A, Yildiz A. Hepatitis C virus associated glomerulopathies. World J Gastroenterol 2014;20(24):7544–54.

84. D'Amico G. Renal involvement in hepatitis C infection: cryoglobulinemic glomerulonephritis. Kidney Int 1998;54(2):650–71.

85. Rodriguez-Inigo E, Casqueiro M, Bartolome J, et al. Hepatitis C virus RNA in kidney biopsies from infected patients with renal diseases. J viral Hepat 2000;7(1):23–9.

86. Pouteil-Noble C, Maiza H, Dijoud F, et al. Glomerular disease associated with hepatitis C virus infection in native kidneys. Nephrol Dial Transplant 2000;15(suppl 8):28–33.

87. Sinico RA, Winearls CG, Sabadini E, et al. Identification of glomerular immune deposits in cryoglobulinemia glomerulonephritis. Kidney Int 1988;34(1):109–16.

88. D'Amico G, Colasanti G, Ferrario F, et al. Renal involvement in essential mixed cryoglobulinemia. Kidney Int 1989;35(4):1004–14.

89. Ferri C, Sebastiani M, Giuggioli D, et al. Mixed cryoglobulinemia: demographic, clinical, and serologic features and survival in 231 patients. Seminars in arthritis and rheumatism 2004;33(6):355–74.

90. Stehman-Breen C, Alpers C, Couser W, et al. Hepatitis C virus associated membranous glomerulonephritis. Clin Nephrol 1995;44(3):141–7.

91. Johnson RJ, Gretch DR, Couser WG, et al. Hepatitis C virus-associated glomerulonephritis. Effect of α-interferon therapy. Kidney Int 1994;46(6):1700–4.

92. Coroneos E, Truong I, Olivero J. Fibrillary glomerulonephritis associated with hepatitis C viral infection. Am J Kidney Dis 1997;29(1):132–5.

93. Markowitz G, Cheng J, Colvin R, et al. Hepatitis C viral infection is associated with fibrillary glomerulonephritis and immunotactoid glomerulopathy. J Am Soc Nephrol 1998;9(12):2244–52.

94. Rosenstock JL, Markowitz GS, Valeri AM, et al. Fibrillary and immunotactoid glomerulonephritis: distinct entities with different clinical and pathologic features. Kidney Int 2003;63(4):1450–61.

95. Monga G, Mazzucco G, Motta M, et al. Immunotactoid glomerulopathy (ITGP): a not fully defined clinicopathologic entity. Ren Fail 1993;15(3):401–5.

96. Duffy JL, Khurana E, Susin M, et al. Fibrillary renal deposits and nephritis. Am J Pathol 1983;113(3):279.

97. Alpers CE, Rennke HG, Hopper J, et al. Fibrillary glomerulonephritis: an entity with unusual immunofluorescence features. Kidney Int 1987;31(3):781–9.

98. Iskandar SS, Falk RJ, Jennette JC. Clinical and pathologic features of fibrillary glomerulonephritis. Kidney Int 1992;42(6):1401–7.

99. Roccatello D, Picciotto G, Torchio M, et al. Removal systems of immunoglobulin A and immunoglobulin A containing complexes in IgA nephropathy and cirrhosis patients. The role of asialoglycoprotein receptors. Lab Invest 1993;69(6):714–23.

100. Johnson RJ, Gretch DR, Yamabe H, et al. Membranoproliferative glomerulonephritis associated with hepatitis C virus infection. N Engl J Med 1993;328(7):465–70.

101. Misiani R, Bellavita P, Fenili D, et al. Interferon alfa-2a therapy in cryoglobuline-mia associated with hepatitis C virus. N Engl J Med 1994;330(11):751–6.
102. Casato M, Agnello V, Pucillo LP, et al. Predictors of long-term response to high-dose interferon therapy in type II cryoglobulinemia associated with hepatitis C virus infection. Blood 1997;90(10):3865–73.
103. Ferri C, Marzo E, Longombardo G, et al. Interferon-alpha in mixed cryoglobuli-nemia patients: a randomized, crossover-controlled trial. Blood 1993;81(5):1132–6.
104. Naarendorp M, Kallemuchikkal U, Nuovo GJ, et al. Longterm efficacy of interferon-alpha for extrahepatic disease associated with hepatitis C virus infec-tion. J Rheumatol 2001;28(11):2466–73.
105. Mazzaro C, Zorat F, Caizzi M, et al. Treatment with peg-interferon alfa-2b and ribavirin of hepatitis C virus-associated mixed cryoglobulinemia: a pilot study. J Hepatol 2005;42(5):632–8.
106. Hadziyannis SJ, Sette H, Morgan TR, et al. Peginterferon-α2a and ribavirin com-bination therapy in chronic hepatitis C: a randomized study of treatment dura-tion and ribavirin dose. Ann Intern Med 2004;140(5):346–55.
107. Cacoub P, Saadoun D, Sene D, et al. Treatment of hepatitis C virus-related sys-temic vasculitis. J Rheumatol 2005;32(11):2078–82.
108. Dammacco F, Tucci FA, Lauletta G, et al. Pegylated interferon-α, ribavirin, and rituximab combined therapy of hepatitis C virus–related mixed cryoglobuline-mia: a long-term study. Blood 2010;116(3):343–53.
109. Cacoub P, Lidove O, Maisonobe T, et al. Interferon-α and ribavirin treatment in patients with hepatitis C virus–related systemic vasculitis. Arthritis Rheumatol 2002;46(12):3317–26.
110. Cacoub P, Saadoun D, Limal N, et al. PEGylated interferon alfa-2b and ribavirin treatment in patients with hepatitis C virus–related systemic vasculitis. Arthritis Rheumatol 2005;52(3):911–5.
111. Saadoun D, Resche-Rigon M, Thibault V, et al. Antiviral therapy for hepatitis C virus–associated mixed cryoglobulinemia vasculitis: a long-term followup study. Arthritis Rheumatol 2006;54(11):3696–706.
112. Alric L, Plaisier E, Thébault S, et al. Influence of antiviral therapy in hepatitis C virus-associated cryoglobulinemic MPGN. Am J Kidney Dis 2004;43(4):617–23.
113. Bruchfeld A, Lindahl K, Ståhle L, et al. Interferon and ribavirin treatment in pa-tients with hepatitis C-associated renal disease and renal insufficiency. Nephrol Dial Transplant 2003;18(8):1573–80.
114. Sansonno D, De Re V, Lauletta G, et al. Monoclonal antibody treatment of mixed cryoglobulinemia resistant to interferon α with an anti-CD20. Blood 2003;101(10):3818–26.
115. Zaja F, Vianelli N, Sperotto A, et al. Anti-CD20 therapy for chronic lymphocytic leukemia-associated autoimmune diseases. Leuk Lymphoma 2003;44(11):1951–5.
116. Roccatello D, Baldovino S, Rossi D, et al. Long-term effects of anti-CD20 mono-clonal antibody treatment of cryoglobulinaemic glomerulonephritis. Nephrol Dial Transplant 2004;19(12):3054–61.
117. Quartuccio L, Soardo G, Romano G, et al. Rituximab treatment for glomerulone-phritis in HCV-associated mixed cryoglobulinaemia: efficacy and safety in the absence of steroids. Rheumatology 2006;45(7):842–6.
118. Saadoun D, Rigon MR, Pol S, et al. PegIFNα/ribavirin/protease inhibitor combi-nation in severe hepatitis C virus-associated mixed cryoglobulinemia vasculitis. J Hepatol 2015;62(1):24–30.

119. Saadoun D, Resche-Rigon M, Sene D, et al. Rituximab combined with Peg-interferon-ribavirin in refractory hepatitis C virus-associated cryoglobulinaemia vasculitis. Ann Rheum Dis 2008;67(10):1431–6.
120. Cacoub P, Delluc A, Saadoun D, et al. Anti-CD20 monoclonal antibody (rituximab) treatment for cryoglobulinemic vasculitis: where do we stand? Ann Rheum Dis 2008;67(3):283–7.
121. Saadoun D, Rigon MR, Sene D, et al. Rituximab plus Peg-interferon-α/ribavirin compared with Peg-interferon-α/ribavirin in hepatitis C–related mixed cryoglobulinemia. Blood 2010;116(3):326–34.
122. De Vita S, Quartuccio L, Isola M, et al. A randomized controlled trial of rituximab for the treatment of severe cryoglobulinemic vasculitis. Arthritis Rheumatol 2012;64(3):843–53.
123. Sneller MC, Hu Z, Langford CA. A randomized controlled trial of rituximab following failure of antiviral therapy for hepatitis C virus–associated cryoglobulinemic vasculitis. Arthritis Rheumatol 2012;64(3):835–42.
124. Gordon CE, Balk EM, Becker BN, et al. KDOQI US commentary on the KDIGO clinical practice guideline for the prevention, diagnosis, evaluation, and treatment of hepatitis C in CKD. Am J Kidney Dis 2008;52(5):811–25.
125. AASLD-IDSA. HCV guidance: recommendations for testing, managing, and treating hepatitis C. 2017. Available at: http://www.hcvguidelines.org. Accessed July 2, 2017.
126. Pockros PJ, Reddy KR, Mantry PS, et al. Efficacy of direct-acting antiviral combination for patients with hepatitis C virus genotype 1 infection and severe renal impairment or end-stage renal disease. Gastroenterology 2016;150(7):1590–8.
127. Gane EJ, Lawitz E, Pugatch D, et al. EXPEDITION-IV: safety and efficacy of GLE/PIB in adults with renal impairment and Chronic Hepatitis C Virus Genotype 1 – 6 Infection. Hepatology 2016;64(6):1125A.
128. Roth D, Nelson DR, Bruchfeld A, et al. Grazoprevir plus elbasvir in treatment-naive and treatment-experienced patients with hepatitis C virus genotype 1 infection and stage 4-5 chronic kidney disease (the C-SURFER study): a combination phase 3 study. Lancet 2015;386(10003):1537–45.
129. Saxena V, Koraishy FM, Sise ME, et al. Safety and efficacy of sofosbuvir-containing regimens in hepatitis C-infected patients with impaired renal function. Liver Int 2016;36(6):807–16.
130. Kalyan Ram B, Frank C, Adam P, et al. Safety, efficacy and tolerability of half-dose sofosbuvir plus simeprevir in treatment of Hepatitis C in patients with end stage renal disease. J Hepatol 2015;63(3):763–5.
131. Nazario HE, Ndungu M, Modi AA. Sofosbuvir and simeprevir in hepatitis C genotype 1-patients with end-stage renal disease on haemodialysis or GFR< 30 ml/min. Liver Int 2016;36(6):798–801.
132. Li T, Qu Y, Guo Y, et al. Efficacy and safety of direct-acting antivirals-based antiviral therapies for hepatitis C virus patients with stage 4-5 chronic kidney disease: a meta-analysis. Liver Int 2017;37(7):974–81.
133. Feld JJ, Jacobson IM, Hezode C, et al. Sofosbuvir and velpatasvir for HCV genotype 1, 2, 4, 5, and 6 infection. N Engl J Med 2015;373(27):2599–607.
134. Saadoun D, Pol S, Ferfar Y, et al. Efficacy and safety of sofosbuvir plus daclatasvir for treatment of HCV-associated cryoglobulinemia vasculitis. Gastroenterology 2017;153(1):49–52.e5.
135. Emery JS, Kuczynski M, La D, et al. Efficacy and safety of direct acting antivirals for the treatment of mixed cryoglobulinemia. Am J Gastroenterol 2017;112(8):1298–308.

136. Bonacci M, Lens S, Londoño M-C, et al. Virologic, clinical, and immune response outcomes of patients with hepatitis C virus–associated cryoglobuline-mia treated with direct-acting antivirals. Clin Gastroenterol Hepatol 2017;15(4): 575–83.e1.

137. Cerretelli G, Gragnani L, Monti M, et al. FRI-216-Sofosbuvir/Ribavirin treatment in patients with genotype 2, Hepatitis C Virus infection and symptomatic mixed cryoglobulinemia: an interim analysis on safety, efficacy and impact on quality of life. J Hepatol 2017;66(1):S505.

138. Gragnani L, Piluso A, Urraro T, et al. Virological and clinical response to interferon-free regimens in patients with HCV-related mixed cryoglobulinemia: preliminary results of a prospective pilot study. Curr Drug Targets 2017;18(7): 772–85.

139. Saadoun D, Thibault V, Ahmed SNS, et al. Sofosbuvir plus ribavirin for hepatitis C virus-associated cryoglobulinaemia vasculitis: VASCUVALDIC study. Ann Rheum Dis 2016;75(10):1777–82.

140. Comarmond C, Garrido M, Pol S, et al. Direct-acting antiviral therapy restores immune tolerance to patients with hepatitis c virus–induced cryoglobulinemia vasculitis. Gastroenterology 2017;152(8):2052–62.e2.

141. Mauro E, Quartuccio L, Ghersetti M, et al. Direct acting antiviral (DAA) therapy of HCV, effects on the cryoglobulinemic vasculitis: a multi center open label study. Dig Liver Dis 2017;49(1):e32.

142. Gragnani L, Visentini M, Fognani E, et al. Prospective study of guideline-tailored therapy with direct-acting antivirals for hepatitis C virus-associated mixed cryo-globulinemia. Hepatology 2016;64(5):1473–82.

143. Sise ME, Bloom AK, Wisocky J, et al. Treatment of hepatitis C virus–associated mixed cryoglobulinemia with direct-acting antiviral agents. Hepatology 2016; 63(2):408–17.

144. Diakite M, Hartig-Lavie K, Miailhes P, et al. FRI-265-Benefit of direct-acting anti-viral therapy in hepatitis C virus (HCV) monoinfected and HIV-HCV coinfected patients with mixed cryoglobulinemia. J Hepatol 2017;66(1):S528–9.

145. Sollima S, Milazzo L, Peri AM, et al. Persistent mixed cryoglobulinaemia vascu-litis despite hepatitis C virus eradication after interferon-free antiviral therapy. Rheumatology 2016;55(11):2084–5.

146. Cacoub P, Vautier M, Desbois AC, et al. Effectiveness and cost of hepatitis C virus cryoglobulinemia vasculitis treatment: from interferon-based to direct acting antivirals era. Liver Int 2017;37(12):1805–13.

147. Cornella SL, Stine JG, Kelly V, et al. Persistence of mixed cryoglobulinemia despite cure of hepatitis C with new oral antiviral therapy including direct-acting antiviral sofosbuvir: a case series. Postgrad Med 2015;127(4):413–7.

148. Gragnani L, Fabbrizzi A, Triboli E, et al. Triple antiviral therapy in hepatitis C virus infection with or without mixed cryoglobulinaemia: a prospective, controlled pilot study. Dig Liver Dis 2014;46(9):833–7.

149. KDIGO. KDIGO 2017 clinical practice guideline on the prevention, diagnosis, evaluation and treatment of hepatitis C in CKD. 2017. Accessed February 8, 2017. Available at: https://kdigo.org/clinical_practice_guidelines/Hep%20C/ KDIGO%202017%20Hep%20C%20GL%20Public%20Review%20Draft%20 FINAL.pdf

150. Matsumoto S, Nakajima S, Nakamura K, et al. Interferon treatment on glomeru-lonephritis associated with hepatitis C virus. Pediatr Nephrol 2000;15(3):271–3.

151. Ji F, Li Z, Ge H, et al. Successful interferon-α treatment in a patient with IgA nephropathy associated with hepatitis C virus infection. Intern Med 2010;49(22): 2531–2.

152. GBD 2015 HIV Collaborators. Estimates of global, regional, and national incidence, prevalence, and mortality of HIV, 1980-2015: the Global Burden of Disease Study 2015. Lancet HIV 2016;3(8):e361–87.

153. Lucas S, Nelson AM. HIV and the spectrum of human disease. J Pathol 2015; 235(2):229–41.

154. WHO. Number of deaths due to HIV. 2018. Available at: http://www.who.int/gho/hiv/epidemic_status/deaths/en/. Accessed April 18, 2018.

155. Palella FJ Jr, Delaney KM, Moorman AC, et al. Declining morbidity and mortality among patients with advanced human immunodeficiency virus infection. HIV Outpatient Study Investigators. N Engl J Med 1998;338(13):853–60.

156. Freiberg MS, Chang CC, Kuller LH, et al. HIV infection and the risk of acute myocardial infarction. JAMA Intern Med 2013;173(8):614–22.

157. Butt AA, Chang CC, Kuller L, et al. Risk of heart failure with human immunodeficiency virus in the absence of prior diagnosis of coronary heart disease. Arch Intern Med 2011;171(8):737–43.

158. Drelichowska J, Kwiatkowska W, Knysz B, et al. Metabolic syndrome in HIV-positive patients. HIV & AIDS Review 2015;14(2):35–41.

159. Winston J, Deray G, Hawkins T, et al. Kidney disease in patients with HIV infection and AIDS. Clin Infect Dis 2008;47(11):1449–57.

160. Nadkarni GN, Patel AA, Yacoub R, et al. The burden of dialysis-requiring acute kidney injury among hospitalized adults with HIV infection: a nationwide inpatient sample analysis. AIDS 2015;29(9):1061–6.

161. Sise ME, Hirsch JS, Canetta PA, et al. Nonalbumin proteinuria predominates in biopsy-proven tenofovir nephrotoxicity. AIDS 2015;29(8):941–6.

162. Rosenberg AZ, Naicker S, Winkler CA, et al. HIV-associated nephropathies: epidemiology, pathology, mechanisms and treatment. Nat Rev Nephrol 2015; 11(3):150–60.

163. Rao TK, Filippone EJ, Nicastri AD, et al. Associated focal and segmental glomerulosclerosis in the acquired immunodeficiency syndrome. N Engl J Med 1984;310(11):669–73.

164. Sise ME, Lo GC, Goldstein RH, et al. Case 12-2017-A 34-year-old man with nephropathy. N Engl J Med 2017;376(16):1575–85.

165. Razzak Chaudhary S, Workeneh BT, Montez-Rath ME, et al. Trends in the outcomes of end-stage renal disease secondary to human immunodeficiency virus-associated nephropathy. Nephrol Dial Transplant 2015;30(10):1734–40.

166. Bige N, Lanternier F, Viard JP, et al. Presentation of HIV-associated nephropathy and outcome in HAART-treated patients. Nephrol Dial Transplant 2012;27(3): 1114–21.

167. Bruggeman LA, Dikman S, Meng C, et al. Nephropathy in human immunodeficiency virus-1 transgenic mice is due to renal transgene expression. J Clin Invest 1997;100(1):84–92.

168. Kopp JB, Nelson GW, Sampath K, et al. APOL1 genetic variants in focal segmental glomerulosclerosis and HIV-associated nephropathy. J Am Soc Nephrol 2011;22(11):2129–37.

169. Papeta N, Kiryluk K, Patel A, et al. APOL1 variants increase risk for FSGS and HIVAN but not IgA nephropathy. J Am Soc Nephrol 2011;22(11):1991–6.

170. Lucas GM, Eustace JA, Sozio S, et al. Highly active antiretroviral therapy and the incidence of HIV-1-associated nephropathy: a 12-year cohort study. AIDS 2004; 18(3):541–6.

171. Schwartz EJ, Szczech LA, Ross MJ, et al. Highly active antiretroviral therapy and the epidemic of HIV+ end-stage renal disease. J Am Soc Nephrol 2005; 16(8):2412–20.

172. Lescure FX, Flateau C, Pacanowski J, et al. HIV-associated kidney glomerular diseases: changes with time and HAART. Nephrol Dial Transplant 2012;27(6): 2349–55.

173. Lucas GM, Ross MJ, Stock PG, et al. Clinical practice guideline for the management of chronic kidney disease in patients infected with HIV: 2014 update by the HIV Medicine Association of the Infectious Diseases Society of America. Clin Infect Dis 2014;59(9):e96–138.

174. Atta MG, Gallant JE, Rahman MH, et al. Antiretroviral therapy in the treatment of HIV-associated nephropathy. Nephrol Dial Transplant 2006;21(10):2809–13.

175. Burns GC, Paul SK, Toth IR, et al. Effect of angiotensin-converting enzyme inhibition in HIV-associated nephropathy. J Am Soc Nephrol 1997;8(7):1140–6.

176. Post FA, Campbell LJ, Hamzah L, et al. Predictors of renal outcome in HIV-associated nephropathy. Clin Infect Dis 2008;46(8):1282–9.

177. Stock PG, Barin B, Murphy B, et al. Outcomes of kidney transplantation in HIV-infected recipients. N Engl J Med 2010;363(21):2004–14.

178. Foy MC, Estrella MM, Lucas GM, et al. Comparison of risk factors and outcomes in HIV immune complex kidney disease and HIV-associated nephropathy. Clin J Am Soc Nephrol 2013;8(9):1524–32.

179. Szczech LA, Gupta SK, Habash R, et al. The clinical epidemiology and course of the spectrum of renal diseases associated with HIV infection. Kidney Int 2004; 66(3):1145–52.

180. Peyriere H, Reynes J, Rouanet I, et al. Renal tubular dysfunction associated with tenofovir therapy: report of 7 cases. J Acquir Immune Defic Syndr 2004;35(3): 269–73.

181. Cote HC, Magil AB, Harris M, et al. Exploring mitochondrial nephrotoxicity as a potential mechanism of kidney dysfunction among HIV-infected patients on highly active antiretroviral therapy. Antivir Ther 2006;11(1):79–86.

182. Herlitz LC, Mohan S, Stokes MB, et al. Tenofovir nephrotoxicity: acute tubular necrosis with distinctive clinical, pathological, and mitochondrial abnormalities. Kidney Int 2010;78(11):1171–7.

183. Pozniak A, Arribas JR, Gathe J, et al. Switching to tenofovir alafenamide, coformulated with elvitegravir, cobicistat, and emtricitabine, in HIV-infected patients with renal impairment: 48-week results from a single-arm, multicenter, open-label phase 3 study. J Acquir Immune Defic Syndr 2016;71(5):530–7.

184. Nishijima T, Hamada Y, Watanabe K, et al. Ritonavir-boosted darunavir is rarely associated with nephrolithiasis compared with ritonavir-boosted atazanavir in HIV-infected patients. PLoS One 2013;8(10):e77268.

185. Izzedine H, M'Rad MB, Bardier A, et al. Atazanavir crystal nephropathy. AIDS 2007;21(17):2357–8.

186. Izzedine H, Lescure FX, Bonnet F. HIV medication-based urolithiasis. Clin Kidney J 2014;7(2):121–6.

187. Liaw YF. Results of lamivudine trials in Asia. J Hepatol 2003;39(Suppl 1):S111–5.

188. Igarashi T, Shimizu A, Igarashi T, et al. Seroconversion of hepatitis B envelope antigen by entecavir in a child with hepatitis B virus-related membranous nephropathy. J Nippon Med Sch 2013;80(5):387–95.

Renal Manifestations of Inflammatory Bowel Disease

Josephine M. Ambruzs, MD, MPH*, Christopher P. Larsen, MD

KEYWORDS

- Inflammatory bowel disease • Crohn disease • Ulcerative colitis • Kidney disease
- Renal biopsy • Glomerulonephritis • Tubulointerstitial nephritis • Aminosalicylates

KEY POINTS

- Renal and urinary involvement has been reported to occur in 4% to 23% of inflammatory bowel disease (IBD) patients, manifested primarily as urinary calculi, fistulas, and obstruction. Parenchymal renal disease is rare but has been well documented and presents most commonly as glomerulonephritis or tubulointerstitial nephritis.
- IgA nephropathy is the most frequent finding on renal biopsy in IBD and has a significantly higher diagnostic prevalence compared with all non-IBD renal biopsies. This may reflect a common pathogenic mechanism.
- Although several cases of tubulointerstitial nephritis have been related to drug exposure, there is increasing evidence that this finding may represent a true extraintestinal manifestation of IBD itself.
- A high index of clinical suspicion is needed for the early diagnosis and prevention of IBD-related renal manifestations and complications. Optimal screening and monitoring protocols, however, have yet to be established.

INTRODUCTION

Inflammatory bowel disease (IBD) is a condition characterized by chronic inflammation of the gastrointestinal tract with the 2 most common types Crohn disease (CD) and ulcerative colitis (UC). The inciting agent and exact underlying mechanism of IBD is not entirely known; however, there is convincing evidence that it is mediated by abnormal T-cell function in genetically susceptible individuals.[1,2] Despite these etiologic similarities, the 2 diseases are characterized by different T-cell responses with CD driven mainly by a T helper (T_h)1/ T_h17 cell response in which interleukin (IL)-12 and IL-23 cytokines play key roles, whereas UC is driven mainly by a T_h2 cell-like response with natural killer T cells producing IL-13 and IL-5.[3] Epidemiologic studies have shown an overall greater incidence of CD among women compared with men, although

No disclosures to report.

Nephropathology, Arkana Laboratories, 10810 Executive Center Drive, Suite 100, Little Rock, AR 72211, USA

* Corresponding author.

E-mail address: josephine.ambruzs@arkanalabs.com

https://doi.org/10.1016/j.rdc.2018.06.007   **rheumatic.theclinics.com**
0889-857X/18/© 2018 The Author(s). Published by Elsevier Inc. This is an open access article under the CC BY-NC-ND license (http://creativecommons.org/licenses/by-nc-nd/4.0/).

this varies by geographic region and age, whereas no significant gender difference is seen in UC.[4] Involvement of other organs outside primary intestinal disease is seen in both CD and UC, although the reasons for this are not entirely clear.

EXTRAINTESTINAL MANIFESTATIONS

Extraintestinal manifestations (EIMs) of IBD are common, occurring in 6% to 47% of patients, and can involve nearly every organ system.[5–7] Some EIMs may precede IBD, although the majority accompany the underlying intestinal disease and are influenced by its activity.[8] The development of one EIM seems to increase the susceptibility of developing others, and there is a high concordance of EIMs in siblings and first-degree relatives with IBD.[9,10] The most common organs involved include the skin, eyes, joints, and hepatobiliary tract and their involvement is dependent on different mechanisms.[11] These include

- Systemic reactive manifestations often directly related to intestinal inflammation and disease activity, reflecting a common pathogenic mechanism[11]
- Autoimmune diseases independent of IBD but reflecting an overall susceptibility to autoimmunity due to genetic risk factors and systemic immune dysregulation, such as aberrant self-recognition and generation of autoantibodies[12]
- Deposition of circulating immune complexes or in situ formation of immune complexes leading to an increased risk of glomerulonephritis and perhaps tubulointerstitial nephritis (TIN)[13,14]
- Manifestations secondary to the metabolic and anatomic derangements commonly present as a direct result of intestinal disease and/or its treatment, also referred to as complications rather than manifestations[10,12]

Renal and urinary involvement has been reported to occur in 4% to 23% of IBD patients manifested primarily as urinary calculi, fistulas, and ureteral obstruction.[15,16] Parenchymal renal disease is rare but has been well documented in the worldwide literature. This has been in the form of case reports and small series describing glomerulonephritis,[17–23] minimal change disease,[24–29] secondary amyloidosis,[30–32] and TIN[33–36] (**Box 1**). The morbidity and even mortality associated

---

Box 1
Renal manifestations of inflammatory bowel disease

Nephrolithiasis
  Calcium oxalate
  Uric acid

Glomerulopathy
  IgAN
  Membranoproliferative glomerulonephritis
  Membranous glomerulopathy
  Antiglomerular basement membrane glomerulonephritis
  Minimal change disease

AA amyloidosis

Tubulointerstitial disease
  Acute tubular injury
  TIN
    Acute
    Chronic
    Granulomatous

with renal EIMs are significant, and a high index of clinical suspicion is often needed for early recognition, as is continued surveillance to minimize recurrences and complications.

RENAL INSUFFICIENCY IN INFLAMMATORY BOWEL DISEASE

Renal EIMs and IBD-related therapy are potential risk factors for the development of renal insufficiency (both acute and chronic) in patients with CD and UC. There is a lack of large, population-based studies, however, looking at actual incidence and prevalence of renal insufficiency in IBD patients. Two retrospective studies examined the frequency of renal insufficiency and its associated risk factors in IBD patients admitted to a tertiary care center.[37,38] In Primas and colleagues' study,[38] 775 patients with IBD were analyzed and only 11 (2%) had renal insufficiency, all patients with CD. Significant risk factors identified were duration of disease, length of resected small bowel, and recurrent nephrolithiasis and the number of interventions due to stones. They extrapolated that this suggests an annual prevalence of 1.63/ 100,000 IBD patients (per year). A separate study by Lewis and colleagues[37] also retrospectively examined 251 admitted patients with IBD and found a higher 15.9% frequency of renal insufficiency, two-thirds of them chronic. This frequency was not statistically different between patients with CD and UC. They also found, however, that risk factors for renal insufficiency included older age and duration of disease as well as history of nephrolithiasis. They determined that for every 5-year increase in age, the likelihood of having renal insufficiency increased by 30%. Despite multiple reports of 5-aminosalicylate (5-ASA)-related nephrotoxicity, neither of the studies found 5-ASA therapy a significant risk factor for renal insufficiency. Both studies conclude that renal function should be routinely monitored in patients with IBD, particularly in elderly patients.

Renal biopsy is not frequently performed on patients with IBD, although it should be considered in patients presenting with renal insufficiency, proteinuria, or hematuria, particularly if other comorbid conditions are absent or renal insufficiency persists despite removal of nephrotoxic agents. In the largest case series of IBD patients referred for renal biopsy, the most common indication was acute and/or chronic renal insufficiency followed by proteinuria (**Table 1**).[13] A cross-sectional national survey conducted among private gastroenterologists found that only 59% screen for renal insufficiency before initiating treatment with 5-ASA, a potential nephrotoxic agent.[39] If impairment is found, however, 80% report consulting a nephrologist prior to commencing treatment.

NEPHROLITHIASIS

Nephrolithiasis is the most common urinary complication in IBD patients, most often the result of metabolic and anatomic derangements directly related to intestinal disease. Although large epidemiologic studies are lacking, smaller studies have estimated a lifetime risk for nephrolithiasis of 9% to 18% in IBD patients, higher than in the general population.[15,40] The risk has been found to be higher in adult patients than pediatric patients, higher in CD than UC, and higher in those patients who have had surgical bowel resection, particularly of the terminal ileum (up to 28%).[15,16,40,41] The overall morbidity is often significant secondary to repeated recurrences requiring medical and surgical interventions, obstruction and hydronephrosis, and infection. As discussed previously, it has also been shown that recurrent nephrolithiasis and the number of interventions for its treatment are 2 risk factors for the development of chronic kidney disease in IBD patients.[38,40]

Table 1
Demographic and clinical characteristics of patients with inflammatory bowel disease referred for renal biopsy

Characteristic	Data
Patients (n)	83
Men, n (%)	51 (61)
Mean age ± SD (y)	46 ± 18
UC, n (%)	38 (46)
CD, n (%)	45 (54)
Median serum creatinine (mg/dL) (25th, 75th percentiles)	2.7 (1.7, 4.3)
Indications for renal biopsy, n (%)	
Acute kidney injury	26 (31)
Chronic kidney disease	9 (11)
Acute on chronic kidney disease	17 (21)
Nephrotic-range proteinuria	13 (16)
Subnephrotic proteinuria	12 (14)
Isolated hematuria	6 (7)

Adapted from Ambruzs JM, Walker PD, Larsen CP. The histopathologic spectrum of kidney biopsies in patients with inflammatory bowel disease. Clin J Am Soc Nephrol 2014;9(2):266; with permission.

Kidney stones in IBD patients are composed primarily of calcium oxalate or uric acid. Calcium oxalate is more commonly seen in patients with CD, particularly as a result of ileocolonic disease with subsequent bile salt and fatty acid malabsorption. This malabsorption results in increased oxalate intestinal absorption, termed enteric hyperoxaluria. There is also increased permeability of the colonic mucosa and decreased numbers of colonic oxalate-metabolizing bacteria (*Oxalobacter formingens*).[16,42] These factors, along with low urinary volume and low concentration of stone inhibitors (ie, magnesium and citrate), all likely promote lithogenesis in IBD patients.[43,44] Uric acid stones often result from loss of volume and bicarbonate through frequent diarrhea or small bowel ostomies resulting in concentrated and acidic urine.[16] Pediatric IBD patients may have predominantly calcium phosphate stones.[16,45] Finally, sulfasalazine-induced crystalluria and nephrolithiasis resulting in obstructive uropathy has rarely been reported.[46,47]

Early recognition and management of nephrolithiasis in IBD patients are imperative and often involve a dietary, medical, and surgical approach.[48] This includes patient counseling regarding risks, increased hydration and control of fluid losses from diarrhea and ostomy output, reduction in dietary oxalate and fat, and urinary alkalization.[40] Some investigators have also advocated for imaging of the upper urinary tract at regular intervals as well as early elective surgical intervention for detected stones.[40,49,50]

GLOMERULOPATHY

Glomerular involvement in IBD is rare, although several morphologic patterns of glomerular injury have been described (**Fig. 1**). These include

- IgA nephropathy (IgAN)[20,51–70]
- Membranoproliferative glomerulonephritis[21,22,71]
- Minimal change disease[24–29]

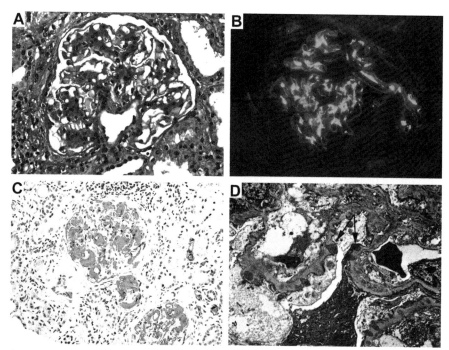

Fig. 1. Glomerular lesions associated with inflammatory bowel disease. (*A*) Glomerulus with mesangial matrix expansion and hypercellularity in a patient with IgAN and CD (periodic acid–Schiff; original magnification ×400). (*B*) Positive IgA staining of the glomerular mesangium by immunofluorescence (fluorescein conjugated antihuman IgA; original magnification ×400). (*C*) Glomerular and vascular amyloid deposits show positive staining for AA in this case of AA amyloidosis and CD (immunoperoxidase; original magnification ×200). (*D*) Transmission electron photomicrograph showing a glomerulus with numerous subepithelial electron dense deposits (*arrows*) from a case of membranous glomerulopathy and CD (original magnification ×2000). Tissue staining for the phospholipase A2 receptor (PLA2R) and thrombospondin (THSD7A) were both negative (not shown here).

- Membranous glomerulopathy[17,72,73]
- Antiglomerular basement membrane glomerulonephritis[18,19,74,75]
- C3 glomerulopathy[76]

The etiology of glomerular involvement in IBD is not entirely understood and may involve a common pathogenic mechanism or genetic susceptibility, deposition of intestine derived immune complexes as a result of increased mucosal permeability and antigenic exposure, and finally an effect of drug therapy, particularly in the case of minimal change disease. The fact that many reports show presentation or exacerbation of glomerulonephritis coincident with bowel disease activity, as well as subsequent resolution after successful IBD treatment, bolsters the consideration of glomerular injury as an EIM of IBD.[12]

The most common reported glomerulonephritis in patients with IBD, by a wide margin, is IgAN. The largest cases series of renal biopsy findings in IBD patients also showed that IgAN was the most common diagnosis, present in 43% of all biopsies.[13] Given the relative frequency of subclinical IgAN in otherwise healthy populations, it has been suggested that this high frequency of IgAN found in IBD patients is coincidental.[52,77] When Ambruzs and colleagues[13] compared their IBD cohort to all native renal biopsies from patients without IBD, however, they found the prevalence of IgAN in patients with IBD significantly higher. Hubert and colleagues[51] reported the first cases of IBD-associated IgAN in 1984. They described both clinical and pathologic remission of renal disease concomitant with the symptomatic treatment of intestinal disease. There have been numerous subsequent case reports in the literature of IgAN in IBD, as discussed previously. A majority of these patients had occurrence of IgAN during onset or exacerbation of IBD as well as clinical remission of renal disease in conjunction with successful treatment of bowel inflammation. Elevated serum IgA levels were not consistently measured but were reported to be elevated in several patients. Repeat renal biopsy confirming histologic remission of glomerulonephritis was rare. When a biopsy was repeated, however, it showed resolution of both mesangial proliferation and IgA deposits.[51]

Secondary forms of IgAN have been described most commonly in the setting of liver disease. There has been increasing literature, however, associating mucosal inflammation and/or infection with IgAN.[53,77] This is perhaps not surprising given the important immunologic role IgA plays in the defense against environmental and microbial antigenic exposures occurring at mucosal sites, in particular the gastrointestinal tract. Antibodies to various dietary antigens have also been detected both in sera as well as in IgA immune complexes and renal eluates in patients with IgAN.[78] Secondary IgAN in IBD, therefore, is likely to represent a complex interplay of mucosal inflammation, loss of antigenic exclusion and tolerance, chronic immune stimulation, and dysregulated IgA production and transport.[77] Given that intestinal mucosal immune responses are highly dependent on costimulation, the role of T-cell dysfunction in this process has also been implicated.[79] In their study of transgenic mice, Wang and colleagues[79] showed that T-cell–mediated mucosal immunity was critical in intestinal inflammation and in the pathogenesis of IgAN. Localized gastrointestinal immunosuppression (ie, enteric budesonide) as a potential treatment of primary IgAN likewise alludes to a pathogenic role of gut immune responses in the development of glomerulonephritis.[80,81] Genetic susceptibility has also been investigated and an association with HLA-DR1 has been described in both IgAN and IBD.[60,61] More recently, new risk loci for IgAN have been identified with most implicating genes either directly associated with risk of IBD or maintenance of the intestinal epithelial barrier and response to mucosal pathogens.[7,82] Together, these findings support a pathogenic link between immune mechanisms operating in IBD and IgAN rather than the idea that IBD serves only to exacerbate primary IgAN as has been previously suggested.

AMYLOIDOSIS

Amyloid A (AA) amyloidosis, so-called secondary amyloidosis, is a rare but serious complication of IBD. It involves the deposition of amyloid fibrils derived from serum AA (SAA) protein, an acute-phase reactant protein resulting from chronic inflammatory or infectious diseases. CD is the fourth leading cause[83] of AA amyloidosis worldwide. Early reports of amyloidosis associated with IBD were largely from autopsy series. The kidneys are frequently involved (up to 90% of cases) with deposits predominantly involving the glomerular tuft and vessels. This results in not only significant patient morbidity with progressive renal impairment, proteinuria, and often end-stage kidney disease but also mortality.[84] A recent systematic review of amyloidosis in IBD reported an overall estimated frequency of 0.53%; however, when stratified, prevalence of amyloidosis in patients with CD was significantly higher than UC (1.05% vs 0.08%).[83] Several studies have shown a clear predilection of AA amyloidosis in men, and it more commonly presents in those with long-standing disease, in particular those with fistulizing-stenotic forms, suppurative complications, and ileocolonic involvement, although cases of early presentation have also been reported.[12,30–32,85] Patients with IBD and amyloidosis also frequently have other EIMs.

The most common clinical presentation of amyloidosis in IBD is that of renal insufficiency (up to 70%) and nephrotic range proteinuria.[83] Up to 15.3% of cases, however, show no evidence of renal injury or proteinuria at diagnosis, although this likely represents an overestimation.[83] In terms of outcome, one prospective series found progression to end-stage renal disease in 15 of 22 (68%) patients with CD and AA amyloidosis, 6 of whom subsequently underwent renal transplantation.[86] Recurrence of amyloidosis occurred in only 1 graft after 14.5 years in a patient with sustained chronic active disease. Diagnosis of amyloidosis is most commonly made through tissue biopsy of the affected organ, typically a renal biopsy. Specific amyloid typing can be performed by immunohistochemistry testing or mass spectrometry.

Treatment of AA amyloidosis in IBD focuses on controlling the underlying inflammatory state, decreasing the formation and circulating levels of SAA protein, and potentially reversing the amyloid deposits already present in affected organs.[7,30] There are currently no prospective, randomized control trials on treatment of amyloidosis in IBD. Corticosteroids and other immunosuppressive drugs (such as azathioprine, methotrexate, and cyclosporine), colchicine, dimethylsulfoxide, and elemental diet have all been used, although their effectiveness has not been established.[87–89] Several studies with infliximab, a tumor necrosis factor (TNF)-α inhibitor, have been more promising and have demonstrated a decrease in SAA circulating levels, decrease in proteinuria, and stabilization of renal function, although it is unclear if reversibility of established damage can be achieved.[83,85,90–92] Newer treatments, such as tocilizumab, a humanized monoclonal antibody to the IL-6 receptor, have also shown promising results.[83,93,94] The administration of the drug (R)-1-[6-[(R)-2-carboxy-pyrrolidin 1-yl]-6-oxo-hexanoyl]pyrrolidine-2-carboxylic acid, followed by a fully humanized monoclonal IgG1 antiserum amyloid P antibody, has been shown to effectively clear amyloid deposits from target organs, including kidney.[83,95,96] Further prospective trials are needed.

Acute Tubular Injury

Renal tubular injury has been reported as both an EIM of IBD as well as a complication of IBD-related therapy.[97] Specifically, renal tubular injury, in the form of proteinuria and enzymuria, has been frequently observed in IBD and is more strongly correlated with disease activity than therapy.[98–100] Kreisel and colleagues[100] measured enzymuria as an early marker of renal tubular damage in 147 consecutive patients with IBD. They found that pathologic enzymuria occurred in 28% of patients with UC and 19% of patients with CD. In UC, elevated enzymes were present almost exclusively in patients with active disease, with the highest levels measured before the start of therapy, and there was subsequent normalization in a subset of patients during the course of treatment with 5-ASA or sulfasalazine. Two subsequent studies looking at tubular proteinuria in IBD patients with normal renal function found pathologic proteinuria in essentially half of the patients and this correlated with disease activity and not 5-ASA treatment.[98,99] These reports suggest that renal tubular injury in IBD may often be subclinical and represent a true EIM of active disease rather than a toxic drug effect. More sensitive markers for kidney injury are needed given the shortcomings of serum creatinine as an indication of renal function.

TUBULOINTERSTITIAL NEPHRITIS

There have been several case reports of both acute and chronic TIN occurring in CD and UC patients, particularly in the setting of 5-ASA drug therapy and its derivatives.[33,34,101–104] This perhaps represents a complication rather than true manifestation of IBD; however, there are increasing reports of TIN presenting concurrently with IBD diagnosis in drug-naïve patients.[36,105] Both sulfasalazine and 5-ASA have proved efficacy in inducing and maintaining disease remission in IBD patients, particularly in UC, so frequent and long-term drug exposures are not uncommon.[106] Epidemiologic studies have shown that 5-ASA–related nephrotoxicity among IBD patients is rare with a mean overall risk and incidence that seems less than 0.5%.[106,107] In their case series of renal biopsies in IBD patients, Ambruzs and colleagues[13] found TIN the second most common finding after IgAN (**Fig. 2**). This included cases of both acute and chronic TIN and it was more frequently seen in UC patients (69%, (Ambruzs et al, unpublished data ,2014)). In a subset of patients with granulomatous interstitial nephritis, all of them had current or recent past exposure to aminosalicylates.

The pathogenesis of 5-ASA–related nephrotoxicity is unknown, although it is believed to represent a delayed-type hypersensitivity reaction that is dose independent.[108–110]

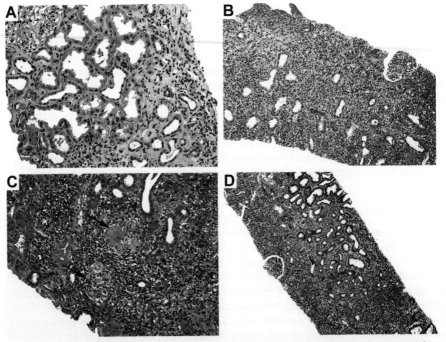

Fig. 2. Tubulointerstitial lesions associated with IBD. (*A*) Tubular profiles show simplification, reactive nuclei, and apical cytoplasmic blebbing in this case of acute tubular injury (hematoxylin-eosin; original magnification ×200). (*B*) Interstitial edema with an intense mixed inflammatory infiltrate and prominent tubulitis diagnostic of acute TIN in a patient with UC (hematoxylin-eosin; original magnification ×100). (*C*) Intense interstitial inflammation, including epithelioid histiocytes and multinucleated giant cells forming noncaseating granulomata (*arrows*) from a case of granulomatous TIN in a patient with CD (periodic acid–Schiff; original magnification ×200). (*D*) The renal interstitium is expanded by fibrosis and has an associated inflammatory infiltrate with severe tubular atrophy in this case of chronic TIN in a patient with UC (Masson trichrome; original magnification ×100).

A strong predilection in men has previously been reported and a recent genome-wide association study identified a genetic predisposition in the HLA region.[9,111] Onset of renal injury is typically within the first 12 months of treatment but delayed onset after several years has also been reported.[106,111] Unfortunately, the most frequent form of 5-ASA–related TIN is that of severe, chronic, and progressive renal injury, which often escapes early clinical detection.[106,108,109] Complete recovery of renal function has been reported if TIN is diagnosed within 10 months from the start of treatment. If diagnosis is delayed beyond 18 months, only one-third of cases show recovery of renal function, and this is usually only partial.[7,109,110] Steroid therapy, along with drug withdrawal, may help hasten renal recovery.[34,108,110,112,113] Given the lack of sensitive markers for early detection of renal injury, a high index of clinical suspicion is needed and routine monitoring of renal function in IBD patients has been emphasized, particularly in those undergoing treatment with aminosalicylates. There are currently no standardized or optimal algorithms for monitoring IBD patients, and there is no evidence that such screening or monitoring improves patient outcomes.[106] However, there appears to be general consensus that renal function should be assessed prior to initiation of drug therapy, with ongoing monitoring of renal function every 3 months to 6 months the first year, followed by annual to semiannual monitoring thereafter.[109,110,113]

The association between TIN in IBD patients and drug therapy is bolstered by those reports demonstrating a strong temporal relationship to drug exposure, recovery of renal function after withdrawal of the drug, and recurrence of renal injury upon rechallenge.[103,104,114] There have been several reports, however, of acute and chronic TIN occurring simultaneously with the diagnosis of IBD or in patients with no known exposure to nephrotoxic agents.[14,35,36,115–119] This seems particularly true in cases of granulomatous interstitial nephritis and CD.[105,120–123] Additionally, TIN was most commonly found during active intestinal disease. These findings strongly implicate TIN as a true EIM of IBD with potentially serious consequences because renal impairment has been reported to persist despite initial response to treatment of the underlying bowel disease, with most showing chronic kidney disease, to include end-stage renal disease, in 30% by 3 years.[14] Possible mechanisms for nondrug-related TIN include systemic immune dysregulation and cytokine activation, immunopathogenetic autoantibodies and immune complexes against organ-specific epitopes shared by colon and extracolonic sites (such as the tubular basement membrane), and possibly molecular mimicry[8,14]

Although well described in association with anti–TNF-α therapy, development of granulomatous TIN has also been reported in association with vedolizumab, a newer therapeutic monoclonal antibody that selectively binds to the $\alpha4/\beta7$ integrin.[114] The exact mechanism is unknown, although likely involves a similar delayed-type hypersensitivity as seen in other drug classes rather than a specific biologic effect of the monoclonal antibody.[114]

RENAL MANIFESTATIONS IN PEDIATRIC INFLAMMATORY BOWEL DISEASE PATIENTS

EIMs also occur in the pediatric IBD population in 20% to 35% of children with CD and 15% of children with UC.[7,105,124] They can also precede the onset of gastrointestinal symptoms in 25% to 35% of cases.[105] Although the actual frequency of renal involvement in pediatric IBD is not well described, there have been several reports of nephrolithiasis,[125–127] glomerulonephritis (in particular, IgAN),[17,61,63,64] TIN,[14,35,105,108,112,117,128] and rarely AA amyloidosis.[129] A recent literature review by Corica and Romano[7] identified 50 reported cases of renal involvement in the pediatric IBD population and found a strong predilection in boys (72%) as well as a majority occurring in patients with CD (80%). The most common occurrence was nephrolithiasis (58%) followed by TIN (30%), the latter occurring in two-thirds of all UC patients reported. Similar to adults, no standard guidelines for routine surveillance of renal function have been established, although screening and more frequent monitoring has been recommended.[112]

SUMMARY

Although renal and urinary involvement in IBD is not uncommon, renal parenchymal disease is rare and most commonly affects the glomerular and tubulointerstitial compartments. The most common findings on renal biopsy of IBD patients are IGAN and TIN, and this occurrence may represent a common pathogenic mechanism. The overall morbidity of IBD-related renal manifestations is significant, and there is often only a short window of injury reversibility. This, along with an often subtle clinical presentation, requires a high index of suspicion and likely routine monitoring of renal function in patients, in particular the elderly and those with other comorbidities. There are currently no established guidelines for the optimal screening and routine monitoring of renal function in IBD patients.

REFERENCES

1. Marsal J, Agace WW. Targeting T-cell migration in inflammatory bowel disease. J Intern Med 2012;272:411–29.
2. Sartor RB. Mechanisms of disease: pathogeneis of chrone's disease and ulcerative colitis. Nat Clin Pract Gastroenterol Hepatol 2006;3(7):390–407.
3. Strober W, Fuss IJ. Pro-inflammatory cytokines in the pathogenesis of IBD. Gastroenterology 2011;140(6):1756–67.
4. Brant SR, Nguyen GC. Is there a gender difference in the prevalence of Crohn's disease or ulcerative colitis? Inflamm Bowel Dis 2008;14(Suppl 2):S2–3.
5. Bernstein CN, Blanchard JF, Rawsthorne P, et al. The prevalence of extraintestinal diseases in inflammatory bowel disease: a population-based study. Am J Gastroenterol 2001;96(4):1116–22.
6. Mendoza JL, Lana R, Taxonera C, et al. Extraintestinal manifestations in inflammatory bowel disease: differences between Crohn's disease and ulcerative colitis. Med Clin (Barc) 2005;125(8):297–300.
7. Corica D, Romano C. Renal involvement in inflammatory bowel diseases. J Crohns Colitis 2016;10(2):226–35.
8. Das KM. Relationship of extraintestinal involvements in inflammatory bowel disease: new insights into autoimmune pathogenesis. Dig Dis Sci 1999; 44(1):1–13.
9. Sato H, Umemura K, Yamamoto T, et al. Interstitial nephritis associated with ulcerative colitis in monozygotic twins. BMJ Case Rep 2017;2017 [pii: bcr2016218346].
10. Rothfuss KS, Stande EF, Herrlinger KR. Extraintestinal manifestations and complications in inflammatory bowel diseases. World J Gastroenterol 2006;12(30): 4813–31.
11. Danese S, Semeraro S, Papa A, et al. Extraintestinal manifestations in inflammatory bowel disease. World J Gastroenterol 2005;11(46):7227–36.
12. Oikonomou K, Kapsoritakis A, Eleftheriadis T, et al. Renal manifestations and complications of inflammatory bowel disease. Inflamm Bowel Dis 2011;17(4): 1034–45.

13. Ambruzs JM, Walker PD, Larsen CP. The histopathologic spectrum of kidney biopsies in patients with inflammatory bowel disease. Clin J Am Soc Nephrol 2014;9(2):265–70.

14. Waters AM, Zachos M, Herzenberg AM, et al. Tubulointerstitial nephritis as an extraintestinal manifestation of Crohn's disease. Nat Clin Pract Nephrol 2008; 4(12):693–7.

15. Shield DE, Lytton B, Weiss RM, et al. Urologic complications of inflammatory bowel disease. J Urol 1976;115(6):701–6.

16. Pardi DS, Tremaine WJ, Sandborn WJ, et al. Renal and urologic complications of inflammatory bowel disease. Am J Gastroenterol 1998;93(4):504–14.

17. Ridder RM, Kreth HW, Kiss E, et al. Membranous nephropathy associated with familial chronic ulcerative colitis in a 12-year-old girl. Pediatr Nephrol 2005; 20(9):1349–51.

18. Shaer AJ, Stewart LR, Cheek DE, et al. IgA antiglomerular basement membrane nephritis associated with Crohn's disease: a case report and review of glomerulonephritis in inflammatory bowel disease. Am J Kidney Dis 2003;41(5): 1097–109.

19. Plaisier E, Borradori L, Hellmark T, et al. Anti-glomerular basement membrane nephritis and bullous pemphigoid caused by distinct anti-a3(IV)NC1 and anti-BP180 antibodies in a patient with Crohn's disease. Am J Kidney Dis 2002; 40(3):649–54.

20. Peeters AJ, van den Wall Bake AW, Daha MR, et al. Inflammatory bowel disease and ankylosing spondylitis associated with cutaneous vasculitis, glomerulonephritis, and circulating IgA immune complexes. Ann Rheum Dis 1990;49(8): 638–40.

21. Schofield PM, Williams PS. Proliferative glomerulonephritis associated with Crohn's disease. Br Med J (Clin Res Ed) 1984;20:1039.

22. Hellwege HH, Bläker F, Gebbers JO. Hypocomplementemic membranoproliferative glomerulonephritis in a child with ulcerative colitis. Monatsschr Kinderheilkd 1976;124(10):706–11.

23. Koçak E, Köklü S, Akbal E, et al. Development of glomerulonephritis early in the course of Crohn's disease. Inflamm Bowel Dis 2010;16(4):548–9.

24. Barbour VM, Williams PF. Nephrotic syndrome associated with sulphasalazine. BMJ 1990;301(6755):818.

25. Fornaciari G, Maccari S, Borgatti PP, et al. Nephrotic syndrome from 5-ASA for ulcerative colitis? Complicated by carcinoma of the colon and sclerosing cholangitis. J Clin Gastroenterol 1997;24(1):37–9.

26. Skhiri H, Knebelmann B, Martin-Lefevre L, et al. Nephrotic syndrome associated with inflammatory bowel disease treated by mesalazine. Nephron 1998;79(2):236.

27. Firwana BM, Hasan R, Chalhoub W, et al. Nephrotic syndrome after treatment of Crohn's disease with mesalamine: case report and literature review. Avicenna J Med 2012;2(1):9–11.

28. Molnár T, Farkas K, Nagy F, et al. Sulfasalazine-induced nephrotic syndrome in a patient with ulcerative colitis. Inflamm Bowel Dis 2010;16(4):552–3.

29. Novis BH, Korzets Z, Chen P, et al. Nephrotic syndrome after treatment with 5-aminosalicylic acid. Br Med J (Clin Res Ed) 1988;296(6634):1442.

30. Guardiola-Arévalo A, Alcántara-Torres M, Valle-Muñoz J, et al. Amyloidosis and Crohńs disease. Rev Esp Enferm Dig 2011;103(5):268–74.

31. Wester AL, Vatn MH, Fausa O. Secondary amyloidosis in inflammatory bowel disease: a study of 18 patients admitted to Rikshospitalet University Hospital, Oslo, from 1962 to 1998. Inflamm Bowel Dis 2001;7(4):295–300.

32. Greenstein AJ, Sachar DB, Panday AK, et al. Amyloidosis and inflammatory bowel disease. A 50-year experience with 25 patients. Medicine (Baltimore) 1992;71(5):261–70.

33. Tadic M, Grgurevic I, Scukanec-Spoljar M, et al. Acute interstitial nephritis due to mesalazine. Nephrology (Carlton) 2005;10(2):103–5.

34. Margetts PJ, Churchill DN, Alexopoulou I. Interstitial nephritis in patients with inflammatory bowel disease treated with mesalamine. J Clin Gastroenterol 2001; 32(2):176–8.

35. Tokuyama H, Wakino S, Konishi K, et al. Acute interstitial nephritis associated with ulcerative colitis. Clin Exp Nephrol 2010;14(5):483–6.

36. Izzedine H, Simon J, Piette AM, et al. Primary chronic interstitial nephritis in Crohn's disease. Gastroenterology 2002;123(5):1436–40.

37. Lewis B, Mukewar S, Lopez R, et al. Frequency and risk factors of renal insufficiency in inflammatory bowel disease inpatients. Inflamm Bowel Dis 2013;19(9): 1846–51.

38. Primas C, Novacek G, Schweiger K, et al. Renal insufficiency in IBD–prevalence and possible pathogenetic aspects. J Crohns Colitis 2013;7(12):e630–4.

39. Zallot C, Billioud V, Frimat L, et al. CREGG (Club de Reflexion des cabinets et Groupes d'Hépato-Gastroentérologie). 5-Aminosalicylates and renal function monitoring in inflammatory bowel disease: a nationwide survey. J Crohns Colitis 2013;7(7):551–5.

40. Gkentzis A, Kimuli M, Cartledge J, et al. Urolithiasis in inflammatory bowel disease and bariatric surgery. World J Nephrol 2016;5(6):538–46.

41. Andersson H, Bosaeus I, Fasth S, et al. Cholelithiasis and urolithiasis in Crohn's disease. Scand J Gastroenterol 1987;22(2):253–6.

42. Allison MJ, Cook HM, Milne DB, et al. Oxalate degradation by gastrointestinal bacteria from humans. J Nutr 1986;116(3):455–60.

43. Parks JH, Worcester EM, O'Connor RC, et al. Urine stone risk factors in nephrolithiasis patients with and without bowel disease. Kidney Int 2003;63(1):255–65.

44. McConnell N, Campbell S, Gillanders I, et al. Risk factors for developing renal stones in inflammatory bowel disease. BJU Int 2002;89(9):835–41.

45. Clark JH, Fitzgerald JF, Bergstein JM. Nephrolithiasis in childhood inflammatory bowel disease. J Pediatr Gastroenterol Nutr 1985;4(5):829–34.

46. Russinko PJ, Agarwal S, Choi MJ, et al. Obstructive nephropathy secondary to sulfasalazine calculi. Urology 2003;62(4):748.

47. Durando M, Tiu H, Kim JS. Sulfasalazine-induced crystalluria causing severe acute kidney injury. Am J Kidney Dis 2017;70(6):869–73.

48. Gaspar SR, Mendonca T, Oliveira P, et al. Urolithiasis and Crohn's disease. Urol Ann 2016;8(3):297–304.

49. Ishii G, Nakajima K, Tanaka N, et al. Clinical evaluation of urolithiasis in Crohn's disease. Int J Urol 2009;16(5):477–80.

50. Varda BK, McNabb-Baltar J, Sood A, et al. Urolithiasis and urinary tract infection among patients with inflammatory bowel disease: a review of US emergency department visits between 2006 and 2009. Urology 2015;85(4):764–70.

51. Hubert D, Beaufils M, Meyrier A. Immunoglobulin a glomerular nephropathy associated with inflammatory colitis. Apropos of 2 cases. Presse Med 1984; 13(17):1083–5.

52. Filiopoulos V, Trompouki S, Hadjiyannakos D, et al. IgA nephropathy in association with Crohn's disease: a case report and brief review of the literature. Ren Fail 2010;32(4):523–7.

53. Pipili C, Michopoulos S, Sotiropoulou M, et al. Is there any association between IgA nephropathy, Crohn's disease and Helicobacter pylori infection? Ren Fail 2012;34(4):506–9.
54. Ku E, Ananthapanyasut W, Campese VM. IgA nephropathy in a patient with ulcerative colitis, Graves' disease and positive myeloperoxidase ANCA. Clin Nephrol 2012;2012(77):2.
55. Choi JY, Yu CH, Jung HY, et al. A case of rapidly progressive IgA nephropathy in a patient with exacerbation of Crohn's disease. BMC Nephrol 2012;13:84.
56. Lee JM, Lee KM, Kim HW, et al. Crohn's disease in association with IgA nephropathy. Korean J Gastroenterol 2008;52(2):115–9.
57. Onime A, Agaba EI, Sun Y, et al. Immunoglobulin a nephropathy complicating ulcerative colitis. Int Urol Nephrol 2006;38(2):349–53.
58. Youm JY, Lee OY, Park MH, et al. Crohn's disease associated with IgA nephropathy. Korean J Gastroenterol 2006;47(4):324–8.
59. de Moura CG, de Moura TG, de Souza SP, et al. Inflammatory bowel disease, ankylosing spondylitis, and IgA nephropathy. J Clin Rheumatol 2006;12(2): 106–7.
60. Forshaw MJ, Guirguis O, Hennigan TW. IgA nephropathy in association with Crohn's disease. Int J Colorectal Dis 2005;20(5):463–5.
61. Takemura T, Okada M, Yagi K, et al. An adolescent with IgA nephropathy and Crohn disease: pathogenetic implications. Pediatr Nephrol 2002;17(10):863–6.
62. Trimarchi HM, Lotti A, Lotti R, et al. Immunoglobulin a nephropathy and ulcerative colitis. a focus on their pathogenesis. Am J Nephrol 2001;21(5):400–500.
63. McCallum D, Smith L, Harley F, et al. IgA nephropathy and thin basement membrane disease in association with Crohn disease. Pediatr Nephrol 1997;11(5): 637–40.
64. Dabadie A, Gié S, Taque S, et al. Glomerular nephropathy with IgA mesangium deposits and Crohn disease. Arch Podiatr 1996;3(9):884–7.
65. Hirsch DJ, Jindal KK, Trillo A, et al. Acute renal failure in Crohn's disease due to IgA nephropathy. Am J Kidney Dis 1992;20(2):189–90.
66. López Barbarín JM, Lafuente Martínez P, García Campos F, et al. Crohn's disease associated with Berger's disease. A rare complication. Rev Esp Enferm Dig 1990;78(4):233–5.
67. Iida H, Asaka M, Izumino K, et al. IgA nephropathy complicated by ulcerative colitis. Nephron 1989;53(3):285–6.
68. Soejima A, Nakabayasi K, Kitamoto K. Iga nephropathy in a patient with ulcerative colitis. Nihon Naika Gakkai Zasshi 1988;77:685–9.
69. Kammerer J, Genin I, Michel P, et al. Glomerulonephritis caused by mesangial deposits of immunoglobulins A associated with Crohn disease. Gastroenterol Clin Biol 1994;18(3):293.
70. Terasaka T, Uchida HA, Umebayashi R, et al. The possible involvement of intestine-derived IgA1: a case of IgA nephropathy associated with Crohn's disease. BMC Nephrol 2016;17(1):122.
71. Moayyedi P, Fletcher S, Hamden P, et al. Mesangiocapillary glomerulonephritis associated with ulcerative colitis: case reports of two patients. Nephrol Dial Transplant 1995;10(10):1923–4.
72. Casella G, Perego D, Baldini V, et al. A rare association between ulcerative colitis (UC), celiac disease (CD), membranous glomerulonephritis, leg venous thrombosis, and heterozygosity for factor V Leiden. J Gastroenterol 2002; 37(9):761–2.

73. Warling O, Bovy C, Co DO, et al. Overlap syndrome consisting of PSC-AIH with concomitant presence of a membranous glomerulonephritis and ulcerative colitis. World J Gastroenterol 2014;20(16):4811–6.

74. Hibbs AM, Bznik-Cizman B, Guttenberg M, et al. Ulcerative colitis in a renal transplant patient with previous Goodpasture disease. Pediatr Nephrol 2001; 16(7):543–6.

75. Nakamura T, Suzuki Y, Koide H. Granulocyte and monocyte adsorption apheresis in a patient with antiglomerular basement membrane glomerulonephritis and active ulcerative colitis. Am J Med Sci 2003;325(5):296–8.

76. Marques da Costa P, Correia L, Correia LA. The complexity of renal involvment in IBD-C3 glomerulopathy in ulcerative colitis. Inflamm Bowel Dis 2018. https://doi.org/10.1093/ibd/izy070.

77. Pouria S, Barratt J. Secondary IgA nephropathy. Semin Nephrol 2008;28(1): 27–37.

78. Coppo R. The pathogenetic potential of environmental antigens in IgA nephropathy. Am J Kidney Dis 1988;12(5):420–4.

79. Wang J, Anders RA, Wu Q, et al. Dysregulated LIGHT expression on T cells mediates intestinal inflammation and contributes to IgA nephropathy. J Clin Invest 2004;113(6):826–35.

80. Filiopoulos V, Vlassopoulos D. Steroids with local enteric action in IgA nephropathy and the association between kidney and bowel disease. Nephrol Dial Transplant 2012;27(3):1265–6.

81. Smerud HK, Barany P, Lindstrom K, et al. New treatment for IgA nephropathy: enteric budesonide targeted to the ileocecal region ameliorates proteinuria. Nephrol Dial Transplant 2011;26(10):3237–42.

82. Kiryluk K, Li Y, Scolari F, et al. Discovery of new risk loci for IgA nephropathy implicates genes involved in immunity against intestinal pathogens. Nat Genet 2014;46(11):1187–96.

83. Tosca Cuquerella J, Bosca-Watts MM, Anton Ausejo R, et al. Amyloidosis in inflammatory bowel disease: a systematic review of epidemiology, clinical features, and treatment. J Crohns Colitis 2016;10(10):1245–53.

84. Efstratiadis G, Mainas A, Leontsini M. Renal amyloidosis complicating Crohn's disease. Case report and review of the literature. J Clin Gastroenterol 1996; 22(4):308–10.

85. Pukitis A, Zake T, Groma V, et al. Effect of infliximab induction therapy on secondary systemic amyloidosis associated with Crohn's disease: case report and review of the literature. J Gastrointestin Liver Dis 2013;22(3):333–6.

86. Sattianayagam PT, Gillmore JD, Pinney JH, et al. Inflammatory bowel disease and systemic AA amyloidosis. Dig Dis Sci 2013;58(6):1689–97.

87. Ebert EC, Nagar M. Gastrointestinal manifestations of amyloidosis. Am J Gastroenterol 2008;103(3):776–87.

88. Cucino C, Sonnenberg A. The comorbid occurrence of other diagnoses in patients with ulcerative colitis and Crohn's disease. Am J Gastroenterol 2001; 96(7):2107–12.

89. Saitoh O, Kojima K, Teranishi T, et al. Renal amyloidosis as a late complication of Crohn's disease: a case report and review of the literature from Japan. World J Gastroenterol 2000;6(3):461–4.

90. Park YK, Han DS, Eun CS. Systemic amyloidosis with Crohn's disease treated with infliximab. Inflamm Bowel Dis 2008;14(3):431–2.

91. Said Y, Debbeche R, Hamzaoui L, et al. Infiximab for treatment of systemic amyloidosis associated with Crohn's disease. J Crohns Colitis 2011;5(2):171–2.

92. Iizuka M, Sagara S, Etou T. Efficacy of scheduled infliximab maintenance therapy on systemic amyloidosis associated with crohn's disease. Inflamm Bowel Dis 2011;17(7):E67–8.

93. Ito H, Takazoe M, Fukuda Y, et al. A pilot randomized trial of a human anti-interleukin-6 receptor monoclonal antibody in active Crohn's disease. Gastroenterology 2004;126(4):989–96.

94. Brulhart L, Nissen MJ, Chevallier P, et al. Tocilizumab in a patient with ankylosing spondylitis and Crohn's disease refractory to TNF antagonists. Joint Bone Spine 2010;77(6):625–6.

95. Richards DB, Cookson LM, Berges AC, et al. Therapeutic clearance of amyloid by antibodies to serum amyloid P component. N Engl J Med 2015;373(12):1106–14.

96. Richards DB, Cookson LM, Barton SV, et al. Repeat doses of antibody to serum amyloid P component clear amyloid deposits in patients with systemic amyloidosis. Sci Transl Med 2018;10(422) [pii:eaan3128].

97. Schreiber S, Hämling J, Zehnter E, et al. Renal tubular dysfunction in patients with inflammatory bowel disease treated with aminosalicylate. Gut 1997;40(6):761–6.

98. Fraser JS, Muller AF, Smith DJ, et al. Renal tubular injury is present in acute inflammatory bowel disease prior to the introduction of drug therapy. Aliment Pharmacol Ther 2001;15(8):1131–7.

99. Herrlinger KR, Noftz MK, Fellermann K, et al. Minimal renal dysfunction in inflammatory bowel disease is related to disease activity but not to 5-ASA use. Aliment Pharmacol Ther 2001;15(3):363–9.

100. Kreisel W, Wolf LM, Grotz W, et al. Renal tubular damage: an extraintestinal manifestation of chronic inflammatory bowel disease. Eur J Gastroenterol Hepatol 1996;8(5):461–8.

101. Agharazii M, Marcotte J, Boucher D, et al. Chronic interstitial nephritis due to 5-aminosalicylic acid. Am J Nephrol 1999;19(3):373–6.

102. De Broe ME, Stolear JC, Nouwen EJ, et al. 5-Aminosalicylic acid (5-ASA) and chronic tubulointerstitial nephritis in patients with chronic inflammatory bowel disease: is there a link? Nephrol Dial Transplant 1997;12(9):1839–41.

103. Manenti L, De Rosa A, Buzio C. Mesalazine-associated interstitial nephritis: twice in the same patient. Nephrol Dial Transplant 1997;12(9):2031.

104. Witte T, Olbricht CJ, Koch KM. Interstitial nephritis associated with 5-aminosalicylic acid. Nephron 1994;67(4):481–2.

105. Marcus SB, Brown JB, Melin-Aldana H, et al. Tubulointerstitial nephritis: an extraintestinal manifestation of Crohn disease in children. J Pediatr Gastroenterol Nutr 2008;46(3):338–41.

106. Gisbert JP, Gonzalez-Lama Y, Mate J. 5-Aminosalicylates and renal function in inflammatory bowel disease: a systematic review. Inflamm Bowel Dis 2007;13(5):629–38.

107. Elseviers MM, D'Haens G, Lerebours E, et al. Renal impairment in patients with inflammatory bowel disease: association with aminosalicylate therapy? Clin Nephrol 2004;61(2):83–9.

108. Arend LJ, Springate JE. Interstitial nephritis from mesalazine: case report and literature review. Pediatr Nephrol 2004;19:550–3.

109. Corrigan G, Stevens PE. Review article: interstitial nephritis associated with the use of mesalazine in inflammatory bowel disease. Aliment Pharmacol Ther 2000;14:1–6.

110. World MJ, Stevens PE, Ashton MA, et al. Mesalazine-associated interstitial nephritis. Nephrol Dial Transplant 1996;11(4):614–21.
111. Heap GA, So K, Weedon M, et al. Clinical features and HLA association of 5-aminosalicylate (5-ASA)-induced nephrotoxicity in inflammatory bowel disease. J Crohns Colitis 2016;10(2):149–58.
112. Co ML, Gorospe EC. Pediatric case of mesalazine-induced interstitial nephritis with literature review. Pediatr Int 2013;55(3):385–7.
113. Calviño J, Romero R, Pintos E, et al. Mesalazine-associated tubulo-interstitial nephritis in inflammatory bowel disease. Clin Nephrol 1998;49(4):265–7.
114. Bailly E, Von Tokarski F, Beau-Salinas F, et al. Interstitial nephritis secondary to vedolizumab treatment in Crohn disease and safe rechallenge using steroids: a case report. Am J Kidney Dis 2018;71(1):142–5.
115. Semjén D, Fábos Z, Pakodi F, et al. Renal involvement in Crohn's disease: granulomatous inflammation in the form of mass lesion. Eur J Gastroenterol Hepatol 2011;23(12):1267–9.
116. Zeier M, Schmidt R, Andrassy K, et al. Idiopathic interstitial nephritis complicating ulcerative colitis. Nephrol Dial Transplant 1990;5(10):901.
117. Shahrani Muhammad HS, Peters C, Casserly LF, et al. Relapsing tubulointerstitial nephritis in an adolescent with inflammatory bowel disease without aminosalicylate exposure. Clin Nephrol 2010;73(3):250–2.
118. Khosroshahi HT, Shoja MM. Tubulointerstitial disease and ulcerative colitis. Nephrol Dial Transplant 2006;21(8):2340.
119. Tovbin D, Kachko L, Hilzenrat N. Severe interstitial nephritis in a patient with renal amyloidosis and exacerbation of Crohn's disease. Clin Nephrol 2000; 53(2):147–51.
120. Archimandritis AJ, Weetch MS. Kidney granuloma in Crohn's disease. BMJ 1993;307(6903):540–1.
121. Unal A, Sipahioglu MH, Akgun H, et al. Crohn's disease complicated by granulomatous interstitial nephritis, choroidal neovascularization, and central retinal vein occlusion. Intern Med 2008;47(2):103–7.
122. Colvin RB, Traum AZ, Taheri D, et al. Granulomatous interstitial nephritis as a manifestation of Crohn disease. Arch Pathol Lab Med 2014;138(1):125–7.
123. Timmermans SA, Christiaans MH, Abdul-Hamid MA, et al. Granulomatous interstitial nephritis and Crohn's disease. Clin Kidney J 2016;9(4):556–9.
124. Mamula P, Markowitz JE, Baldassano RN. Inflammatory bowel disease in early childhood and adolescence: special considerations. Gastroenterol Clin North Am 2003;32(3):967–95.
125. Hueppelshaeuser R, von Unruh GE, Habbig S, et al. Enteric hyperoxaluria, recurrent urolithiasis, and systemic oxalosis in patients with Crohn's disease. Pediatr Nephrol 2012;27(7):1103–9.
126. Torio M, Ishimura M, Ohga S, et al. Nephrolithiasis as an extra-intestinal presentation of pediatric inflammatory bowel disease unclassified. J Crohns Colitis 2010;4(6):674–8.
127. Yamamoto Y, Kurokawa Y, Oka N, et al. A pediatric case of ammonium acid urate lithiasis with ulcerative colitis. Nihon Hinyokika Gakkai Zasshi 2002;93(5): 652–5.
128. Frandsen NE, Saugmann S, Marcussen N. Acute interstitial nephritis associated with the use of mesalazine in inflammatory bowel disease. Nephron 2002;92(1): 200–2.
129. Kirschner BS, Samowitz WS. Secondary amyloidosis in Crohn's disease of childhood. J Pediatr Gastroenterol Nutr 1986;5(5):816–21.

UNITED STATES POSTAL SERVICE®

Statement of Ownership, Management, and Circulation (All Periodicals Publications Except Requester Publications)

1. Publication Title	2. Publication Number		3. Filing Date
RHEUMATIC DISEASE CLINICS OF NORTH AMERICA	006 – 272		9/18/2018

4. Issue Frequency	5. Number of Issues Published Annually	6. Annual Subscription Price
FEB, MAY, AUG, NOV	4	$355.00

7. Complete Mailing Address of Known Office of Publication (Not printer) (Street, city, county, state, and ZIP+4®)

ELSEVIER INC.
230 Park Avenue, Suite 800
New York, NY 10169

Contact Person
STEPHEN R. BUSHING

Telephone (Include area code)
215-239-3688

8. Complete Mailing Address of Headquarters or General Business Office of Publisher (Not printer)

ELSEVIER INC.
230 Park Avenue, Suite 800
New York, NY 10169

9. Full Names and Complete Mailing Addresses of Publisher, Editor, and Managing Editor (Do not leave blank)

Publisher (Name and complete mailing address)

TAYLOR E BALL, ELSEVIER INC.
1600 JOHN F KENNEDY BLVD. SUITE 1800
PHILADELPHIA, PA 19103-2899

Editor (Name and complete mailing address)

LAUREN BOYLE, ELSEVIER INC.
1600 JOHN F KENNEDY BLVD. SUITE 1800
PHILADELPHIA, PA 19103-2899

Managing Editor (Name and complete mailing address)

PATRICK MANLEY, ELSEVIER INC.
1600 JOHN F KENNEDY BLVD. SUITE 1800
PHILADELPHIA, PA 19103-2899

10. Owner (Do not leave blank. If the publication is owned by a corporation, give the name and address of the corporation immediately followed by the names and addresses of all stockholders owning or holding 1 percent or more of the total amount of stock. If not owned by a corporation, give the names and addresses of the individual owners. If owned by a partnership or other unincorporated firm, give its name and address as well as those of each individual owner. If the publication is published by a nonprofit organization, give its name and address.)

Full Name	Complete Mailing Address
WHOLLY OWNED SUBSIDIARY OF REED/ELSEVIER, US HOLDINGS	1600 JOHN F KENNEDY BLVD. SUITE 1800 PHILADELPHIA, PA 19103-2899

11. Known Bondholders, Mortgagees, and Other Security Holders Owning or Holding 1 Percent or More of Total Amount of Bonds, Mortgages, or Other Securities. If none, check box ▶ ☐ None

Full Name	Complete Mailing Address
N/A	

12. Tax Status (For completion by nonprofit organizations authorized to mail at nonprofit rates) (Check one)
The purpose, function, and nonprofit status of this organization and the exempt status for federal income tax purposes:
☒ Has Not Changed During Preceding 12 Months
☐ Has Changed During Preceding 12 Months (Publisher must submit explanation of change with this statement)

PS Form **3526**, July 2014 (Page 1 of 4 (see instructions page 4)) PSN: 7530-01-000-9931   PRIVACY NOTICE: See our privacy policy on www.usps.com

---

13. Publication Title	14. Issue Date for Circulation Data Below
RHEUMATIC DISEASE CLINICS OF NORTH AMERICA	MAY 2018

15. Extent and Nature of Circulation			Average No. Copies Each Issue During Preceding 12 Months	No. Copies of Single Issue Published Nearest to Filing Date
a. Total Number of Copies (Net press run)			155	240
b. Paid Circulation (By Mail and Outside the Mail)	(1)	Mailed Outside-County Paid Subscriptions Stated on PS Form 3541 (Include paid distribution above nominal rate, advertiser's proof copies, and exchange copies)	68	103
	(2)	Mailed In-County Paid Subscriptions Stated on PS Form 3541 (Include paid distribution above nominal rate, advertiser's proof copies, and exchange copies)	0	0
	(3)	Paid Distribution Outside the Mails Including Sales Through Dealers and Carriers, Street Vendors, Counter Sales, and Other Paid Distribution Outside USPS®	38	57
	(4)	Paid Distribution by Other Classes of Mail Through the USPS (e.g., First-Class Mail®)	0	0
c. Total Paid Distribution (Sum of 15b (1), (2), (3), and (4))		▶	106	160
d. Free or Nominal Rate Distribution (By Mail and Outside the Mail)	(1)	Free or Nominal Rate Outside-County Copies included on PS Form 3541	40	65
	(2)	Free or Nominal Rate In-County Copies Included on PS Form 3541	0	0
	(3)	Free or Nominal Rate Copies Mailed at Other Classes Through the USPS (e.g., First-Class Mail)	0	0
	(4)	Free or Nominal Rate Distribution Outside the Mail (Carriers or other means)	40	65
e. Total Free or Nominal Rate Distribution (Sum of 15d (1), (2), (3) and (4))		▶		
f. Total Distribution (Sum of 15c and 15e)		▶	146	225
g. Copies not Distributed (See Instructions to Publishers #4 (page 83))		▶	9	15
h. Total (Sum of 15f and g)		▶	155	240
i. Percent Paid (15c divided by 15f times 100)		▶	72.6%	71.11%

* If you are claiming electronic copies, go to line 16 on page 3. If you are not claiming electronic copies, skip to line 17 on page 3.

16. Electronic Copy Circulation		Average No. Copies Each Issue During Preceding 12 Months	No. Copies of Single Issue Published Nearest to Filing Date
a. Paid Electronic Copies	▶	0	0
b. Total Paid Print Copies (Line 15c) + Paid Electronic Copies (Line 16a)	▶	106	160
c. Total Print Distribution (Line 15f) + Paid Electronic Copies (Line 16a)	▶	146	225
d. Percent Paid (Both Print & Electronic Copies) (16b divided by 16c × 100)	▶	72.6%	71.11%

☒ I certify that 50% of all my distributed copies (electronic and print) are paid above a nominal price.

17. Publication of Statement of Ownership

☒ If the publication is a general publication, publication of this statement is required. Will be printed in the NOVEMBER 2018 issue of this publication. ☐ Publication not required.

18. Signature and Title of Editor, Publisher, Business Manager, or Owner	Date
STEPHEN R. BUSHING - INVENTORY DISTRIBUTION CONTROL MANAGER	9/18/2018

I certify that all information furnished on this form is true and complete. I understand that anyone who furnishes false or misleading information on this form or who omits material or information requested on the form may be subject to criminal sanctions (including fines and imprisonment) and/or civil sanctions (including civil penalties).

PS Form **3526**, July 2014 (Page 3 of 4)   PRIVACY NOTICE: See our privacy policy on www.usps.com

Moving?

Make sure your subscription moves with you!

To notify us of your new address, find your **Clinics Account Number** (located on your mailing label above your name), and contact customer service at:

Email: journalscustomerservice-usa@elsevier.com

800-654-2452 (subscribers in the U.S. & Canada)
314-447-8871 (subscribers outside of the U.S. & Canada)

Fax number: 314-447-8029

Elsevier Health Sciences Division
Subscription Customer Service
3251 Riverport Lane
Maryland Heights, MO 63043

*To ensure uninterrupted delivery of your subscription, please notify us at least 4 weeks in advance of move.

Printed and bound by CPI Group (UK) Ltd, Croydon, CR0 4YY

08/05/2025

01864735-0002